Microbiology

for the Health Sciences

Fourth Edition

Gwendolyn R. W. Burton, Ph.D.

Professor, Emeritus
Department of Science
Front Range Community College
Westminster, Colorado

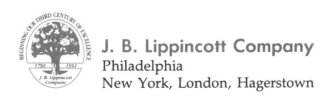

J. B. Lippincott Company
Philadelphia
New York, London, Hagerstown

Sponsoring Editor: Andrew Allen
Designer: Charles Field
Production Supervisor: Robert D. Bartleson
Production Service: Caslon, Inc.
Compositor: Digitype, Inc.
Printer/Binder: R. R. Donnelley & Sons Company
Cover Designer: Lou Fuiano
Cover Printer: John P. Pow Co.

Fourth Edition

6   5   4   3   2

Library of Congress Cataloging-in-Publication Data

Burton, Gwendolyn R. W. (Gwendolyn R. Wilson)
    Microbiology for the health sciences / Gwendolyn R.W. Burton, —
4th ed.
      p.   cm.
    Includes bibliographical references and index.
    ISBN 0-397-54886-9
    1. Microbiology.   2. Medical microbiology.   I. Title.
    [DNLM: 1. Allied Health Personnel.   2. Microbiology.   QW 4 B974m]
    QR41.2.B88   1992
    616'.01 — dc20
    DNLM/DLC   91-41873
    for Library of Congress   CIP

The author and publisher have exerted every effort to ensure that drug
selection and dosage set forth in this text are in accord with current
recommendations and practice at the time of publication. However, in view
of ongoing research, changes in government regulations, and the constant
flow of information relating to drug therapy and drug reactions, the reader
is urged to check the package insert for each drug for any change in
indications and dosage and for added warnings and precautions. This is
particularly important when the recommended agent is a new or infrequently
employed drug.

For Cindy, Gary, Alan, Earl,
Robin, Penny, Rae, Austin, and Kelsey

Preface

Microbiology, the study of microbes, is a fascinating topic to those of us who feel its importance in our daily lives. Others find it necessary to learn the microbiological concepts and vocabulary in order to function well in their chosen vocations. For example, those who plan to work in any area of health care, such as prevention of disease or care and treatment of the diseased, must be aware of the principles of sterilization, disease causation, and disease prevention.

Microbiology for the Health Sciences will aid those who want to learn the basic microbiological concepts that apply to the health care field. It is also intended for students who have little or no science background and for mature students returning to school after several years' absence.

There is a need for a "simplified" microbiology text that presents the major concepts clearly and concisely for people entering the health care occupations. This book is appropriate for use in a one-term allied health microbiology class or as one unit in a basic science class for health-oriented students.

Microbiology is an enormous and complex subject with many interrelated facets and hundreds of scientific terms. I have attempted a very fundamental approach to the subject matter by presenting at the beginning of each chapter the basic information necessary for understanding the more complex concepts with which the chapters conclude. Specialized vocabulary has been kept to a minimum. Key terms are italicized and are defined at the beginning of each chapter for easy reference. A complete glossary can also be found in the back of the book. The glossaries also include aids to pronunciation. The objectives are clearly stated at the beginning of each chapter to enable the student to survey the topics to be covered. A study outline, discussion questions, and self tests are included for review at the end of each chapter.

In this fourth edition some chapters have been combined and rearranged for better continuity and length. The whole book has been updated and partially rewritten for clarity. Insight boxes have been added to some chapters. These provide a more detailed look at an aspect of the topic being discussed in the chapter.

The student workbook has been incorporated into each chapter to encourage students to review the material and to take the self test while learning the information. In this way the student may have more insight into the important facts to be stressed on exams.

Although this book is intended primarily for non-science majors, it is not an "easy" text, because microbiology is not an "easy" topic. As the student will discover, the concise nature of this text has made each sentence significant. Thus, the reader will be intellectually challenged to learn each new concept as it is presented. It is my hope that the students will enjoy their study of microbiology and be motivated to further explore this fascinating field, especially as it relates to their occupations.

I am deeply indebted to those colleagues, friends, family members, and students who provided illustrations used in the text or who served as sources of advice and encouragement, especially Dr. Paul Engelkirk, Penny Anderson, Dr. Sam Langstaff, Ursi Chappelle, and my husband and children. I particularly wish to acknowledge Andrew Allen, sponsoring editor, and Miriam Benert, editorial assistant at J. B. Lippincott Company, for their editorial assistance in the preparation of this manuscript, and Charles Field of Caslon, Inc., for designing and coordinating the production of this book.

Gwendolyn R. W. Burton

Contents

Chapter 1

Introduction to Microbiology

Objectives

After studying this chapter, you should be able to

1. Define microbiology
2. List some important functions of microbes in the environment
3. Explain the relevance of microbiology to the health professions
4. List some areas of microbiological study
5. Outline some contributions of Leeuwenhoek, Pasteur, and Koch to microbiology
6. Explain the biological theory of fermentation
7. Explain the germ theory of disease
8. Learn Koch's postulates and give some circumstances in which they may not apply
9. Describe the difference between light microscopes and electron microscopes and the applications of both
10. List the metric units used in microscopic measurements and indicate their relative sizes

New Words

Algae (al'-gee), sing. *alga*. Primitive plants capable of producing their own food

Bacteria (back-tier'-ee-uh), sing. *bacterium*. Primitive, mostly unicellular organisms that do not have membrane-enclosed nuclei

Fungi (fun'-ji), sing. *fungus*. Microorganisms that live on decaying organic material

Immunology (im-mew-noll'-oh-gee). The science that deals with immunity from disease and the immune process

Microorganism (my'-kro-or'-gan-izm). Microscopic organisms, usually single cells, sometimes called microbes

Opportunist (op-poor-tune'-ist). A microbe that causes disease in susceptible persons with lowered resistance

Pathogen (path'-o-jen). Disease-causing microorganism

Protozoa (pro-toe-zoe'-ah), sing. *protozoan*. Single-celled microscopic animals found in water and soil; a few are pathogens

Tyndallization (tin-dal-i-zay'-shun). A process of boiling and cooling in which spores are allowed to germinate and then are killed by boiling again

Virology (vi-rol'oh-gee). The study of viruses and the diseases they cause

Virus (vir'-rus). An infective agent smaller than a bacterium

Microbiology, the Science

What is microbiology? *Micro-* means very small, anything so small that it must be viewed with a microscope; *-bio* means "living organisms"; and *-ology* means "the study of." Therefore, microbiology is the study of very small living organisms. These microorganisms include the *bacteria, algae, protozoa, fungi,* and *viruses* (Fig. 1–1). They are often called *microbes,* single-celled organisms, and germs.

You cannot see microorganisms without the aid of a microscope, and you may not be aware of the effect they have on your daily life. Occasionally, you may become conscious of their effect on your body when a cut or a burn becomes infected or when you have a sore throat. Have you ever been very sick after a picnic and wondered which of the foods you ate contained harmful germs? Most of us are aware of *pathogens,* or disease-causing microorganisms, only when we are affected by them. Actually, only a small percentage of microbes are pathogenic, that is, are able to cause disease (Fig. 1–2). The others are considered beneficial or harmless, or they cause disease only if they accidentally invade the "wrong" place at the "right time," such as when the host's resistance is low and the growth conditions are right. These microbes are considered opportunistic. Normally, these *opportunists* are harmless microorganisms, consisting of the indigenous microflora that live on the skin, in the mouth, and in the intestine.

Microorganisms can be found nearly everywhere as normal inhabitants of the earth, and with few exceptions, they contribute to the welfare of humans. The indigenous microflora that live on and within our bodies actually inhibit the growth of pathogens in those areas by occupying the space, using the food supply, and secreting materials (waste products, toxins, antibiotics) that may prevent or reduce the growth of pathogens. Other nonpathogens make it possible to produce yogurt, cheese, raised bread, beer, wine, and many other foods and drinks.

Many bacteria and fungi are *saprophytes,* which aid in fertilization by returning inorganic nutrients to the soil; they break down dead organic materials (plants and animals) into nitrates, phosphates, carbon dioxide, water, and other chemicals necessary for plant growth (Fig. 1–3). These saprophytes also destroy paper, feces, and other biodegradable substances, although they cannot break down

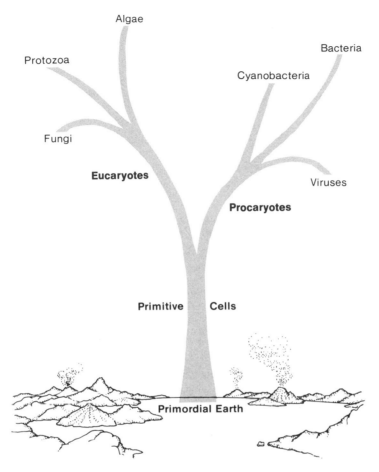

Figure 1–1. Family tree of microorganisms. The primitive cells are divided into eucaryotes (organisms with a true nucleus), such as fungi, protozoa, and most algae, and procaryotes (organisms without a bound nucleus), such as bacteria, cyanobacteria, and viruses (see Chapter 2).

most plastics and glass. The nitrogen-fixing bacteria, which live with those plants called legumes (peas, peanuts, alfalfa, clover), are able to return nitrogen from the air to the soil in the form of nitrates for use by other plants. This knowledge is important to the farmer who practices crop rotation to replenish his fields and to the gardener who keeps a compost pit as a source of natural fertilizer. In each case, the dead organic material is broken down into the inorganic nutrient, (nitrates and phosphates) by microorganisms.

The purification of waste water is partially accomplished by bacteria in the holding tanks of sewage disposal plants, where feces, garbage, and other organic materials are collected and reduced to harmless waste. Some microorganisms

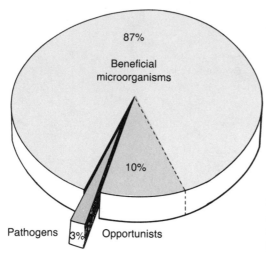

Figure 1–2. Pathogens comprise about 3% of all the microorganisms. Another 10% are opportunistic microbes that may cause disease if they land in the appropriate place.

such as the iron- and sulfur-utilizing bacteria even break down metals and minerals. The beneficial activities of microbes affect every part of our environment, in the land, water, and air.

Those who work in the health professions must be particularly aware of pathogens, their sources, and how they may be transmitted from one person to another. Physicians' assistants, dental assistants, nurses, laboratory technicians, respiratory therapists, orderlies, nurses' aides, and all others associated with patient care must take precautions to prevent the spread of pathogens. Harmful microorganisms may be transferred from health workers to patients; from patient to patient; from contaminated mechanical devices, instruments, and syringes to pa-

Figure 1–3. Saprophytes break down dead, decaying organic material into inorganic nutrients in the soil.

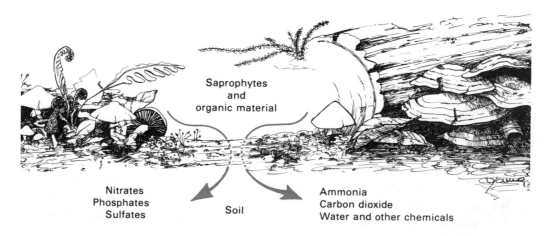

tients; from contaminated bedding, clothes, dishes, and food to patients; and from patients to health workers and other susceptible people.

The Scope of Microbiology

There are many fields of study within microbiology. One may specialize in the study of many different types of microorganisms. For example, the bacteriologist concentrates on *bacteriology*, the study of structure, functions, and activities of bacteria. *Phycology* is the study of the various types of algae by scientists called phycologists. Those who specialize in the study of fungi, or *mycology*, are called mycologists. Protozoologists explore the area of *protozoology*, the study of protozoa and their activities. *Virology* encompasses the study of viruses and their effects on living cells of all types. Virologists and cell biologists may become genetic engineers who manipulate the genetic material (DNA) from one cell to another.

Within the general field of microbiology there are many specialized areas in which the knowledge of all types of microorganisms and of their applications is important. These areas include medical, veterinary, and agricultural microbiology as well as applications in sewage disposal, industrial production, space research, microbial ecology, biodegradation, and genetic engineering.

General Microbiology   The study and classification of microorganisms and how they function is known as general microbiology. It encompasses all areas of microbiology.

Medical Microbiology   The field of medical microbiology involves the study of pathogens, the diseases caused by them, and the body's defenses against disease. This field is concerned with epidemiology, transmission of pathogens, disease-prevention measures, aseptic techniques, treatment of infectious diseases, immunology, and the production of vaccines to protect against infectious diseases. The almost complete eradication of smallpox and diphtheria, the safety of modern surgery, and the treatment of victims of acquired immunodeficiency syndrome (AIDS) are due to the many technological advances in this field.

Veterinary Microbiology   The spread and control of diseases among animals is the concern of veterinary microbiologists. The production of food from livestock, the raising of other agriculturally important animals, the care of pets, and the transmission of diseases from animals to humans are areas of major importance in this field.

Agricultural Microbiology   Included in the field of agricultural microbiology are studies of the beneficial and harmful roles of microbes in soil formation and fertility; in carbon, nitrogen, phosphorus, and sulfur cycles; in diseases of plants; in the digestive processes of cows and other ruminants; and in the production of crops and foods (Fig. 1-4). The *food microbiologist* is concerned with the production, processing, storage, cooking, and serving of food, as well as the prevention of food spoilage, food poisoning, and food toxicity. The *dairy microbiologist* oversees the grading, pasteurization, and processing of milk and cheeses to prevent con-

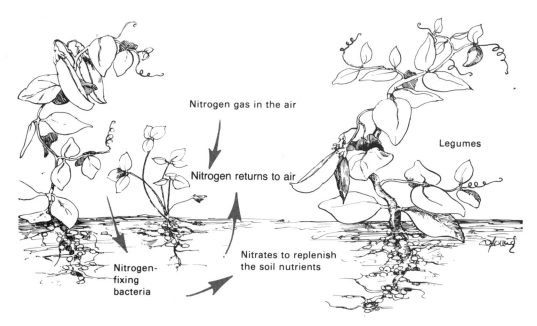

Nitrogen gas in the air

Nitrogen returns to air

Legumes

Nitrogen-
fixing
bacteria

Nitrates to replenish
the soil nutrients

Figure 1–4. Nitrogen fixation. The nitrogen-fixing bacteria that live on or near the roots of legumes convert free nitrogen from the air into nitrates to replenish the soil nutrients.

tamination, spoilage, and transmission of diseases from environmental, animal, and human sources.

Sanitary Microbiology   The field of *sanitary microbiology* includes the processing and disposal of garbage and sewage wastes, as well as the purification and processing of water supplies to ensure that no pathogens are carried to the consumer by the water. Sanitary microbiologists also inspect food processing installations and eating establishments to ensure the enforcement of proper food handling procedures.

Industrial Microbiology   Many businesses and industries depend on the proper growth and maintenance of certain microbes to produce beer, wine, alcohol, and organic materials such as enzymes, vitamins, and antibiotics. *Industrial microbiologists* monitor and maintain the essential microorganisms for these commercial enterprises. *Applied microbiologists* conduct research aimed at producing new products and more effective antibiotics. The scope of microbiology, indeed, has broad, far-reaching effects on humans, on pathogens, and on their relationship to the environment.

Microbial Physiology and Genetics   Research in microbial physiology has contributed greatly to a clearer understanding of the function of microorganisms, the structure of DNA, and the science of genetics in general. Genetic manipulation is much easier and faster with viruses and bacteria than with more complex cells;

thus, everyday organisms such as the intestinal *Escsherichia coli* are invaluable tools in this study.

Environmental Microbiology   The field of environmental microbiology, or microbial ecology, has become important because of increased concern about the environment. This field encompasses the areas of soil, air, water, sewage, food, and dairy microbiology, as well as the cycling of the elements by microbial, environmental, and geochemical processes (see Fig. 1–4). In addition, the biodegradation of toxic chemicals by various microorganisms is being researched as a new method for cleaning up these hazardous materials found in soil and water.

Milestones of Microbiology

Before the beginning of humanity, parasites lived on or in other living organisms. We know human pathogens have been present for ages because damage caused by these pathogens has been observed in the bones of mummies and early humans, indicating that diseases such as osteomyelitis and syphilis were present.

In the ancient civilizations of Egypt and China, the people kept clean by washing with water in an effort to prevent disease. They also knew that some diseases were easily transmitted from one person to another, and they learned to isolate the sick to prevent the spread of these diseases, which we recognize as being contagious. The Egyptians were aware of the effectiveness of biological warfare. They often used the blood and bodies of their diseased dead to contaminate the water supplies of their enemies and to spread diseases among them.

The Book of Leviticus in the Bible was probably the first recording of laws concerning public health. The Hebrew people were told to practice personal hygiene by washing and keeping clean. They were also instructed to bury their waste material away from their campsites, to isolate those who were sick, and to burn soiled dressings. They were prohibited from eating animals that had died of natural causes. The procedure for killing an animal was clearly described, and the edible parts were so designated.

Most of the knowledge about public sanitation and transmission of disease was lost in Europe during the Middle Ages when there was a general stagnation of culture and learning for almost 1,000 years. However, during the Renaissance, widespread epidemics of smallpox, syphilis, rabies, and other diseases prompted physicians and alchemists to search for explanations as to how the contraction and transfer of diseases occurred. Most people believed that diseases were caused by curses of the gods, and as a result, many bizarre treatments (bleeding, drilling holes in the head, attaching leeches) were used to drive the devils or evil spirits away and relieve the symptoms.

An Italian physician, Girolamo Fracastorius, having observed the syphilis epidemic of the 1500s, proposed in 1546 that the agents of communicable diseases were living germs that could be transmitted by direct contact with humans and animals and indirectly by objects. Proof for vague theories such as this was long

Insight: Leeuwenhoek's Discoveries

The discovery of various microorganisms by Antony van Leeuwenhoek, using his primitive simple microscope over 300 years ago, has long been an area for study and discussion. How did he build the microscope and use it effectively to observe the "wee beasties," especially the bacteria? Some believe he may have used polished clear glass beads of various sizes for lenses and various intensities of outdoor light to view the bacteria and smaller protista. By changing the direction and intensity of the sunlight, he could have developed the darkfield capability to enable him to observe microbial movement. See Insight Figure 1–1 for an idea of what the microscope looked like and what Leeuwenhoek saw.

Perhaps it was curiosity about the sense of taste that led him to the discovery of bacteria on peppercorns as he searched for an explanation for why pepper has such a potent taste. After he steeped the peppercorns for 3 weeks to soften them, he examined the water, and on April 24, 1676, described the "incredibly small organisms" (now known as bacteria) and reported that 100 of them arranged lengthwise (possibly they were rod-shaped organisms) would not equal the length of a grain of coarse sand. This has been acknowledged as the first recorded observation of

Insight Figure 1–1. (A) Leeuwenhoek used a microscope with a single biconvex lens to view bacteria suspended in a drop of liquid placed on a moveable pin. (B) Although his microscope was capable of only 200- to 300-fold magnification, Leeuwenhoek was able to achieve these remarkable drawings of different bacteria types, which he submitted to the Royal Society of London. (Volk WA, et al.: Essentials of Medical Microbiology, 4th ed. Philadelphia, JB Lippincott, 1990)

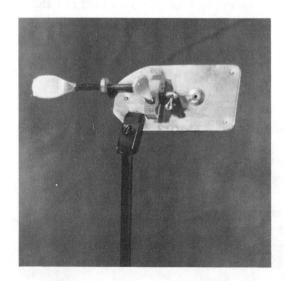

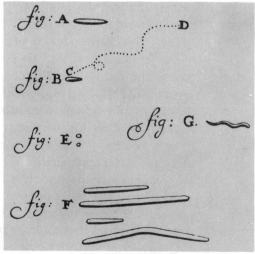

bacteria. However, definitive evidence for the discovery of bacteria was not provided until he wrote a letter to the Royal Society of London dated September 17, 1686, in which he described his regimen for keeping his teeth clean and detailed his examination of the white matter (plaque) that grew between his teeth. When he added this white matter to saliva (which he thought was free of microorganisms) and examined it microscopically, he described the "many very small living animals that moved very prettily."

Of course, all of this is speculation drawn from his letters and by experimentation because Leeuwenhoek, determined to keep his microscopic methods to himself, shared his techniques with no one.

delayed because the agents of disease could not be observed and experimental evidence was lacking.

Until the development of magnifying lenses and microscopes that could sufficiently magnify microorganisms to allow them to be visualized, the discovery of disease-causing agents was impossible. Actually, it is not known who built the first microscope, but *compound microscopes*, which use two lenses to increase the magnification, were developed by Johannes Janssen (1590), Galileo Galilei (1609), and Robert Hooke (1660). When Antony van Leeuwenhoek first described bacteria in 1667, he used a small, simple microscope with one lens the size of a large pinhead and observed the material placed on the point of a pin. Leeuwenhoek is called the "Father of Microbiology" because he described the three shapes of bacteria as well as protozoa, sperm, and blood cells as a result of his microscopic observations of pepper water, tooth scrapings, gutter water, semen, blood, urine, and feces. His letters to the Royal Society of London convinced the scientists of the late 17th century of the existence of microorganisms, which Leeuwenhoek called "animalcules." He did not speculate on the origin of these microbes nor did he associate them with the cause of disease. These relationships were not established until the work of Louis Pasteur and Robert Koch in the late 19th century. Leeuwenhoek's fine art of grinding a single lens that would magnify an object to 300 times its size was lost at his death, for he had not taught this skill to anyone.

Detailed descriptions of microorganisms were delayed until the development of better microscopes in the 19th and 20th centuries. Modern microscopy is discussed at the end of this chapter.

Although Leeuwenhoek was probably not concerned about the origin of microorganisms, many other scientists were searching for an explanation of the spontaneous appearance of living creatures in decaying meat, stagnating ponds, fermenting grain, and infected wounds. On the basis of observation, many of the so-called scientists of that time believed that life could develop spontaneously

from decomposing nonliving material. This is the theory of spontaneous generation or *abiogenesis*. For over 2 centuries, from 1650 to 1850, this theory was debated and tested. Following the work of many others, Pasteur and John Tyndall
finally disproved the theory of spontaneous generation and proved that life must
arise from preexisting life; this is called the theory of *biogenesis*.

The experiments devised by Louis Pasteur and other scientists in the
mid-1800s resulted in several major advances in the field of microbiology: (1) the
concept that life must arise from preexisting life; (2) the techniques of sterilization
and pasteurization; (3) understanding of the biological process of fermentation;
(4) the germ theory of disease; and (5) the development of vaccines from killed
bacteria for anthrax and from attenuated, or weakened, viruses for rabies.

The sterilization techniques used by Pasteur showed that boiled broth remains
sterile until it is contaminated by particles in the air. While repeating Pasteur's ex-
periment, Tyndall found bacterial fragments, called endospores, that were not
destroyed by the first boiling and that germinated into reproducing (vegetative)
bacteria. This discovery led to the development of the fractional sterilization process, often called *tyndallization*, in which the endospores of bacteria are destroyed
by boiling and cooling three times, allowing the spores to germinate between
boilings.

When Pasteur was investigating the reasons for the spoilage of beer and wine,
he developed the *biological theory of fermentation*, which states that a specific microbe produces a specific change in the substance on which it grows or a specific
microorganism produces a specific fermentation process. Just as yeasts ferment
sugar in grape juice to produce ethyl alcohol in wine, some contaminating bacteria, such as *Acetobacter*, may change the alcohol to acetic acid (vinegar), which, of
course, ruins the taste of the wine. To eliminate the harmful contaminating bacteria from beer and wines, Pasteur heated them up to 50° to 60°C (122° to 140°F).
This process, now called *pasteurization*, has been adapted to destroy the pathogens in milk by heating it to 63°C (145.4°F) for 30 minutes or to 72°C (161.6°F)
for 15 seconds.

By extending the biological theory of fermentation to animals and humans,
Pasteur developed the *germ theory of disease*, which states that a specific disease is
caused by a specific type of microorganism (Fig. 1–5). After isolating the causative pathogens of chicken cholera, anthrax, and rabies, he prepared vaccines
against these diseases. He used the attenuated or weakened pathogen, which was
no longer pathogenic but which made the injected animal immune to the disease.
For example, Pasteur found the rabies virus in the brain and spinal cord of rabid
dogs. He discovered that by transferring the virus from rabbit to rabbit many
times, the virus became so weakened it no longer caused rabies in rabbits or dogs.
It was this attenuated virus that he used to immunize animals and people against
rabies.

Actually, the beginnings of immunology occurred in ancient China, where a
type of vaccination against smallpox was practiced in which healthy people in-

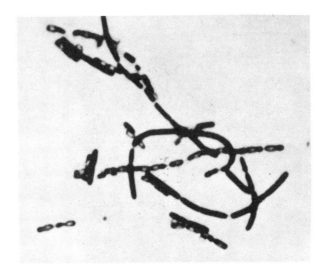

Figure 1 – 5. *Bacillus anthracis*, from a 48-hr culture, showing endospores. This bacterium causes anthrax and was used by Pasteur and Koch in many experiments on disease causation (original magnification × 1,200). (Burrows W: Textbook of Microbiology. Philadelphia, WB Saunders, 1963)

haled a powder made from the scabs of healing pustules of smallpox. Although many Chinese developed the disease as a result of this custom, others became immune. This method is called *variolation*, because the dying smallpox virus was used. In the late 1700s, Edward Jenner used the cowpox virus to vaccinate people against smallpox after he observed that milkmaids who caught cowpox, a mild disease transmitted to them from cows, were protected against smallpox, a far more serious disease.

Although Pasteur employed the technique of isolating a microorganism and growing it in a pure culture in nutrient media in the laboratory, Robert Koch, a German physician, is usually given credit for most pure-culture research methods in microbiology. He and his assistant, Julius Petri, developed the *petri dish*, which is still in use today, for microbial growth on solid media. At the suggestion of an associate's wife, Frau Hesse, they used agar, an extract from a marine seaweed used at that time to make jelly, to solidify the growth medium so that distinct colonies of bacteria could be observed.

In addition, Robert Koch, in 1876, established an experimental procedure to prove the germ theory of disease, which states that *a specific disease is caused by a specific pathogen*. This scientific procedure is known as *Koch's postulates* (Fig. 1 – 6).

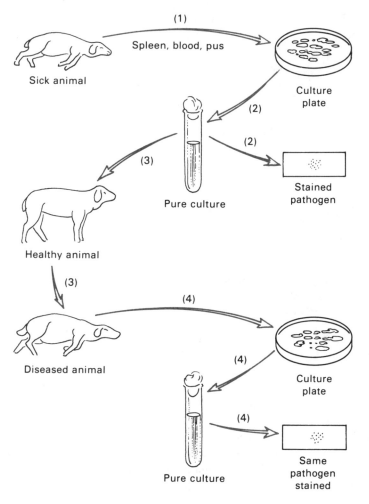

Figure 1 – 6. Koch's postulates: proof of the germ theory of disease.

Koch's Postulates

1. The causative agent must be present in every case of the disease and must not be present in healthy animals.
2. The pathogen must be isolated from the diseased host animal and must be grown in pure culture.
3. The same disease must be produced when microbes from the pure culture are inoculated into healthy susceptible animals.
4. The same pathogen must be recoverable once again from this artificially infected host animal, and it must be able to be grown again in pure culture.

Koch's postulates not only proved the germ theory of disease but also gave a tremendous boost to the development of microbiology by stressing laboratory culture and identification of microorganisms. However, some circumstances exist in which these postulates may not be easy to apply, as outlined below:

Exceptions to Koch's Postulates

1. Many healthy people carry pathogens but do not exhibit symptoms of the disease. These "carriers" may transmit the pathogens to others who then may become diseased. This is usually the circumstances with epidemics of certain hospital (nosocomial) infections, gonorrhea, typhoid fever, diphtheria, pneumonia, and AIDS.
2. Some microbes are very difficult or impossible to grow in the laboratory in artificial media, such as most viruses and the bacteria that cause leprosy and syphilis. Thus, pure cultures of those pathogens are difficult to obtain. However, many of these fastidious pathogens may now be grown in tissue cultures of living cells of various types, in egg embryos, or in certain animals. The leprosy pathogen thrives in armadillos; the spirochetes of syphilis grow well in the testes of rabbits and chimpanzees; and human immunodeficiency virus (HIV), also known as AIDS virus, proliferates in human lymphocyte cultures.
3. To induce a disease from a pure culture, the experimental animal must be susceptible to that pathogen. Many animals, such as rats, are very resistant to microbial infections. Many pathogens are species-specific, which means that they grow in only one species of animal; for example, the pathogen that causes cholera in humans does not cause hog cholera, and *vice versa*. Because human volunteers are difficult to find and ethical reasons limit their use, the researcher may only be able to observe the changes caused by the pathogen in human cells that can be grown in tissue cultures in the laboratory.
4. Certain diseases develop only when an opportunistic pathogen invades a weakened host. These secondary invaders or opportunists cause disease in a weakened person who is ill or is recovering from another disease. Examples are pneumonia and ear infections, which may follow influenza. If researchers were looking for the influenza virus, they might be misled by isolating the bacteria that caused the pneumonia.

It is also important to remember that not all diseases are caused by microorganisms. Many diseases, such as rickets and scurvy, result from diet deficiencies. Some diseases are inherited or are caused by an abnormality in the chromosomes, as in sickle cell anemia. Others, such as diabetes, result from malfunction of a body organ or system, and still others, such as cancer of the lungs and skin, are influenced by environmental factors. The infectious diseases are caused by microorganisms.

The period of rapid development of microbiological techniques in the late 1800s is known as the "Golden Age of Microbiology." Efficient surgical techniques based on Pasteur's fermentation theories and sterilization techniques were developed. During this period Ignaz Semmelweis, a physician, showed that puerperal sepsis (infection following childbirth) was caused by infectious agents present in the mother and on the hands of doctors and midwives. In 1847, he demonstrated that washing and disinfecting the hands greatly reduced the number of infections following childbirth. However, this work was not widely accepted. It was nearly 20 years later (1865) when Joseph Lister showed there were less complications from infections following surgery and childbirth if the instruments were boiled and if the hands of the surgeon and the wound were disinfected with carbolic acid (phenol). Refer to Table 1–1.

This technique of using disinfectants to prevent microorganisms from entering a surgical wound became known as *antiseptic surgery*. The application of antiseptic principles to surgery paved the way for many advances in surgical techniques, including *sterile techniques* and *aseptic techniques* (techniques that exclude pathogens), which are practiced throughout the modern world in operating theaters and research laboratories.

Modern nursing techniques logically followed a better understanding of the concepts of disease causation, transmission, and sterilization. Florence Nightingale, an English nurse of the 19th century, developed modern principles of nursing, methods of training nurses, and procedures for organizing hospitals to reduce the spread of disease.

The Tools of Microbiology

Microscopes

Because microorganisms cannot be seen without the aid of powerful magnifying lenses or a microscope, the expansion of the field of microbiology beyond the advances made during the 19th century depended on the development of better microscopes to properly observe these organisms. Although submicroscopic infectious agents, such as rabies and smallpox viruses, were known to exist, they could not be seen until the electron microscope was developed.

Light Microscope

A single magnifying glass usually magnifies the image of an object from about 3 to 20 times the object's actual size. The *light microscope* used today is a compound brightfield microscope with two lenses and a visible light source that passes through the specimen and lenses to the observer's eye (hence the term "bright-

Table 1–1. Major Contributors to the Development of Microbiology as a Science before 1900

Contributor	Contribution	Date(s)
Antony van Leeuwenhoek	First to observe microorganisms with simple microscope.	1685
Francisco Redi	Demonstrated that animals do not arise spontaneously from dead organic matter.	1660
Abbe Spallanzani	One of the first to demonstrate that heated broth, in the absence of air, did not support spontaneous generation.	1770
Schröder and von Dusch	Demonstrated that broth heated in the presence of filtered air did not support spontaneous generation.	1854
John Tyndall	Demonstrated that open tubes of broth remained free of bacteria if air was free of dust.	1860
Louis Pasteur	Disproved the theory of spontaneous generation (1861). Contributed to understanding of fermentation (1858). Technique for selective destruction of microorganisms (pasteurization) (1866). Study of diseases of wine (1866) and silkworms (1868). Attenuated vaccines for anthrax (1881) and chicken cholera. Immunization against rabies (1885).	1855–1890s
Joseph Lister	Contributed to concept of aseptic technique and pure culture concept.	1865–1870
Robert Koch	Developed postulates for proving the cause of infectious disease (1884). Observed anthrax bacilli (1876). Developed solid culture media (1882). Discovered organisms causing tuberculosis (1882).	1870s to 1890s
Paul Ehrlich	Formulated humoral theory of resistance. Developed new staining techniques. Developed first chemotherapeutic agent.	1890s to 1900
Elie Metchnikoff	Formulated cellular theory of resistance.	1890s
Emil von Behring	Developed method for producing immunity by using antitoxin against diphtheria.	1890s

field") (Fig. 1–7). The eyepiece contains the ocular lens; the second lens is in the objective, near the object to be viewed.

The two-lens system of the compound microscope can magnify 40 to 1,200 times. The magnification is usually indicated by a numeral followed by an $\times$, such as "1,200$\times$," in which $\times$ means *times*. The total magnification of a compound microscope is obtained by multiplying the magnifying power of the ocular lens (usually 10$\times$) by the magnifying power of the objective lens (usually 10, 40, or 100$\times$). Thus, with the low-power objective, the total magnification is 10 multi-

Figure 1–7. A modern light microscope. (Photograph courtesy Carl Zeiss, Inc.)

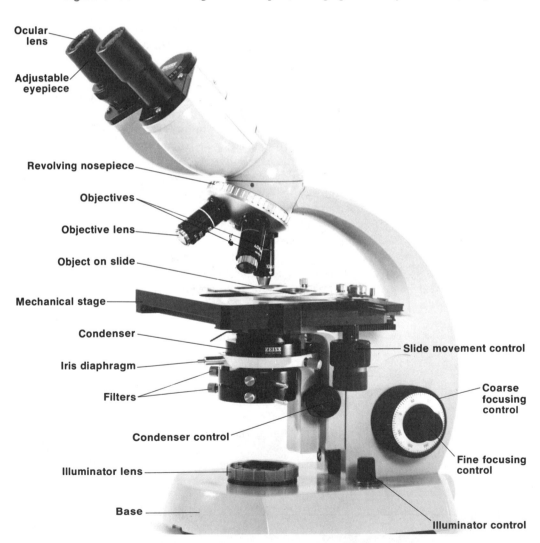

plied by 10, or 100X. Usually this objective is used to locate the microorganism to be studied. With the high-dry lens, the total magnification is 10 multiplied by 40, or 400X, which is used to study algae, protozoa, and other large microorganisms. With the oil-immersion objective (100X), a total magnification of 1000X is obtained, which is useful for observing the general characteristics of bacteria.

The oil-immersion objective must be used only with a drop of immersion oil between the slide and the objective lens; the oil reduces the scattering of light. For clear observation of the specimen, the light must be properly adjusted and focused. The condenser under the stage focuses the light on the specimen, adjusts the amount of light, and shapes the cone of light entering the objective. Generally, the higher the magnification, the more light that is needed.

Magnification alone is of little value unless the enlarged image possesses increased detail and clarity. The image clarity depends on the microscope's *resolving power*, which is the ability of the lens to distinguish two adjacent points or objects at a particular distance apart. The resolving power depends on the wavelength of the light source and the numerical aperture (NA) of the microscope. The greater the numerical aperture, the greater the resolving power will be. The resolving power of a compound microscope is approximately $0.2\,\mu m$ when oil immersion is used at a maximum numerical aperture (focus). This means that two bacteria could be distinguished as separate entities if they are separated by $0.2\,\mu m$ or more.

Other light microscopes are built and adjusted for darkfield techniques, phase-contrast microscopy, and fluorescence. In darkfield microscopy, the light is directed toward the specimen from the side so that the only light to reach the objective is reflected from the bacteria or object to be studied. Thus, the microbe appears as a bright object on a dark background. This technique is frequently used to study very small bacteria like the spirochete *Treponema pallidum*, which causes syphilis. The phase-contrast microscope may be used to observe living microbes without staining because the light refracted by living cells is different from the surrounding medium, and thus they are more easily seen. The microscope used for fluorescence microscopy has an ultraviolet (UV) light source that illuminates the object but does not pass into the objective of the microscope. When UV light strikes certain dyes and pigments they emit a certain type of light; for example, different types of chlorophyll emit green, yellow, or orange light that can be seen in the microscope against a dark background. The UV light microscope is often used in immunology laboratories to show that antibodies stained with a fluorescent dye combine with the specific antigens on bacteria. The fluorescent antibody technique is frequently used as a diagnostic test in medical bacteriology.

Electron Microscope

The *electron microscope* uses an electron beam instead of visible light and magnets instead of lenses to focus the beam. The electrons pass through the dry specimen, which is mounted in wax or plastic, and the image is seen on a fluorescent screen.

The picture may then be photographed and enlarged to magnify the object several hundred thousand times, much more than with light microscopes. Thus, very tiny microbes and viruses may be observed. Also, by using thin sections of cells mounted in plastic, in the transmission microscope, the internal structure of the cells can be studied. A recent modification of this scope is the scanning electron microscope, which is very useful for observing the surfaces and the three-dimensional image of an object. Figures 1–8, 1–9, and 1–10 show the difference in magnification and detail between electron and light photomicrographs and Table 1–2 lists the characteristics of various types of microscopes.

Units of Measurement

In microbiology, several common metric units are used to describe the size of the microorganisms. The meter, the basic unit, is equivalent to approximately 39 inches. It is divided into 10 decimeters or 100 centimeters or 1,000 millimeters or 1 million micrometers or 1 billion nanometers, and so forth. The relationship among these units may be observed in Figure 1–11.

It should be noted that the old term *micron* (μ) has been replaced by the term *micrometer* (μm); the term *millimicron* ($m\mu$) has been replaced by the term *nanometer* (*nm*); and the *angström* (Å) is 0.1 nanometer (0.1 nm), according to the International System adopted by scientists worldwide. On this scale, red blood cells are about 100 μm in diameter. Bacteria vary in width and length from about 0.20

Figure 1–8. *Staphylococcus aureus*, as seen by light microscopy magnified 1,000 times. (Photograph courtesy W. L. Wong)

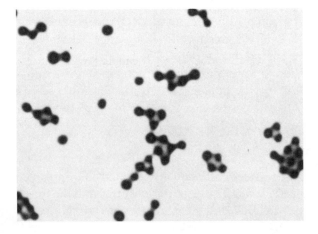

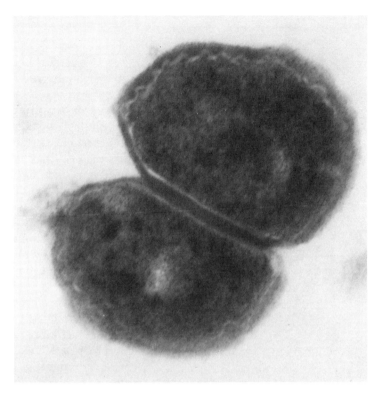

Figure 1-9. *Staphylococcus aureus*, as seen by transmission electron microscopy magnified 40,000 times. (Photograph courtesy Ray Rupel)

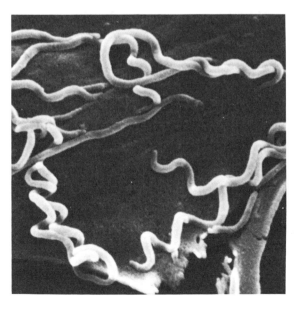

Figure 1-10. The three-dimensional qualities of scanning electron microscopy clearly reveal the corkscrew shape of cells of the syphilis-causing spirochete, *Treponema pallidum*, attached here to rabbit testicular cells grown in culture (original magnification × 8,000). (Volk WA, et al.: Essentials of Medical Microbiology, 4th ed. Philadelphia, JB Lippincott, 1991)

Table 1 – 2. Characteristics of the Various Types of Microscopes

Type	Resolving Power	Useful Magnification	Characteristics
Brightfield	0.2000 μm	1,000	Use to observe morphology of microorganisms, such as bacteria, protozoa, fungi, and algae in living (unstained) and nonliving (stained) state. Cannot resolve organisms less than 0.2 μm, such as spirochetes and viruses.
Darkfield	0.2000 μm	1,000	Background is dark, and unstained organisms can be seen. Useful for examining spirochetes. Slightly more difficult to operate than brightfield.
Phase contrast	0.2000 μm	1,000	Can observe dense structures in living procaryotic and eucaryotic microorganisms.
Fluorescent	0.2000 μm	1,000	Fluorescent dye attached to organism. Primarily a diagnostic technique (immuno-fluorescence) to detect organisms in cells, tissue, and clinical specimens. Training required in specimen preparation and microscope operation.
Transmission electron microscope (TEM)	0.0005 μm	200,000	Specimen can be viewed on screen. Excellent resolution. Allows examination of cellular ultrastructure, as well as viruses. Specimen is nonliving. Image is two dimensional.
Scanning electron microscope (SEM)	0.0200 μm	10,000	Specimen can be viewed on screen. Three-dimensional view of specimen. Useful in examining surface structure of cells and viruses. Specimen is nonliving. Resolution limited compared with TEM.

(Adapted from Boyd, 1988)

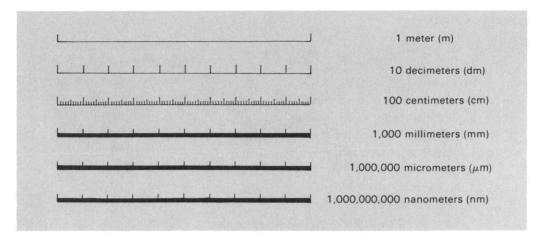

Figure 1-11. Representation of some metric units.

to 10 μm, and viruses from about 0.02 to 0.35 μm. Some very large protozoa reach the length of 2,000 μm, or 2 mm.

The sizes of microorganisms are calculated by using a microscope stage measuring device, called a stage micrometer, to determine the distance between the marks on another measuring device known as the ocular micrometer (a small ruler on a glass disk), which is placed in the eyepiece of the microscope. This procedure is known as calibration. The ocular micrometer is then used to measure the length and width of the microbe on the specimen slide, using the same objective as was used during the calibration process.

Each type of microscope has its limits of visibility. The light microscope can be used for observation of cells larger than 0.2000 μm, whereas the electron microscope can discern objects as small as 0.5000 nm (0.0005 μm) in diameter.

Summary

In this chapter the field of microbiology is introduced to illustrate the importance of all the microorganisms around you. Many of the areas of study that are included in this science are explained. As you read the milestones of the historical development, you should realize that this is a relatively new field of study that could only be developed with refined microscopes and techniques. These microscopic and biochemical discoveries enabled the microbiologists to explore and understand more about the characteristics of these organisms that cannot be seen with the unaided eye.

Study Outline

I. Microbiology, the science
    A. Microbiology: the study of very
        small living organisms
        1. Occurrence of microbes
        2. Relevance to health sciences
    B. The scope of microbiology
        1. General microbiology
        2. Medical microbiology
        3. Veterinary microbiology
        4. Agricultural microbiology
            a. Food microbiology
            b. Dairy microbiology
        5. Sanitary microbiology
        6. Industrial and applied
            microbiology
        7. Microbial genetics

    8. Environmental microbiology
    C. Milestones of microbiology
        1. Discovery of microorganisms
        2. Spontaneous generation
        3. Theory of biogenesis
        4. Biological theory of
            fermentation
        5. Germ theory of disease
        6. Koch's postulates
        7. Sterilization and disinfection
            techniques
II. The tools of microbiology
    A. Microscopes
        1. Light microscopy
        2. Electron micoscopy
    B. Units of measurement

Problems and Questions

1. What does the study of microbiology include? What types of organisms?
2. Why is the study of microbiology important to people working in
    health occupations?
3. Why is Leeuwenhoek called the "Father of Microbiology"?
4. Why was the theory of spontaneous generation debated for 200 years?
5. What contributions did Pasteur make to microbiology?
6. What did Pasteur do to save the wine industry in France?
7. What contributions to microbiology were made by Semmelweis, Lister,
    Jenner, and Nightingale?
8. What did Koch's postulates prove?
9. List Koch's postulates and the circumstances under which they might
    not be easily applied.
10. What types of microscopes are used to observe bacteria and viruses?
11. What units of measurement are used to describe the size of bacteria?

Self Test

After you have read Chapter 1, examined the objectives, studied the new words,
reviewed the study outline and answered the questions at the end of the chapter,
complete the following self test.

Matching Exercises

Complete each statement from the list of words provided within each section.

Historical Milestones of Microbiology

Leeuwenhoek   Tyndall   Lister
Fracastorius   Nightingale   Hesse
Janssen   Pasteur   Petri
Jenner   Koch   Semmelweis

1. Modern nursing techniques that reduce the spread of disease were developed by _Florence Nightingale_
2. The man who proved the germ theory of disease by animal and laboratory procedures followed by a list of postulates was _Koch_.
3. The chemist who stated the biological theory of fermentation and the germ theory of disease and who disproved the theory of spontaneous generation was _Pasteur_.
4. The physician who demonstrated the effectiveness of hand washing in reducing infections following childbirth was _Semmelweis_.
5. The "Father of Microbiology," who first described microorganisms, was _Leeuwenhoek_.
6. The physician who described the transmission of diseases in 1546 was _Fracastorius_.
7. An early compound microscope was built by _Janssen_.
8. The process of boiling and cooling repeatedly to destroy spores, which is called tyndallization, was discovered by _Tyndall_.
9. The person who developed vaccines for anthrax and chicken cholera and rabies was _Pasteur_.
10. The antiseptic surgical technique was proved effective by _Semmelweis_. _Lister_
11. The small, flat glass dish for the growth of microorganisms was developed by _Petri_.
12. The wife of a researcher in Koch's laboratory who suggested the use of agar growth medium was _Hesse_.
13. The physician who demonstrated that the cowpox virus could be used to vaccinate against smallpox was _Jenner_.
14. The technique for pure culture research methods is attributed to the laboratory group led by _Lister_. _Koch_

Some Types of Microbes

pathogenic   indigenous microflora   nitrogen-fixing microbes
opportunists   saprophytes   iron-utilizing microbes

1. The microorganisms usually found on or within a person are called _indigenous microflora_.

2. The microbes that are usually harmless but that may cause disease when a person's normal resistance is low are called _opportunists_.

3. The soil microbes that return nitrogen from the air to the soil are _nitrogen-fixing microbes_.

4. Those bacteria and fungi that break down decaying organic materials to return plant nutrients to the soil are called _saprophytes_.

5. The microorganisms that cause diseases are known as _pathogenic_.

6. Those bacteria that can destroy metal filters in water wells are _iron-utilizing microbes_.

7. The legumes are plants that have microbes living on or near their roots, such as clover, alfalfa, and peanuts. Some of these microbes replenish the soil because they are _nitrogen-fixing microbes_.

Theories and Terms

abiogenesis   biological theory of   pure culture
sterile technique   fermentation   saprophytes
biogenesis   medium   spontaneous
contaminant   micrometer   generation
fermentation   pasteurization   sterilization
germ theory of disease   pathogen   vaccination

1. The procedure for killing all microorganisms is _sterilization_.

2. The process used to destroy the harmful microbes in milk and beer is _pasteurization_.

3. The surgical technique in which all microorganisms are excluded from the surgical field is _sterile technique_.

4. The theory stating that a specific disease is caused by a specific pathogen is the _germ theory of disease_.

5. The theory stating that a specific microorganism produces a specific change in the material on which it grows is the _biological theory of fermentation_.

6. The theory explaining that life must arise from preexisting life is the theory of _biogenesis_.

7. The technique of isolating and growing one species of microorganisms on a growth medium results in a _pure culture_.
8. For centuries it was believed that living animals could arise spontaneously from nonliving material. This is the theory of _spontaneous generation / abiogenesis_.
9. The artificial process by which people can be made immune to certain diseases is _vaccination_.
10. Unit of measurement equal to 1/1,000 of a millimeter is a _micrometer_.
11. A _pathogen_ is a disease-causing microbe.
12. The breakdown of carbohydrates to produce alcohol is _fermentation_.
13. A culture containing only one species of organisms is a _pure culture_.
14. A substance used to provide nutrients for the growth of microorganisms is a _medium_.
15. Organisms that live on dead organic matter are _saprophytes_.
16. An unwanted organism in an otherwise pure culture is a _contaminant_.
17. The concept of a living organism originating from dead organic matter without prior existence of organisms of its own type is _abiogenesis_.
18. The _germ theory of disease_ is an explanation of the cause of disease based on the existence of pathogenic microorganisms.

True or False (T or F)

_F_   1. Most microorganisms are harmful to humans.
_F_   2. Viruses can be seen with a light microscope.
_F_   3. Pasteurization kills all organisms in milk.
_F_   4. Pasteur believed in abiogenesis.
_F_   5. All bacteria live on living animals.
_T_   6. Sanitary microbiologists are concerned with the microorganisms found in sewage, garbage, water, and food.
_T_   7. Tyndallization is a process of repeated boiling and cooling to destroy spores.
_F_   8. Koch's postulates can be applied when studying animals with viral infections.
_T_   9. Pneumonia and ear infections are usually caused by opportunistic bacteria that invade a weakened host.
_F_   10. Bacteria can be described when using the low-power objective of a light microscope.

Multiple Choice

1. To see viruses one must use
   a. a light microscope.
   b. a phase-contrast microscope.
   c. an electron microscope
   d. Viruses are too small to be seen.
2. Magnification of 1000X would be achieved by
   a. an ocular lens of 10X and an objective lens of 100X.
   b. an ocular lens of 15X and an objective lens of 40X.
   c. an ocular lens of 100X and an objective lens of 100X.
3. Which of the following is an exception to Koch's postulates?
   a. The causative agent is present in every case of the disease.
   b. The causative agent may be present in healthy animals that are carriers.
   c. The pathogen inoculated into a healthy animal produces the disease.
4. The study of algae is
   a. virology.
   b. phycology.
   c. mycology.
   d. algology.

5. Pasteur is credited with all of the following *except*
   a. the development of most pure culture techniques.
   b. germ theory of disease.
   c. sterilization and pasteurization.
   d. the development of vaccines.
6. Attenuated viruses are used
   a. to grow pure cultures.
   b. for vaccines against viral diseases.
   c. to prove Koch's postulates.
   d. during tyndallization.
7. The spirochete *Treponema pallidum* is best seen using
   a. a phase-contrast microscope.
   b. a fluorescence microscope.
   c. a darkfield microscope.
   d. a light microscope.
8. Which of the following are types of light microscopes: (1) ultraviolet; (2) fluorescence; (3) electron; (4) darkfield; (5) phase contrast?
   a. 1,2,4, and 5 only.
   b. 2,3, and 4 only.
   c. 3,4, and 5 only.
   d. 1 and 2 only.
   e. all of the above (1 through 5).

Chapter 2

Types of Microorganisms

Objectives

After studying this chapter, you should be able to

1. State the cell theory
2. Give a function for each part of the eucaryotic animal cell
3. Name a function for each part of the bacterial cell
4. Explain the differences among plant, animal, and bacterial cells.
5. List the characteristics used to classify bacteria
6. State the differences among rickettsias, chlamydias, and mycoplasmas
7. Name several important bacterial diseases
8. List the classes of protozoa and characteristics for classifying them
9. List five pathogenic protozoa
10. State some important characteristics of fungi
11. List five diseases caused by fungi
12. Discuss the important characteristics of procaryotic and eucaryotic algae
13. Discuss the important characteristics that make algae different from protozoa and fungi
14. Describe the characteristics used to classify viruses
15. Compare some of the differences between viruses and bacteria
16. List several important viral diseases

New Words

Amphitrichous (am-fit'-tree-kus). Bacteria with flagella (see flagella) on both ends

Bacillus (bah-sill'-us), pl. *bacilli*. A rod-shaped bacterium; the genus *Bacillus* is made up of aerobic spore-forming rods

Centrosome (sen'-troh-zoam). A eucaryotic cytoplasmic organelle containing two centrioles

Chromosomes (cro'-mo-zoms). The genetic material that contains strands of DNA, which carry the genes of heredity (see *DNA*)

Clostridium (kloss-trid'-ee-um). A genus of anaerobic spore-forming rods

Coccus (cock'-us), pl. *cocci*. A spherical or ball-shaped bacterium

Cytology (sigh-tol'-oh-gee). The study of cells.

Cytoplasm (sigh'-toe-plazm). The protoplasm outside the nucleus of the cell

DNA, deoxyribonucleic acid (de-ox'-e-ri'-bo-nu-clay'-ik). The genetic material in the chromosomes

Eucaryote (you-care'-ee-ote). A cell with a true nucleus

Endoplasmic reticulum (end-oh-plaz'-mick re-tick'-you-lum). A eucaryotic cell organelle for transport and support

Flagella (fluh-gel'-uh), sing. *flagellum*. Protein strands used for movement

Golgi (goal'-gee) **complex**. A eucaryotic cell organelle involved in secretion

Lipopolysaccharide (lip'-o-pol-e-sack'-car-ride). A macromolecule of combined lipid and polysaccharide, often found in gram-negative bacterial cell walls

Lophotrichous (low-fot'-tree-kus). Bacteria with a tuft of flagella

Lysozyme (lie'-so-zime). The cellular digestive enzyme in cytoplasmic organelles called lysosomes (see *organelles*)

Mesosome (me'so-zom). A procaryotic cell organelle involved in cellular respiration

Microtubules (my-croh-tube'-ules). Eucaryotic cell organelle involved in support and secretion

Mitochondria (my-toh-con'-dree-uh). Eucaryotic organelles involved in cellular respiration for the production of energy

Monotrichous (mon-ot'-tree-kus). Bacteria with one flagellum

Motile (mow'-till). Possessing the ability to move

Nucleoid (new'-klee-oid). The nuclear area of procaryotic cells

Nucleolus (new-klee'-oh-lus). The dense portion of the nucleus, containing RNA.

Nucleoplasm (new'-klee-oh-plaz'-um). The protoplasm inside the nucleus

Organelles (or-gan-els'). General term for the various and diverse structures contained within a cell

Peptidoglycan (pep-tid'-o-gly'-can). The rigid component of bacterial cell walls, consisting of polysaccharide chains linked together by peptide chains

Peritrichous (pear-rit'-tree-kus). Bacteria covered by flagella

Primordial (pry-more'-dee-al). Early or first in time

Procaryote (pro-care'-ee-ote). Primitive cells without a true nucleus

Protoplasm (pro'toh-plazum). The semifluid material inside cells

Ribosomes (rye'-boh-zoams). Organelles necessary for protein synthesis

RNA, ribonucleic acid (rye'-boh-new-clay'-ick). Nucleic acids necessary for protein synthesis

Spirochetes (spy'-roh-keets). Spiral-shaped bacteria

Taxonomy (tax-on'-oh-me). A systematic classification of organisms

Teichoic acid (tie-ko'-ick). A chemical in the cell wall of gram-positive bacteria

Vacuoles (vack'-you-oles). Membrane-bound storage spaces in the cell

Cells: Eucaryotes and Procaryotes

In 1665, while peering through his crude microscope, Robert Hooke observed the small empty chambers in the structure of cork. He named them *cells* because they reminded him of the bare rooms in a monastery. More than a century later, when biologists had access to more advanced microscopes, they found that cells are not empty, but rather contain a sticky (viscous) fluid. They learned that the chemical material in the cell enables it to live and reproduce. They called this material *protoplasm*, meaning "the substance of life." Now we know the cell is composed of many different substances and contains tiny particles called *organelles* that have important functions. The living material of the cell is still occasionally called protoplasm. It consists of two parts, the cytoplasm outside the nucleus and the nucleoplasm inside the nucleus.

Two German biologists, Matthias Schleiden and Theodore Schwann, proposed the cell theory in 1838. They theorized that all living things are composed of cells. Rudolf Virchow completed this theory with the idea that cells must arise from preexisting cells. In other words, life must arise from life as it exists on earth.

In biology, the cell is defined as the fundamental living unit of any organism because, like the organism, the cell exhibits the basic characteristics of life. The cell obtains food from the environment to produce energy and nutrients for metabolism (Fig. 2–1). Metabolism is an inclusive term to describe all the chemical reactions by which food is transformed for use by the cells. (See Chapter 4 for a detailed discussion of metabolism.) Through its metabolism, the cell can grow and reproduce. It can respond to changes in its environment such as light, heat, cold, and the presence of chemicals. It can mutate (change) as a result of accidental changes in its genetic material, the DNA (deoxyribonucleic acid), which makes up the genes of the chromosomes, and thus become better or less suited to its environment. As a result of these genetic changes, the mutant organism may be better adapted for survival and development into a new species of organism.

Much evidence exists to indicate that almost 4 billion years ago the first bit of life to appear on earth was a very primitive cell similar to the simple bacteria of today. Bacterial cells exhibit all the characteristics of life, even though they do not have the complex system of membranes and organelles found in the more advanced single-celled organisms. These less complex cells, which include bacteria and cyanobacteria (blue-green algae), are called *procaryotes* or procaryotic cells (Fig. 2–2). The more complex cells, with a nucleus and many organelles, are called *eucaryotes* or eucaryotic cells; these include such organisms as protozoa;

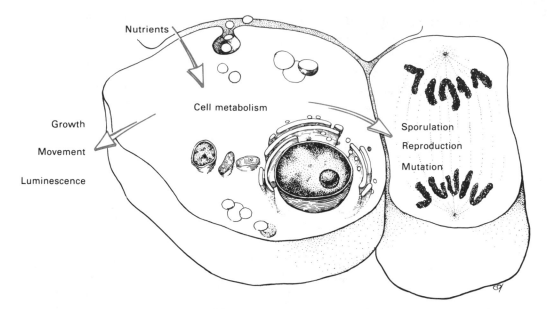

Figure 2–1. Cell metabolism. The metabolic cycles within the cell enable it to use nutrients for growth, movement, luminescence, sporulation, reproduction, and mutation.

fungi; green, brown, and red algae; and all plant and animal cells, including those that make up the human body.

Viruses appear to be the result of regressive, or of what might be termed reverse, evolution, because they are composed of only a few genes protected by a protein coat, a few enzymes, and little other material. Viruses depend on the energy and metabolic machinery of the host cell to live and reproduce. Therefore, because they are not truly viable cells, they are usually placed in a completely separate category and are not classified with the simple procaryotic cells.

For those in the health professions, it is important to understand the structure of different types of cells, not only for purposes of classifying the microorganisms but also to understand the differences in their structure and metabolism. These

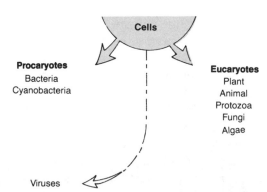

Figure 2–2. Typical cells: procaryotes, the less complex cells, and eucaryotes, the more complex cells. Viruses are not true cells.

factors must be known before we can determine or explain how the chemicals of modern chemotherapy can destroy the pathogens but not the normal human cells.

Cytology, the study of the structure and function of cells has developed during the last 30 years with the aid of the electron microscope and sophisticated biochemical research. Because complete books have been written about the details of these tiny functional factories, only a brief discussion of their structure and activities is presented here.

Eucaryotic Cell Structure

Eucaryotes (*eu* = true; *-karyo* = nut or nucleus) are so named because they have a true nucleus enclosed by a nuclear membrane. Figure 2–3 illustrates a typical eucaryotic animal cell. This illustration is a composite of most of the structures that might be found in the various types of human body cells. The electron photomicrograph in Figure 2–4 is of an actual yeast cell. A discussion of the functional

Figure 2–3. A typical eucaryotic animal cell.

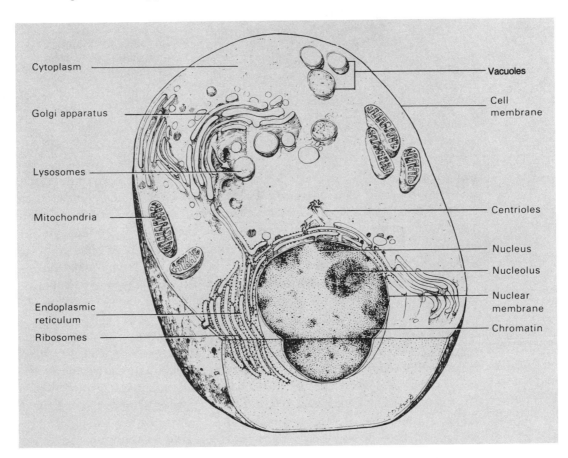

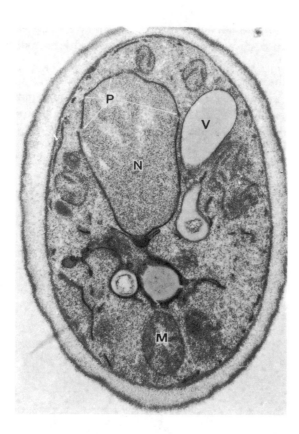

Figure 2–4. Cross section through a yeast cell showing the nucleus (N) with pores (P), mitochondrion (M), and vacuole (V). The cell is surrounded by the cell membrane. The thick, outer portion is the cell wall. (Lechavalier HA, Pramer D: The Microbes. Philadelphia, JB Lippincott, 1970)

parts of eucaryotic cells can be better understood by keeping the illustrated structures in mind.

Cell Membrane   The cell is enclosed and held intact by the cell membrane, which is also often called the plasma membrane or the cellular membrane. Structurally, it is a mosaic composed of large molecules of proteins and phospholipids. These large molecules regulate the passage of nutrients, waste products, and secretions across the cellular membrane. Because the cell membrane has the property of *selective permeability*, only certain substances may enter and leave the cell. The cell membrane is similar in structure and function to all the other membranes that are a part of the organelles of eucaryotic cells.

Nucleus   The organelle within the cell that unifies, controls, and integrates the functions of the entire cell is the nucleus, which is enclosed in the *nuclear membrane*. In this region, the genetic control system lies within the *chromosomes*. The number and composition of chromosomes and the number of genes on each chromosome are characteristic of the organism's species. Different species have different numbers and sizes of chromosomes. Human cells have 46 chromosomes, each consisting of thousands of *genes*. The gene is the unit that codes for, or determines, the traits of an individual organism. When genes are broken apart chemically, they are found to be coiled strands of *deoxyribonucleic acid* (DNA) and proteins. It is the DNA that contains the genetic information for the production of essential proteins that enable the cell to function properly. To understand more about how the base coding of the DNA can chemically control the entire organism, refer to Chapter 3.

Close observation of the nucleus of nondividing cells reveals the *chromatin*, the loosely wound strands of chromosomes that are suspended in the *nucleoplasm*. Nucleoplasm is the nutrient gelatinous matrix or base material of the nucleus. These chromatin strands condense into tightly coiled chromosomes just before the cell divides. In the very dense dark area of the nucleus, called the *nucleolus*, ribosomes are manufactured before they move to the cytoplasmic portion of the cell.

Cytoplasm   The part of the cell that does most of the normal work is the cytoplasm; it is controlled by information carried in the DNA of the nucleus. The cytoplasm is the cellular material outside the nucleus but enclosed by the cell membrane; it is composed of a semifluid gelatinous nutrient matrix and the cytoplasmic organelles, including the endoplasmic reticulum, ribosomes, Golgi apparatus, mitochondria, centrioles, microtubules, lysosomes, and other vacuoles. Each of these organelles has a highly specific function, and all of the functions are interrelated to maintain the cell and allow it to properly perform its activities.

The *endoplasmic reticulum* (ER) is a system of membranes that are interconnected and arranged to form a network of tubules connecting the outside of the cell to the nucleus. The ER transports nutrients to the nucleus and also provides some structural support for the cell. Much of the ER has a rough appearance and is designated as *rough endoplasmic reticulum* (RER). This rough appearance is due to the many *ribosomes* attached to the outer surface of the membranes. The ribosomes consist mainly of ribosomal RNA (*ribonucleic acid*) and play an important part in the synthesis (manufacture) of essential proteins for use in the cell and elsewhere in the organism.

The *Golgi complex*, or *body*, usually connects or communicates with the endoplasmic reticulum. This group of membranes completes the synthesis of secretory products and packages them into small sacs called vesicles for storage or export outside the cell.

The *lysosomes* are small sacs that originate from the Golgi apparatus. They contain *lysozyme* and other digestive enzymes that break down foreign material taken into the cell by *phagocytosis* (the engulfing of large particles by phagocytes). These enzymes also aid in breaking down worn out parts of the cell and may destroy the entire cell by a process called *autolysis* if the cell is damaged or deteriorating.

The energy necessary for cellular function is provided by the formation of high-energy phosphate molecules such as adenosine triphosphate (ATP). The *mitochondria* are the "power plants" of the cell where most of the ATP (energy-carrying) molecules are formed by cellular respiration. During this process, energy is released from glucose and other food nutrients to drive cellular functions (see Chapter 4). The number of mitochondria in the cell varies greatly depending on the activities required of that cell.

Two cylindrical organelles called the *centrioles* lie perpendicular to each other near the nucleus. The centrioles are involved in the formation of spindle fibers for eucaryotic cell division. This process, which results in two daughter cells with the same number of chromosomes as the parent cell, is called *mitosis*, or "the dance of the chromosomes." Eucaryotic cilia and flagella also appear to arise from centriole material because their internal protein fibril configuration is very similar, even though it is quite complex.

Other structures that may be present in the cell include microfilaments, microtubules, granules, and vacuoles containing food, secretory products, and pigments. Always present in plant cells are the *chloroplasts* containing the chlorophyll required for photosynthesis. Photosynthesis is the process in which light energy is used to change carbon dioxide and water into carbohydrates and oxygen.

Cell Wall   The eucaryotic cell wall is an external structure found on plant cells, algae, and fungi. It consists mainly of cellulose but may also contain pectin, lignin, chitin, and some mineral salts (usually found in algae). This eucaryotic cell wall is much simpler and different from the procaryotic bacterial cell wall. The cell wall provides rigidity and protection for these cells.

Procaryotic Cell Structure

The procaryotes are structurally very simple cells when compared with the eucaryotic system of membranes, yet they are able to carry on the normal processes of life. In these cells, division is by binary fission — the simple division of the cell parts with formation of a separating membrane and a cell wall. A generalized bacterium can be considered as a "typical procaryotic cell."

Refer to the composite drawing (Fig. 2–5) of a "typical" gram-positive or gram-negative (explanation follows) bacterial cell and to the electron micrograph in Figure 2–6, as we discuss this cell from internal to external structures. Within the cytoplasm, the nuclear material (nucleoid), mesosomes, polyribosomes, and other cytoplasmic particles can be seen. Note that these cells are not filled with internal membranes as are eucaryotic cells. The cytoplasm is surrounded by cell (plasma or cytoplasmic) membrane, cell wall, and sometimes a capsule or slime layer. These latter three structures make up the bacterial cell envelope. On some of these procaryotes, flagella or pili (see p. 40), or both, may be observed outside the envelope, and spores may be seen inside, depending on the particular genus and species of the bacteria.

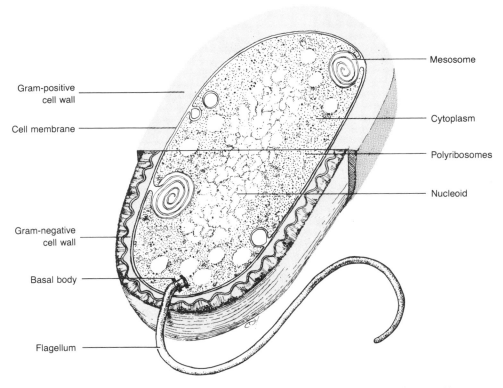

Gram-positive
cell wall

Cell membrane

Gram-negative
cell wall

Basal body

Flagellum

Mesosome

Cytoplasm

Polyribosomes

Nucleoid

Figure 2–5. An illustrated composite procaryotic bacterial cell showing the difference between gram-negative and gram-positive cell walls.

Nucleoid   The procaryotic nucleoid may be considered a primitive nucleus; it is not surrounded by a nuclear membrane, does not have a definite shape, and has little or no protein material. It usually consists of a single, circular chromosome. The chromosome is DNA, which serves as the control center of the bacterial cell, carrying the genetic information needed for producing several thousand enzymes and other proteins. It is capable of duplicating itself, of guiding cell division, and of directing cellular activities.

Cytoplasm   The semiliquid cytoplasm, which surrounds the nucleoid, is contained within the plasma membrane. The cytoplasm consists of water, enzymes, oxygen, waste products, essential nutrients, proteins, carbohydrates, and lipids —a complex mixture of all the materials required by the cell for its metabolic functions.

Cytoplasmic Particles   Within the bacterial cytoplasm, many submicroscopic particles have been observed. Most of these particles are ribosomes, usually occurring in clusters called polyribosomes (*poly* = many). These ribosomes are

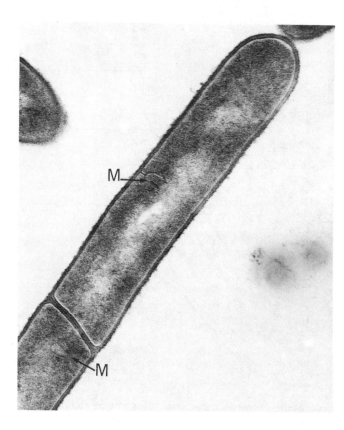

Figure 2–6. Recently divided cells of *Bacillus licheniformis* showing the light nuclear material and mesosomes (*M*). (Lechavalier HA, Pramer D: The Microbes. Philadelphia, JB Lippincott, 1970).

smaller than eucaryotic ribosomes, but their function is the same: the synthesis of proteins.

Cytoplasmic granules occur in certain species of bacteria. These may be stained, by use of a suitable stain, and then identified microscopically. The granules may consist of starch, lipids, sulfur, iron, or other stored substances.

Cell Membrane   Enclosing the cytoplasm is the plasma or cell membrane. This membrane is similar to the eucaryotic cell membrane. Chemically, the plasma membrane consists of proteins and phospholipids, which are discussed further in Chapter 3. Selectively permeable, the membrane controls which substances may enter or leave the cell. It is flexible and so thin it cannot be seen with a light microscope. However, it is frequently observed in electron micrographs of bacteria.

Many metabolic reactions take place on the cell membrane. The *mesosomes* are an inward folding of these membranes, and this is the area in bacteria where cellular respiration takes place. This process is similar to that occurring in the mitochondria of animal cells, in which the food nutrients are broken down to produce energy in the form of ATP molecules to be used in the cell's metabolic activities.

In photosynthetic bacteria and cyanobacteria, some internal membranes, which are derived from the cell membrane, contain chlorophyll and other pigments that serve to trap light energy for photosynthesis. However, bacteria do not have internal membrane systems similar to the endoplasmic reticulum and the Golgi complex of eucaryotic cells.

Bacterial Cell Wall   The rigid exterior cell wall that defines the shape of bacterial cells is chemically complex. Thus, it is quite different from the simple cellulose plant cell wall, although serving the same functions. The main constituent of bacterial cell walls is a complex macromolecular polymer known as *peptidoglycan* (or murein), consisting of many polysaccharide chains linked together by peptide (small protein) chains. The thickness of this wall and its exact composition vary with the species of bacteria. Certain bacteria, grouped as gram-positive (to be explained later) cells, have many layers of peptidoglycan combined with *teichoic acid* components. Gram-negative (also explained later) bacteria have a much thinner layer of peptidoglycan, but this layer is covered with a complex layer of lipid macromolecules, usually referred to as the *outer membrane*, as shown in Figure 2–7. These macromolecules are discussed in Chapter 3.

Figure 2–7. (*A*) A portion of the gram-positive bacterium *Bacillus fastidiosus*; note the cell wall's thick peptidoglycan layer underlaid by the cytoplasmic membrane. (*B*) The gram-negative bacterium *Enterobacter aerogenes*; both the cytoplasmic membrane and the outer membrane are visible along some sections of the cell wall. (Volk WA, et al.: Essentials of Medical Microbiology, 4th ed. Philadelphia, JB Lippincott, 1991)

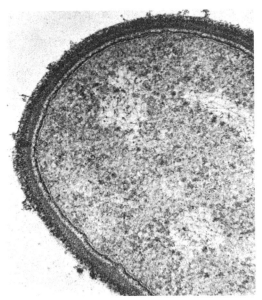

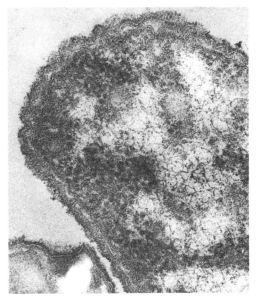

A   B

Capsules   Some bacteria have a layer of material outside the cell wall. This layer is called the capsule or may sometimes be called the slime layer or glycocalyx. It is a thick layer of slimy, gelatinous material produced by the plasma membrane and secreted outside of the cell wall. Capsules usually consist of complex sugars, or polysaccharides, which may combine with lipids and proteins, depending on the species of microorganism. A knowledge of the chemical composition of capsules is useful in identifying different types of bacteria within a species; for example, the type A *Streptococcus pneumoniae*, which can cause pneumonia, is frequently identified by its capsular type. The capsule is usually detected by staining the cell and the surrounding area; the capsule may remain unstained (a negative stain), or be stained a different color and viewed with the light microscope. Antigen-antibody tests may be used to identify specific strains of bacteria by capsular antigens, i.e., the Quellung reaction described in Chapter 9.

Encapsulated bacteria usually produce colonies on nutrient agar that are smooth (S), mucoid, and glistening. Nonencapsulated bacteria tend to grow as dry, rough (R) colonies on nutrient agar growth medium. Capsules on bacteria may serve any of several functions. If it is a thin slime, the cells may be able to glide, slide, or move on the surface of solid material. Some capsules enable the bacterial species to attach to the mucous membranes and tooth surfaces so that they are not flushed away by body secretions. Frequently, encapsulated bacteria are not easily digested by phagocytes (white blood cells); therefore, they can survive longer in the body.

Flagella   Many bacteria have flagella (singular: flagellum), which are threadlike protein appendages whose whiplike motion enables the bacteria to move or be motile. Not all bacteria have flagella; however, for those that do, the number and arrangement of flagella is a characteristic of the species. Thus, the presence of flagella is used for classification purposes.

Those bacteria that have flagella over all of their surface (perimeter) are described as *peritrichous bacteria*. Those with a tuft of flagella in a single location are *lophotrichous*; those having flagella at both ends are *amphitrichous*; and those with a single polar flagellum are *monotrichous* bacteria (Fig. 2–8).

Some spirochetes have two flagellalike fibrils called *axial filaments*, one attached to each end of the bacterium. These axial filaments extend toward the other end of the bacterium, wrap around the organism between the layers of the cell wall, and overlap each other in the midsection. As a result, the spirochetes can move in a spiral, helical, or inch-worm manner.

Bacterial flagella consist of three, four, or more threads of protein twisted like a rope, unlike the eucaryotic flagella and cilia, which have a complex arrangement of protein fibrils enclosed in a membrane. The flagella of bacteria arise from a basal body in the cell membrane and project outwardly through the cell wall and the capsule, as shown in Figure 2–5.

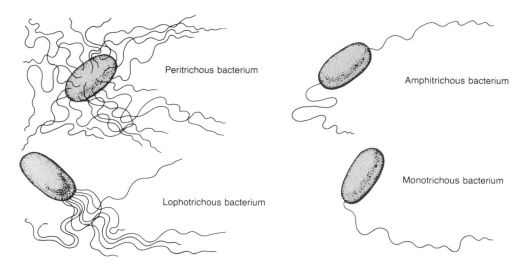

Figure 2-8. The four basic types of flagellation on bacteria: peritrichous, flagella all over surface; lophotrichous, a tuft of flagella; amphitrichous, flagella at each end; and monotrichous, one flagellum.

Pili or Fimbriae   The fimbriae or pili (singular: pilus) are hairlike tubes frequently observed on gram-negative enteric (intestinal) bacteria. They are much smaller than flagella, have a rigid structure, and are not associated with motility. These tiny appendages arise from the cytoplasm and extend through the plasma membrane, cell wall, and capsule. Their many functions vary, depending on the bacterial species. They are believed to (1) enable the bacteria to attach to other bacteria or to other membrane surfaces such as the intestinal lining and red blood cells, (2) provide a site for the attachment of bacterial viruses, and (3) enable bacteria that have a sex pilus to transfer genetic material across a pilus bridge from one to another by a process known as conjugation, which is described in Chapter 4. The pili of *Escherichia coli* can be observed in Figure 2-9.

Spores or Endospores   A few genera of bacteria (*e.g.*, *Bacillus* and *Clostridium*) form endospores as a means of survival when moisture and their nutrient supply are low, a process called *sporulation*. During sporulation, the genetic material is enclosed in several protein coats that are resistant to heat, drying, and most chemicals. Spores have been shown to survive for many years on dust particles. When the dried spore lands on a moist, nutrient surface, it may be activated to develop into a new vegetative bacterial cell. This germination of the spore may be compared with germination of a seed. However, spore formation is related to the survival of the bacterial cell, not to reproduction because usually, only one or two spores are produced in a bacterial cell, and each germinates into only one bacterium. (Fig. 2-10).

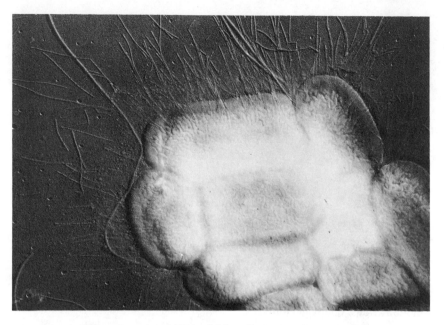

Figure 2–9. Piliated strain of *Escherichia coli*. Each cell possesses hundreds of pili. Some isolated, broken pili are also seen. A few flagella extend from the cells to the edge of the photograph. (Davis BD, et al.: Microbiology, 4th ed. Philadelphia, Harper & Row, 1987)

Differences Between Procaryotic and Eucaryotic Cells

Eucaryotic cells are divided into plant and animal types because animal cells do not have a cell wall, whereas plant cells have a simple cell wall, usually consisting of cellulose. Procaryotic cells have a complex cell wall consisting of proteins, lipids, and polysaccharides. Eucaryotic cells are filled with membrane-bound organelles, such as the endoplasmic reticulum, whereas procaryotic cells have only a few cytoplasmic membranes (mesosomes and photosynthetic membranes), which arise from the plasma membrane. The cytoplasmic ribosomes (involved in

Figure 2–10. A bacillus with a well-defined endospore. (Lechavalier HA, Pramer D: The Microbes. Philadelphia, JB Lippincott, 1970)

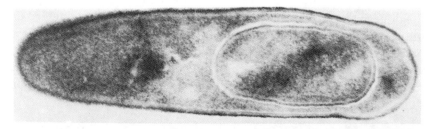

protein synthesis) are larger and more dense (80S) than those found in procaryotes (70S). The fact that 70S ribosomes are found in the mitochondria and chloroplasts of eucaryotes may indicate that these structures are derived from parasitic procaryotes during their evolutionary development. Note the other differences listed in Table 2–1.

Table 2–1. Comparison between Eucaryotic and Procaryotic Cells

	Eucaryotic Cells		Procaryotic Cells
	Plant	*Animal*	
Biological distribution	All plants, fungi, and algae	All animals and protozoa	All bacteria and cyanobacteria
Nuclear membrane	Present	Present	Absent
Membranous structures other than cell membranes	Generally present	Generally present	Generally absent except mesosomes and photosynthetic membranes
Microtubules and centrioles	Present	Present	Absent
Cytoplasmic ribosomes (density)	80S	80S	70S
Chromosomes	Composed of DNA and proteins	Composed of DNA and proteins	Composed of DNA alone
Flagella or cilia	When present, have a complex structure similar to centrioles	When present, have a complex structure similar to centrioles	Flagella, when present, have simple twisted protein structure; no cilia
Cell wall	When present, of simple chemical constitution, usually cellulose	Absent	In bacteria of complex chemical constitution containing peptidoglycan
Active cytoplasmic movements	Present	Present	Absent (not observed)
Photosynthesis (chlorophyll)	Present	Absent	Present in cyanobacteria and some bacteria

Microbial Classification

Since Aristotle's time, naturalists have attempted to classify and name plants, animals, and microorganisms in a meaningful way, on the basis of their appearance and behavior. Thus, the science of taxonomy (biological classification) was devised, based on the binomial system developed in the 18th century by the Swedish scientist, Carolus Linnaeus. In the binomial system, each organism is given two names (*e.g., Homo sapiens* for humans). The first is the *genus* or *genera* (plural), and the second is the *species*.

Each organism is categorized into larger groups based on their similarities and differences. According to the presently popular Whittaker classification scheme, all the living (and extinct) organisms can be placed in five kingdoms: Plantae for plants, Animalia for animals, Fungi for fungi, Protista for algae and protozoa, and Monera for cyanobacteria and bacteria. (However, microbiologists prefer Kingdom Procaryotae to Monera, thus, Procaryotae is used in this book to include bacteria and cyanobactria.) Viruses are usually not included because they are not truly living cells. Note that four of the kingdoms consist of eucaryotic organisms. Each kingdom consists of divisions or phyla divided into *classes, orders, families, genera,* and *species.* Additional subgroups are also fequently used. For an example, see Table 2–2.

Because written reference is often made to genera and species, biologists throughout the world have adopted a standard method of expressing these names that identify a specific organism. To express genus: capitalize the first letter of the word and underline or italicize it—for example, *Escherichia.* To express genus and species together, capitalize the first letter of the genus name (the second word is the species name, which is not capitalized) and then underline or italicize the entire name—for example, *Escherichia coli.* Frequently the genus is designated by an accepted abbreviation; in the example just given, it would read *E. coli,* indicating the genus and species.

Table 2–2. Comparison of Human and Bacterial Classification

	Human	Syphilis Pathogen
Kingdom	Animalia	*Procaryotae*
Phylum/Division	Chordata	*Gracilicutes*
Class	Mammalia	*Scotobacteria*
Order	Primate	*Spirochaetales*
Family	Hominidae	*Spirochaetaceae*
Genus	*Homo*	*Treponema*
Species	*sapiens*	*pallidum*

Bacteria

Characteristics

Bacteria were classified into 19 different categories in *Bergey's Manual of Determinative Bacteriology*, 8th ed. (1974), which was the standard reference of bacterial classification. In 1984, bacterial classification was redesigned because organism identification procedures became more exact. The new comprehensive *Bergey's Manual of Systemic Bacteriology* was published in four volumes, indicating how the taxonomy of bacteria has expanded. An outline of these volumes can be found in Appendix A. Also, by using the computer, microbiologists have established numerical taxonomy systems that not only help to identify bacteria by their characteristics but also can help establish how closely related these organisms are by comparing the composition of the genetic material and other cell substances.

Many characteristics of bacteria are examined to provide data for identification and classification: (1) morphology, (2) staining, (3) motility, (4) growth, (5) nutritional requirements, (6) biochemical and metabolic activities, (7) pathogenicity, (8) amino acid sequencing of proteins, (9) genetic composition.

Morphology   With the light microscope, the size, shape, and cell arrangement of the various bacteria are easily described. Bacteria vary widely in size, ranging from spheres that measure 0.2 μm in diameter to spirals 10.0 μm long. There are three basic shapes: spherical or coccoid — the cocci (singular: coccus); rods or bacilli (singular: bacillus); and spirals or spirilla (singular: spirillum), as shown in Figure 2–11. The cells of cocci are observed in many and various arrangements depending on the species and how they divide (Table 2–3).

Bacilli (rods) may be short or long, thick or thin, pointed or with blunt ends; they may occur singly, in pairs (diplobacilli), or in chains (streptobacilli). Some rods resemble cocci and are often called coccobacilli because they are very short, small bacilli, such as *E. coli*, which is a normal inhabitant of the intestine. Some bacilli stack up next to each other, side by side in a palisade arrangement, which is characteristic of diphtheroids and diphtheria organisms. The vibrios, such as *Vibrio cholerae*, which causes cholera, are rods with a small commalike curve.

Spirilla usually occur singly, but some species may form chains. The different species of spirilla vary in size, length, rigidity, number, and amplitude of their coils. True spirilla have rigid cell walls that maintain the shape of a helix or coil. The spirochetes, *e.g., Treponema pallidum*, the causative agent of syphilis, have a flexible cell wall enabling this coiled bacterium to move readily through tissues (see Fig. 1–10).

Some bacteria may lose their characteristic shape because adverse growth conditions prevent the production of normal cell walls. These wall-deficient bacteria are called *L-forms*. Some revert to their original shape when placed in favorable growth conditions, whereas others do not. Another group of very small bacteria, the genus *Mycoplasma*, characteristically has no cell wall; thus, microscopically

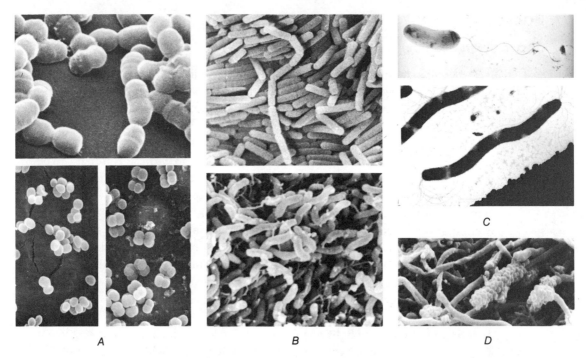

Figure 2–11. Forms of bacteria. (*A*) Cocci. *Top: Streptococcus mutans,* demonstrating pairs and short chains (original magnification ×9,400). *Bottom left:* Single cells and small clusters of *Staphylococcus epidermidis* (original magnification ×3,000). *Bottom right:* Pairs, tetrads, and regular clusters of *Micrococcus luteus* (original magnification ×3,000). (*B*) Bacilli. *Top:* Single cells and short chains of *Bacillus cereus* (original magnification ×1,700). *Bottom:* Flagellated bacilli (unnamed) associated with periodontitis (original magnification ×3,700). (*C*) *Top:* A cell of *Vibrio cholerae;* note curved cell and single flagellum (original magnification ×8,470). *Bottom:* The spirillum *Aquaspirillum bengal;* note polar tufts of flagella (original magnification ×2,870). (*D*) Variety of organisms in dental plaque after 3 days without brushing (original magnification ×1,360). (Volk WA, et al.: Essentials of Medical Microbiology, 4th ed. Philadelphia, JB Lippincott, 1991)

Table 2–3. Arrangement of Cocci

Arrangement	Description	Pathogenic Example	Disease
Diplococci	Pairs of cells	*Neisseria gonorrhoeae*	Gonorrhea
Streptococci	Cocci in chains	*Streptococcus pyogenes*	"Strep" sore throat
Staphylococci	Cocci in clusters	*Staphylococcus aureus*	Boils
Tetrads	Four cocci as in a box	*Micrococcus luteus*	Nonpathogenic
Octads	Eight cocci as in a box	*Sarcina ventriculi*	Nonpathogenic

they appear in various pleomorphic shapes. These bacteria are not genetically related, but they have several properties in common. They have no rigid cell shape; they reproduce slowly; and they are relatively fragile, are very susceptible to changes in osmotic pressure, and are resistant to antibiotics that deter cell wall synthesis.

Staining   Various staining methods have been devised to examine bacteria that have been smeared and dried on a slide. Specific stains and techniques are used to observe bacterial morphology (shape, grouping, type of cell wall, nuclear material, capsules, flagella, spores, flat globules, and various types of granules).

The simple stain is sufficient to determine bacterial shape and grouping characteristics. For this method, as shown in Figure 2 – 12, crystal violet, safranin, carbol fuchsin, or methylene blue is applied to the dried smear on the slide, rinsed, dried, and examined with the oil immersion lens of the microscope. Dr. Hans Gram, in 1884, developed the Gram-staining technique that bears his name. This procedure differentiates between "gram-positive" and "gram-negative" types of bacterial cell walls. The color retained by the bacteria after the staining process

Figure 2 – 12. Bacterial staining techniques. (A) With a flamed loop, smear a loopful of bacteria suspended in broth or water on a slide. (B) Allow slide to air-dry. (C) Pass the slide through the flame to heat-fix the bacteria to the slide. (D) Flood the slide with the stain. (E) Rinse with water. (F) Blot dry with bibulous paper or paper towel. (G) Examine the slide with the 100X microscope objective using a drop of immersion oil directly on the smear.

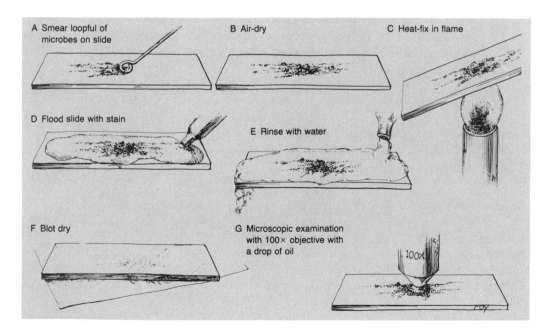

depends on the thickness and chemical composition of the cell wall. This staining process has four steps: (1) flood the smear with crystal violet for 1 minute; (2) rinse with water and cover the slide with Gram's iodine solution; (3) after 1 minute, wash off the iodine with water and decolorize with alcohol or acetone for 20 seconds; then (4) counterstain with safranin for 1 minute, rinse, dry, and examine under oil. The gram-positive bacteria retain the purple color of the crystal violet. In the gram-negative cells, the purple color is removed by the alcohol; thus, the cells are counterstained red by the safranin. Some strains of bacteria are neither consistently purple nor red following this procedure, hence they are called gram-variable bacteria. Most of these cells are members of the genus *Mycobacterium*, such as *M. tuberculosis* and *M. leprae*. They are more easily identified with the acid-fast stain. In this method, carbol fuchsin is driven into the bacterial cell wall with heat so that the acid-alcohol does not remove the red color from the mycobacteria. Most other bacteria are decolorized by the acid-alcohol treatment, and the tuberculosis pathogens can be readily seen in a sputum smear from a tubercular patient as red organisms in a blue background.

The procedures for staining bacteria to observe capsules, spores, flagella, fat globules, granules, and nuclear material are described in most microbiology laboratory manuals. Refer to Table 2–4 for the Gram-staining characteristics of certain pathogens.

Motility   The ability of an organism to move by itself is called motility. Bacterial motility is usually associated with the presence of flagella or axial filaments. Most spiral bacteria and about one half of the bacilli are motile, but cocci are generally nonmotile. Motility can be observed best in a young culture of organisms in a semisolid medium or by the hanging-drop technique. In the latter, motile bacteria suspended in a hanging drop of liquid can be seen darting about in every direction within the drop (Fig. 2–13). Some bacteria exhibit gliding motility on secreted slime on solid agar.

Table 2–4.   Some Important Pathogenic Bacteria

Bacterium	Diseases	Type	Gram-Stain Reaction[a]
Bacillus anthracis	Anthrax	Spore-forming rod	+
Bordetella pertussis	Whooping cough	Rod	−
Brucella abortus and *B. melitensis*	Brucellosis, undulant fever	Rod	−
Chlamydia trachomatis	Lymphogranuloma venereum, trachoma	Coccoid	−

Table 2–4. Some Important Pathogenic Bacteria (*Continued*)

Bacterium	Diseases	Type	Gram-Stain Reaction[a]
Clostridium botulinum	Botulism (food poisoning)	Spore-forming rod	+
Clostridium perfringens	Gas gangrene, wound infections	Spore-forming rod	+
Clostridium tetani	Tetanus (lockjaw)	Spore-forming rod	+
Corynebacterium diphtheriae	Diphtheria	Rod	+
Escherichia coli	Urinary infections	Rod	−
Francisella tularensis	Tularemia	Rod	−
Haemophilus ducreyi	Chancroid	Rod	−
Haemophilus influenzae	Meningitis, pneumonia	Rod	−
Klebsiella pneumoniae	Pneumonia	Rod	−
Mycobacterium leprae	Leprosy	Rod	+/−
Mycobacterium tuberculosis	Tuberculosis	Rod	+/−
Mycoplasma pneumoniae	Atypical pneumonia	Pleomorphic	−
Neisseria gonorrhoeae	Gonorrhea	Diplococcus	−
Neisseria meningitidis	Nasopharyngitis, meningitis	Diplococcus	−
Proteus vulgaris and *P. morgani*	Gastroenteritis, urinary infections	Rod	−
Pseudomonas aeruginosa	Respiratory and urogenital infections	Rod	−
Rickettsia rickettsii	Rocky Mountain spotted fever	Rod	−
Salmonella typhi	Typhoid fever	Rod	−
Salmonella species	Gastroenteritis	Rod	−
Shigella species	Shigellosis (bacillary dysentery)	Rod	−
Staphylococcus aureus	Boils, carbuncles, pneumonia, septicemia	Cocci in clusters	+
Streptococcus pyogenes	Strep throat, scarlet fever, rheumatic fever, septicemia	Cocci in chains	+
Streptococcus pneumoniae	Pneumonia	Diplococcus	+
Treponema pallidum	Syphilis	Spirochete	−
Vibrio cholerae	Cholera	Curved rod	−
Yersinia pestis	Plague	Rod	−

[a]+ = gram-positive; − = gram-negative; +/− = gram-variable

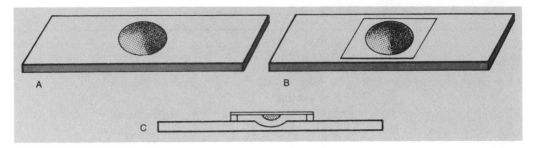

Figure 2–13. Hanging drop preparation for study of living bacteria. (*A*) Depression slide. (*B*) Depression slide with coverglass over the depression area. (*C*) Side view of hanging drop preparation, showing the drop of culture hanging from the center of the coverglass above the depression. (Volk WA, Wheeler MF: Basic Microbiology, 5th ed. Philadelphia, JB Lippincott, 1984)

Growth   The cultural characteristic of bacterial colonies of a single species varies with the type of nutrient agar medium, the nutrients, and the dyes present. The size, color, shape, and consistency of a colony growing on a particular agar medium are characteristic of a given species of bacteria. In a liquid medium, the region in which the organism grows depends on the oxygen needs of that particular species. The rate of growth is also an important characteristic.

Nutritional Requirements   All bacteria need some form of the elements carbon, hydrogen, oxygen, sulfur, phosphorus, and nitrogen for growth. Special elements, such as potassium, calcium, iron, manganese, magnesium, cobalt, copper, zinc, and uranium, are needed by certain bacteria. Some have specific vitamin requirements; others need organic substances secreted by other living microorganisms during their growth. The nutritional needs are characteristic of the species of bacteria. These nutritional requirements are discussed in Chapter 4.

Biochemical and Metabolic Activities   As bacteria grow, they produce many waste products and secretions, some of which are enzymes that enable them to invade their host and cause disease. The pathogenic strains of many bacteria, such as staphylococci and streptococci, can be tentatively identified by the enzymes they secrete. Also, in particular environments, certain bacteria are characterized by the production of carbon dioxide, hydrogen, sulfide, oxygen, or methane.

Pathogenicity   The disease-producing abilities of pathogens are important. Many are able to cause disease because they have capsules or endotoxins (a part of the cell wall) or because they secrete exotoxins and enzymes that damage cells and tissues (see Chapter 7). Frequently, pathogenicity is tested by injecting the pathogen into mice. Some common pathogenic bacteria are listed in Table 2–4.

Amino Acid Sequencing   The proteins found within a bacterium are specific for that species. Thus, by comparing the amino acid sequence of certain bacterial proteins, the species and how closely related it is to other bacteria can be determined.

Genetic Composition   The composition of the genetic material (DNA) is unique to each species. Thus, by determining the base composition and by comparing the cytosine/guanine ratio with the total amount of bases, a numerical ratio can be calculated (see Chapter 3). Also, by identifying or hybridizing a sequence of bases in portions of DNA or RNA, the researcher can determine the degree of relationship between two bacteria and, perhaps, the species, strain, or type of bacteria.

Rudimentary Forms of Bacteria

The rickettsias, chlamydias, and mycoplasmas are bacteria, but they do not possess all of the attributes of typical bacterial cells. Because they are so small and difficult to isolate, they were formerly classified as viruses.

Rickettsias and Chlamydias

This group includes both rickettsias and chlamydias. They are coccoid, rod-shaped, or pleomorphic (irregular) gram-negative bacteria with a bacterial-type cell wall; unlike viruses, they contain both DNA and RNA. Most known forms are intracellular parasites that are pathogenic to humans and other animals.

Most rickettsias are obligate intracellular parasites; because they appear to have leaky cell membranes, they must live inside another cell to retain all the necessary cellular substances. Hence, they are usually transmitted by arthropod vectors. An exception is *Coxiella burnetii*, the cause of Q fever, which may also be airborne or foodborne.

The rickettsias include parasites of arthropods (lice, fleas, ticks). These animals are frequently vectors (carriers) of rickettsial diseases because they transmit pathogens from one host to another by their bites or waste products. Diseases caused by anthropod-borne rickettsias include Rocky Mountain spotted fever and the typhus fevers.

The chlamydias are probably the most primitive of all bacteria because they lack the enzymes to perform many essential metabolic activities, particularly the production of ATP. Thus, they are obligate intracellular parasites and must be transferred by direct contact between hosts, not by insects.

Chlamydias have two forms in their life cycle (Fig. 2 – 14). The infectious form, called the *elementary body*, attaches to the host cell. After it is engulfed by the host cell, the elementary body reorganizes into the larger, less infectious form, called the *reticulate body*. This form finally divides to produce many small infectious elementary bodies that are released to spread and infect surrounding host cells or

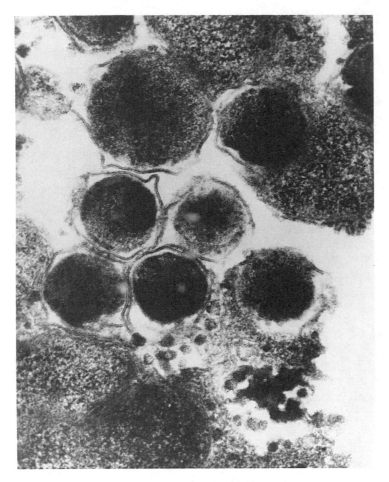

Figure 2–14. Elementary bodies of chlamydia. (Courtesy of S. Koester)

other individuals. Chlamydias are easily transmitted during sexual contact and cause many infections of the urethra (urethritis), bladder, (cystitis), fallopian tubes, prostate (prostatitis), or other complications. They cause many diseases in vertebrate animals (cats, dogs, sheep, cattle, birds, humans), including trachoma (an eye disease), lymphogranuloma venereum (LGV; a venereal disease), and psittacosis (a respiratory infection in humans and birds, often called parrot fever).

Mycoplasmas

The mycoplasmas are the smallest of the cellular microbes (Fig. 2–15). Because they lack cell walls, they assume many pleomorphic shapes, from coccoid to filamentous. Sometimes they are confused with the L-forms of bacteria which were described earlier; however, even in the most favorable growth media, myco-

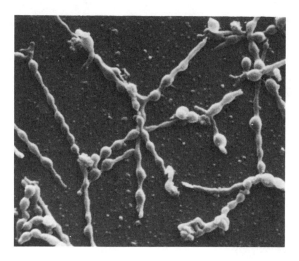

Figure 2–15. Scanning electron micrograph of *Micoplasma pneumoniae;* note the coccoid structures within the filaments (original magnification × 10,000). Volk WA, et al.: Essentials of Medical Microbiology, 4th ed. Philadelphia, JB Lippincott, 1991)

plasmas are not able to produce cell walls, which is not true for the L-forms. Mycoplasmas were formerly called pleuropneumonialike organisms (PPLO) because they were first isolated from cattle with lung infections. These organisms may be free living or parasitic and are pathogenic to many animals and some plants. In humans, the pathogenic mycoplasmas cause primary atypical pneumonia and many secondary infections. Because they have no cell wall, they are resistant to treatment with penicillin and other antibiotics that work by inhibiting cell wall synthesis.

Protozoa

The protozoa are eucaryotic, single-celled, animal-like microorganisms, ranging in length from 3 to 2000 μm. Most of them are free-living organisms found in soil and water. They have no chlorophyll; therefore, they cannot make their own foods by photosynthesis. Some ingest whole algae, yeasts, bacteria, and other smaller protozoans as their source of food (Fig. 2–16); others live on dead, decaying organic matter. The parasitic protozoa break down and absorb the nutrients from the body of the host in which they live. A few parasitic protozoa are pathogens, such as those that cause malaria, giardiasis, and amebic dysentery (see Chapter 10). Other parasitic protozoa exist with the host animal in a symbiotic (living together) relationship, wherein both organisms benefit. A typical example of symbiosis is the termite and its intestinal protozoa, which can digest the wood eaten by the termite; thus, both organisms absorb the nutrients necessary for life. Without the parasitic protozoa, the termite cannot digest wood, its main source of food, and thereby starves to death.

The protozoa are divided into groups according to their method of locomotion or the presence or absence of cilia (short, hairlike structures) and flagella (Table

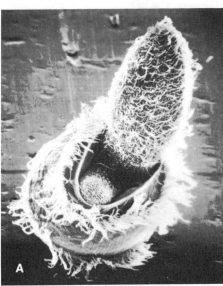

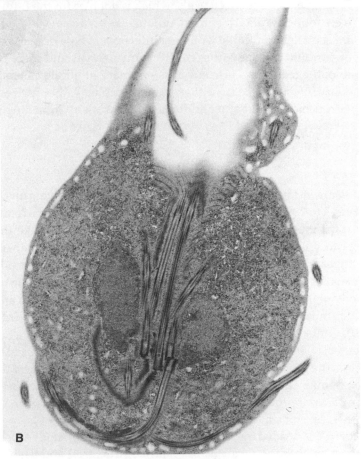

Figure 2–16. Protozoa. (*A*) *Didinium nasutum* with partially ingested prey. (Lechavalier HA, Pramer D: The Microbe. Philadelphia, JB Lippincott, 1970). (*B*) TEM cross section of *Giardia lamblia.* (From S. Koester and P. Engelkirk)

Table 2–5. Characteristics of Major Protozoa

Phylum	Means of Movement	Selected Differentiating Properties (Method of Reproduction)		Representatives
		Asexual	Sexual	
Ciliata	Cilia	Transverse fission	Conjugation	*Balantidium coli, Paramecium, Stentor, Tetrahymena, Vorticella*
Sarcodina	Pseudopodia (false feet)	Binary fission	When present, involves flagellated sex cells	*Amoeba, Diffugia, Entamoeba histolytica*
Mastigophora	Flagella	Binary fission	None	*Chlamydomonas, Giardia lamblia, Trichomonas, Trypanosoma*
Sporozoa	Generally nonmotile except for certain sex cells	Multiple fission	Involves flagellated sex cells	*Plasmodium, Toxoplasma gondii, Cryptosporidium, Pneumocystis carinii*

2–5). The *amebas* (phylum Sarcodina), lacking cilia and flagella, move by pushing forward a bit of cytoplasm (a pseudopodium, or false foot) and slowly flowing into it; this process is called ameboid movement. The ameba engulfs food by surrounding the food particles and enclosing them in a membrane-bounded space called a digestive vacuole, where the particles are digested and used as a source of nutrients. *Phagocytosis* is the engulfment of large particles, whereas *pinocytosis* is the intake of fluids that may contain dissolved food particles. Some white blood cells move through tissues and ingest materials in the same manner. This process is further discussed in Chapter 9, under Phagocytosis. One important pathogenic ameba is *Entamoeba histolytica*, which causes amebic dysentery. This illness is difficult to treat because the pathogen forms resistant cysts deep within the intestinal lining where the amebas live and are protected.

The *flagellates* (phylum Mastigophora) move by means of one or many flagella. A few species are pathogenic. For example, *Trypanosoma gambiense* is carried by the tsetse fly and causes African sleeping sickness in humans; *Trichomonas vagi-*

nalis causes persistent infections of the male and female genital tracts; and *Giardia lamblia* causes a persistent intestinal infection.

Ciliates (phylum Ciliata) move about as a result of large numbers of cilia on their surfaces. They are the most complex of all the protozoa. A pathogenic ciliate, *Balantidium coli*, causes a severe intestinal infection. In underdeveloped countries, it is usually transmitted to man from swine.

The nonmotile protozoa are classified as *Sporozoa*. The most important pathogens are those of the *Plasmodium* species that cause malaria in many areas throughout the world. One of these, *Plasmodium vivax*, causes a mild form of malaria in the United States. These pathogens are carried and transmitted by the female *Anopheles* mosquito. Two Sporozoa that have not previously been recognized as serious pathogens, *Pneumocystis carinii* and *Cryptosporidium*, cause severe secondary infections in immunosuppressed patients, especially those with acquired immunodeficiency syndrome (AIDS) (see Chapter 10).

The protozoa differ from bacteria in that they are eucaryotic, much larger, and do not have a cell wall. They are distinguished from algae by their lack of chlorophyll and from the fungi by their lack of a cellulose or chitin cell wall. Protozoa also have the ability to move.

Fungi

Fungi are found almost everywhere on earth, living on organic matter in water and soil and living on animals and plants. They may be harmful or beneficial. Fungi also live on many unlikely materials, causing deterioration of leather and plastics as well as jams, pickles, and many other foods. Beneficial fungi are important in the production of cheeses, yogurt, beer and wine, and other foods as well as certain drugs and antibiotics.

Characteristics

Fungi are eucaryotic organisms that include mushrooms, molds, and yeasts. As saprophytes, their main source of food is dead, decaying organic mater. Fungi are the "garbage disposers" of nature, the vultures of the microbial world. By secreting digestive enzymes into dead plant and animal matter, they decompose this material into absorbable nutrients for themselves and other living organisms; thus they are the original "recyclers". Imagine living in a world without saprophytes, stumbling through endless piles of decaying debris! Some fungi also live, parasitically, on living animals and plants.

Fungi are often referred to as plants only because they have cellulose or chitin cell walls. They differ from plants and algae in that they are not photosynthetic; they have no chlorophyll or other photosynthetic pigments. Although many fungi are unicellular during some phase of their life cycle (*e.g.*, yeasts), many species grow as filaments called *hyphae* (singular: hypha), which form a mass called the *mycelium* (plural: mycelia); thus, they are different from saprophytic bacteria. Remember, bacteria are procaryotic, whereas fungi are eucaryotic cells.

Reproduction and Spores   Fungal cells can reproduce asexually by budding, by hyphal extension, or by the formation of spores (Fig. 2–17). Sexual reproduction in many fungi involves the nuclear fusion of two gametes and their subsequent division into many sexual spores. Some species of fungi produce both asexual and sexual spores or more than one type of asexual spore. Spores are named after the fungal class or the type of sporulating structure. Figure 2–18 illustrates some typical fungi.

Spores of fungi are very resistant structures that are carried great distances by wind. They are resistant to heat, cold, acids, bases, and other chemicals.

Classification of True Fungi

The mycologists, those who study fungi, have separated the true fungi into five classes: Basidiomycetes, Oomycetes, Zygomycetes, Ascomycetes, and Deuteromycetes. These classes are based on the mode of reproduction and the types of mycelia, spores, and gametes. The characteristics of each of these classes are shown in Table 2–6.

Mushrooms   Mushrooms (Basidiomycetes) are a class of true fungi that consist of a network of filaments or strands, called the mycelium, that grow in the soil or

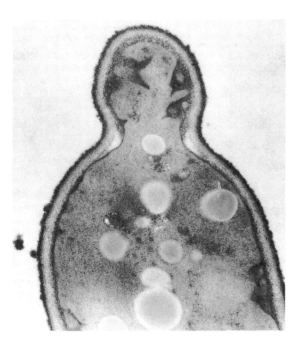

Figure 2–17. Cross section of a budding yeast cell (original magnification ×15,500). (Lechavalier HA, Pramer D: The Microbes. Philadelphia, JB Lippincott, 1970)

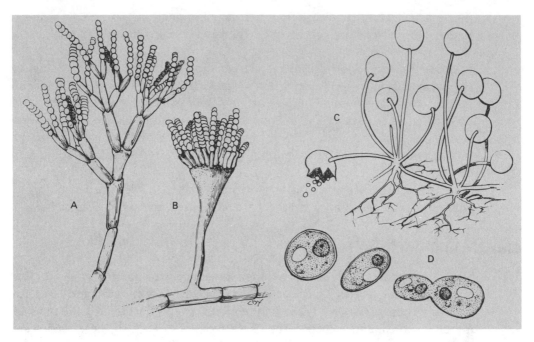

Figure 2–18. Typical fungi. (*A*) *Penicillium* mold, blue-green spores arranged like a brush. (*B*) *Aspergillus*, blue-green with yellow areas. (*C*) *Rhizopus*, white to dark gray with rootlike rhizoids. (*D*) *Saccharomyces cerevisiae*, a yeast.

in a rotting log, and the fruiting body (mushroom) that forms and releases spores. The spore is much like the seed of a plant and germinates into a new organism. Many mushrooms are delicious to eat, but many that resemble edible fungi are extremely toxic and may cause permanent brain damage or death.

Molds   Molds are the filamentous fungi often seen in water and soil and on food. They grow in the form of filaments or hyphae that make up the mycelium of the mold. Reproduction is by spore formation, either sexually or asexually, on the reproductive hyphae. Various species of molds are found in each of the classes of fungi except Basidiomycetes (mushrooms). An interesting mold in class Oomycetes is *Phytophtera*, the potato blight mold that caused a famine in Ireland in the mid-19th century. The black bread mold, *Rhizopus*, is a zygomycete. Both of these genera are primitive molds with aseptate hyphae; this means the hyphae are not divided into individual cells. Although there may be many nuclei in aseptate hyphae, they are not separated by cell walls. Among the Ascomycetes and Deuteromycetes classes are found many antibiotic-producing molds, such as *Penicillium* and *Streptomyces*.

Table 2–6. Selected Characteristics of the Major Classes of Fungi

Class	Type of Mycelium	Site of Spore Formation		Representative Groups
		Asexual	*Sexual*	
Ascomycetes	Septate	Tips of hyphae	Within sacs	Common antibiotic-producing fungi, penicillium, yeasts
Basidiomycetes	Septate	Tips of hyphae	Surface of basidium	Mushrooms, rusts
Deuteromycetes (fungi imperfecti)	Septate	Tips of hyphae	None present	Most human pathogenic molds and yeasts
Oomycetes	Aseptate	In sacs	Within a unicellular female sex organ (oogonium)	Some aquatic forms, mildew, plant blights, fish infections
Zygomycetes	Usually aseptate	In sacs	In mycelium	Bread mold (*Rhizopus nigricans*), aquatic species

Molds have great commercial importance. They are the main source of antibiotics. Many new antibiotics are developed by growing soil cultures and isolating the molds that inhibit the growth of bacteria. The antibiotic penicillin was accidentally discovered when a *Penicillium notatum* mold contaminated an agar plate of staphylococcus and inhibited its growth. Today, antibiotics can be synthesized and chemically changed in the biochemistry laboratory, as has been done with the various penicillins. Some molds are also used to produce large quantities of enzymes (such as amylase, which converts starch to glucose) and of citric acid and other organic acids that are used commercially. The flavor of cheeses such as bleu, roquefort, camembert, and limburger, are the result of the molds grown on them.

Molds also can be harmful. The rusts and molds of crop plants, grains, corn, and potatoes not only destroy crops, but some are also toxic. The aflatoxin from the *Aspergillus* mold on peanuts and cottonseed and the ergot on rye and wheat are extremely toxic to humans and farm animals. Aflatoxins have been shown to be carcinogenic (cancer causing) as well.

Yeasts Yeasts are microscopic eucaryotic single-celled Ascomycetes or Deuteromycetes that lack mycelia. They usually reproduce by budding (see Fig. 2–17), occasionally by spore formation. Yeasts are found in soil and water and on the skins of many fruits and vegetables. People produced wine, beer, and alcoholic beverages for centuries before Pasteur discovered that yeasts, naturally occurring on the skin of grapes and other fruits and grains, were responsible for these fermentation processes. The common yeast *Saccharomyces cerevisiae* ferments sugar to alcohol under anaerobic conditions (without oxygen). In aerobic conditions (with oxygen), this yeast breaks down simple sugars to carbon dioxide and water; for this reason, it has long been used to leaven light bread. (See Chapter 4 for a description of aerobes and anaerobes.) Yeasts are also a good source of nutrients for humans because they produce many vitamins and proteins.

Dimorphism

A few fungi, usually pathogens, can live either as molds or as yeasts depending on growth conditions. When they are isolated from living tissues at body temperature (37°C), they appear in a unicellular parasitic form as yeasts. If they are grown at room temperature (20°C) or isolated from the soil or dust, they grow in the saprophytic form as a mold with hyphae and spore. *Histoplasma*, which causes histoplasmosis, *Sporothrix*, which causes sporotrichosis, *Coccidioides*, which causes coccidioidomycosis, and *Candida albicans*, which causes candidiasis, are examples of dimorphic fungi (Fig. 2–19).

Fungal Diseases

Considering the large number of fungal species, very few are pathogenic for humans, and most of those are found in the class Deuteromycetes, listed in Table

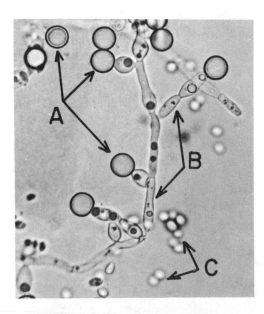

Figure 2–19. Dimorphism shown in a culture of *C. albicans*. (*A*) Chlamydospores. (*B*) Pseudohyphae (elongated yeast cells, linked end to end). (*C*) Budding yeast cells (blastospores) (original magnification × 450). (Davis BD, et al.: Microbiology, 4th ed. Philadelphia, Harper & Row, 1987)

2–6. The diseases caused by fungi are categorized as superficial, deep-seated, or systemic mycotic infections. In some cases the infection may progress through all three of these stages.

Superficial Mycoses   Cutaneous and superficial fungal infections are caused by dermatophytes or other fungi that live on the skin or on the mucous membranes of body openings. Dermatophytes (fungi living on or within the skin) cause athlete's foot, ringworm, and lesions of nails, scalp, and hair follicles.

A yeastlike fungus, *Candida albicans* is an opportunist that normally lives harmlessly on the skin and mucous membranes of the mouth, intestine, and reproductive tract. When the chemical balance (homeostasis) is upset and the number of normal bacteria is reduced, this yeast flourishes to cause infections of the mouth (oral thrush), skin, and vagina (vaginal candidiasis). This type of local infection may become a *focal site* from which it invades the bloodstream to become a generalized or systemic infection in many internal areas.

Deep-seated and Systemic Mycoses   The spores of some pathogenic fungi may be inhaled with dust from contaminated soil and from bird and bat feces, or they may enter through wounds of the hands and feet. If the spores are inhaled into the lungs, they may germinate there to cause a respiratory infection similar to tuberculosis. This type of deep-seated pulmonary infection is caused by species of *Coccidioides* (coccidioidomycosis), *Histoplasma* (histoplasmosis), *Blastomyces* (blastomycosis), and *Cryptococcus* (cryptococcosis). In each case the pathogens may invade further to cause systemic infections, especially in immunosuppressed individuals.

Skin tests for most of these infections are available, but the diseases are difficult to cure. Mycotic diseases are most effectively treated with nystatin, amphotericin B, or 5-fluorocytosine. These chemotherapeutic agents are also toxic to humans and are prescribed with due consideration and caution.

Algae

Algae are photosynthetic organisms that may be multicellular or unicellular. They are arranged in colonies or strands and are found in water and soil and on trees, plants, and rocks. Algae produce their energy by photosynthesis, using energy from the sun, carbon dioxide, water, and inorganic nutrients from the soil to build cellular material. However, a few species use organic nutrients, and others survive with very little sunlight. The blue-green algae (cyanobacteria) are simple procaryotic cells, which are in the kingdom *Procaryotae* with bacteria. The green, brown, and red algae are eucaryotic organisms in the kingdom Protista along with protozoa. Only one genus of algae (*Prototheca*) is a true pathogen, although a few other genera secrete substances that are toxic to humans, fish, and other animals (Table 2–7).

It is easy to find algae. They include the large seaweed and the kelp found

Table 2-7. Characteristics of Algae (Major Groups)

Division	Common Name	General Structural Arrangement	Stored Materials	Motility	Method of Reproduction	Cell Wall Composition	Habitat
Chlorophyta	Green algae	Unicellular to multicellular	Starch, oils	Mostly nonmotile	Asexual by multiple fission; spores sexual	Cellulose and pectin	Fresh water, salt water, soil, lichens
Chrysophyta	Golden algae (includes diatoms)	Mainly unicellular	Oils	Unique movement in diatoms; others have flagella	Asexual and sexual	Pectin, some with silica or calcium	Fresh water, salt water, soil
Euglenophyta	Euglena	Unicellular	Fats	Motile by means of flagella	Asexual only by binary fission	None	Fresh water
Phaeophyta	Brown algae	Multicellular	Fats	Motile	Asexual by motile zoospores; sexual by motile gametes	Cellulose, pectin, algin	Salt water (cool environment)
Pyrrophyta	Dinoflagellates	Unicellular	Starch, oils	Motile	Asexual; sexual rare	Cellulose and pectin	Fresh water, salt water
Rhodophyta	Red algae	Multicellular	Starch, oils	Nonmotile	Asexual by spores; sexual by gametes	Cellulose, pectin, agar, carrageenan	Salt water (warm environment)

along the shores of the ocean, the green scum floating on ponds, and the slippery material on wet rocks. There are also many microscopic forms seen in pond water that differ from the colorless, motile protozoa in that they are photosynthetic, colored, and move very slowly.

Algae are an important source of food, iodine and other minerals, fertilizers, emulsifiers for pudding, and stabilizers for ice cream and salad dressings; they are also used as a gelling agent for jams and nutrient media for bacterial growth. Damage to water systems is frequently caused by algae clogging the filters and pipes where many nutrients are present. Some typical algae are shown in Figure 2–20.

Figure 2–20. Typical algae. (*A*) Vaucheria. (*B*) Diatom. (*C*) Navicula. (*D*) Oocystis. (*E*) Scenedesmus. (*F*) Spirogyra. (*G*) Nostoc. (*H*) Oscillatoria.

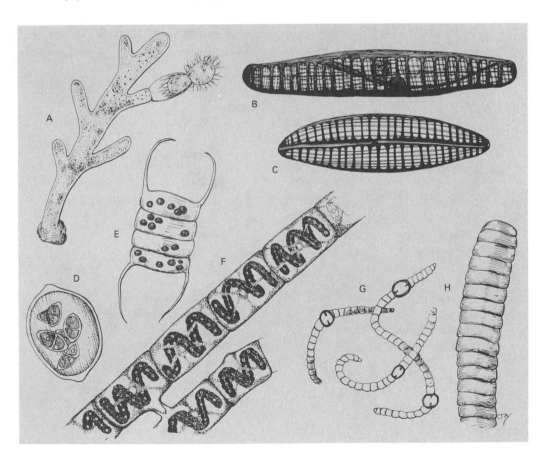

Acellular Infectious Agents

Viruses

Mature virus particles, virions, are so small and simple in structure that they do not fit the living cell classification. They range in size from 0.02 to 0.30 μm in diameter. The smallest is about the size of the large hemoglobin molecule of a red blood cell. Some viruses produce diseases or genetic changes in animals, plants, algae, fungi, protozoa, and bacterial cells (Table 2–8).

Recently, virions have been described as having five specific properties that distinguish them from living cells: (1) they possess either DNA or RNA, never both; (2) their replication (duplication) is directed by the viral nucleic acid within a host cell; (3) they do not divide by binary fission or mitosis; (4) they lack the genes and enzymes necessary for energy production; and (5) they depend on the ribosomes, enzymes and nutrients of the infected cells for protein production.

A typical virus particle has a core containing core protein and the genome (nuclear material) of DNA or RNA surrounded by a capsid (protein coat), sometimes

Table 2–8. Relative Sizes and Shapes of Some Viral Particles (Virions)

Viruses	Nucleic Acid Type	Shape	Size Range (nm)
Animal Viruses			
Vaccinia	DNA	Complex	200 by 300
Mumps	RNA	Helical	150–250
Herpes simplex	DNA	Polyhedral	100–150
Influenza	RNA	Helical	80–120
Retroviruses	RNA	Helical	100–120
Adenoviruses	DNA	Polyhedral	60–90
Reoviruses	RNA	Polyhedral	60–80
Papovaviruses	DNA	Polyhedral	40–60
Polioviruses	RNA	Polyhedral	28
Plant Viruses			
Turnip yellow mosaic	RNA	Polyhedral	28
Wound tumor	RNA	Polyhedral	55–60
Alfalfa mosaic	RNA	Polyhedral	18 by 36–40
Tobacco mosaic	RNA	Helical	18 by 300
Bacteriophages			
T2	DNA	Complex	65 by 210
λ	DNA	Complex	54 by 194
$\phi\chi$-174	DNA	Complex	25

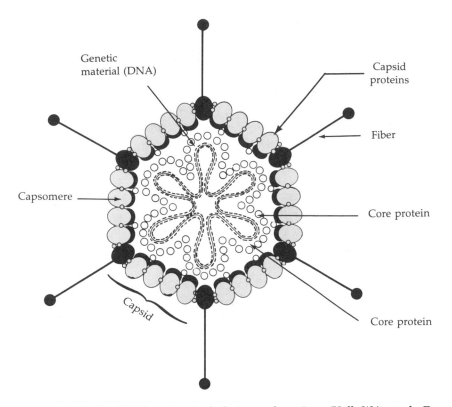

Figure 2–21. Model of an icosahedral virus: adenovirus. (Volk WA, et al.: Essentials of Medical Microbiology, 4th ed. Philadelphia, JB Lippincott, 1991)

consisting of many small units called capsomeres (Fig. 2–21). Some virions have a protective envelope composed of fats and polysaccharides. The bacterial viruses may also have a tail and tail fibers. There are no ribosomes for protein synthesis or sites of energy production, hence the virus must take over a functioning cell to produce new viruses particles.

Viruses are classified by the following characteristics: (1) type of genetic material (either DNA or RNA); (2) shape of the capsid; (3) number of capsomeres; (4) size of capsid (particle); (5) presence or absence of an envelope; (6) host that it infects (plant, animal, or microorganism); (7) the type of disease produced; (8) target cell; and (9) immunological properties.

The genetic material of most viruses is either double-stranded DNA or single-stranded RNA, but a few have single-stranded DNA or double-stranded RNA. Viral genomes are usually circular molecules, but some are linear (with two ends). Capsids of viruses have various shapes and symmetry. They may be polyhedral (many sided), helical (coiled tubes), bullet shaped, spherical, or a complex combination of these shapes. Polyhedral capsids have 20 sides or facets, geometrically referred to as icosahedrons. Each facet consists of several capsomeres; thus, the size of the virus is determined by the size of each facet and the number of capsomeres in each. Frequently, the envelope around the capsid makes the virus appear spherical or irregular in shape in electron micrographs. The envelope is usually acquired by certain animal viruses from the host nuclear or cellular membrane as the new virus particle leaves the cell. Apparently, viruses are able to alter these membranes and add protein fibers, spikes, and knobs that enable the virus to recognize the next host cell to be invaded. A list of some of the viruses, their characteristics, and the diseases they cause is presented in Table 2–9.

The virion usually infects a cell by injecting its DNA or RNA into the cell (Fig. 2–22) or by cellular phagocytosis (Fig. 2–23). The viral genetic material may remain latent or inactive in the cell and be transferred to each daughter cell when it divides. This is the *lysogenic cycle* of viral infection. However, the viral genetic material may be induced by heat (fever), ultraviolet (UV) light, or certain chemical agents to take over the cell and make viruses.

When the genetic material from the virus takes over the metabolic machinery of the cell to produce viruses, it has entered the *lytic cycle* of virus infection. It breaks up the cellular DNA and produces viral DNA or RNA. It then synthesizes viral protein capsids and assembles many new virus particles until the cell bursts (lysis has occurred) and releases the new viruses into the area to infect neighboring cells.

A good example of the lysogenic (latent) and lytic cycles is the ordinary "cold sore," which is caused by the herpes simplex virus. Those persons who get cold sores have the latent or temperature virus genetic material in the nearby nerve ganglion (after the initial infection) in the lysogenic cycle. When a fever develops or the individual is exposed to excessive UV light of the sun, the viral genetic material may be stimulated to take over the cells to produce more viruses (lytic cycle) and the cold sore develops. Such viral infections are usually limited by the body's defenses: the phagocytes and an antiviral protein called interferon that is produced by the virus-infected cells.

Antibiotics are not effective against viral infections because these drugs work by inhibiting certain metabolic reactions within living pathogens. Because viruses are not independent metabolizing cells, agents that affect the synthesis of new virus particles may also cause damage to the host cell. For colds and influenza, antibiotics should be given only to prevent secondary bacterial infections that might occur after the virus infection. However, recently several new chemicals have been developed that interfere with virus-specific enzymes and virus production by either disrupting critical phases in viral cycles or by inhibiting the synthesis of viral DNA or RNA. Refer to Chapter 6 for the discussion of chemotherapy.

Many tumors and cancers are apparently caused by viruses that change the genetic composition of the cell and cause uncontrolled growth of abnormal cells under certain environmental conditions. Some chemotherapeutic drugs used to treat cancer are chemicals that interfere with DNA and RNA synthesis in rapidly

Table 2–9. Selected Important Groups of Viruses and Viral Diseases

Virus Type	Viral Characteristics	Virus	Disease
Poxviruses	Large, brick shape with envelope, double DNA	Poxvirus Poxvirus	Smallpox (variola) Cowpox (vaccinia)
Polyoma-Papilloma	Double DNA, polyhedral	Papillomavirus Polyomavirus	Warts Some tumors, some cancer
Herpesviruses	Polyhedral with envelope, double DNA	Herpes simplex I Herpes simplex II Herpes zoster Varicella	Cold sores or fever blisters Venereal herpes Shingles Chickenpox
Adenoviruses	Double DNA, icosahedral, no envelope		Respiratory infections, pneumonia, conjunctivitis, some tumors
Picornaviruses	Single RNA, tiny icosahedral, with envelope	Rhinovirus Poliovirus Hepatitis types A and B Coxsackievirus	Colds Poliomyelitis Hepatitis Respiratory infections, Meningitis
Reoviruses	Double RNA, icosahedral with envelope	Enterovirus	Intestinal infections
Myxoviruses	RNA, helical with envelope	Orthomyxoviruses types A & B Myxovirus parotidis Paramyxovirus Rhabdovirus	Influenza Mumps Measles (rubeola) Rabies
Arbovirus	Arthropod-borne RNA, cubic	Mosquito-borne type B Mosquito-borne types A and B Tick-borne, corona-virus	Yellow fever Encephalitis (many types) Colorado tick fever
Retrovirus	Double RNA, helical with envelope	RNA tumor virus HTLV virus HIV (Human immunodeficiency virus)	Tumors Leukemia AIDS (Acquired immunodeficiency virus)

dividing cells, thus inhibiting or destroying the tumor cells and some human cells (hair, blood, sperm).

Remnants of viruses are often seen in infected cells and are used as a diagnostic tool to identify certain diseases. These are called *inclusion bodies,* and they may be found in the cytoplasm (cytoplasmic) or within the nucleus (intranuclear), depending on the disease. In rabies, the cytoplasmic inclusion bodies are called Negri bodies. The inclusion bodies of AIDS and the Guarnieri bodies of smallpox are also cytoplasmic. The herpes and poliomyelitis viruses cause intranuclear inclusion bodies. In each case, the inclusion bodies may be merely aggregates or collections of viruses. Some important human viral diseases include the common cold, influenza, mumps, measles, chickenpox, smallpox, rabies, cold sores, venereal herpes, warts, poliomyelitis, encephalitis, and AIDS.

Bacteriophages

The viruses that infect bacteria are called bacteriophages or simply phages. Most bacteriophages are species- and strain-specific. Those that infect the coliform (intestinal) bacteria, such as *Escherichia coli,* are called coliphages. Refer to Figures 2–22 and 2–24 to observe the complexity of the phages. The tail plate, tail fibers, and spikes are used to attach to the bacteria, usually at the site of a *pilus;* and the phage DNA is injected into the bacteria much like water from a syringe (see Figure 2–24).

The phages that lyse the host bacterial cells during the production of new bacteriophages are referred to as *virulent bacteriophages.* However, many DNA

Figure 2–22. A partially lysed cell of *Vibrio cholerae* with attached virions of phage CP-T1. Note the empty capsids, the full head phage capsids, contracted tail sheaths, and base plates and spikes (original magnification × 257,000). (Courtesy of R. W. Taylor and J. E. Ogg, Colorado State University, Fort Collins, Colorado)

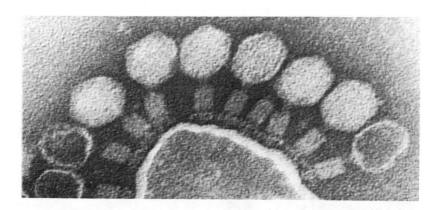

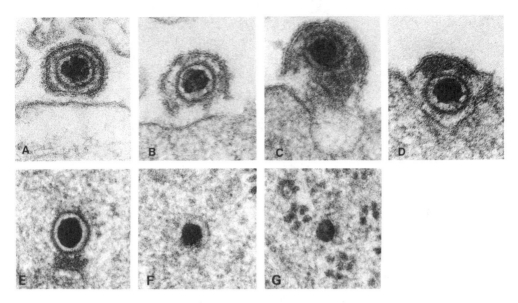

Figure 2-23. Adsorption (A), penetration (B-D), and digestion of the capsid (E-G) of herpes simplex on HeLa cells, as deduced from electron micrographs of infected cell sections. The penetration involves local digestion of the viral and cellular membranes (B,C), resulting in fusion of the two membranes and release of the nucleocapsid into the cytoplasmic matrix (D). The naked nucleocapsid is intact in (E), is partially digested in (F), and has disappeared in (G), leaving a core containing DNA and protein. (Morgan C, et al.: J Virol 2:507, 1968)

Figure 2-24. (A) The bacterial virus T4 is an assembly of protein components. The head is a protein membrane with 20 facets, filled with DNA. It is attached to a tail consisting of a hollow core surrounded by a sheath and based on a spiked end-plate to which six fibers are attached. (B) The sheath contracts, driving the core through the wall, and viral DNA enters the cell. (Volk WA, Wheeler MF: Basic Microbiology, 5th ed. Philadelphia, JB Lippincott, 1984)

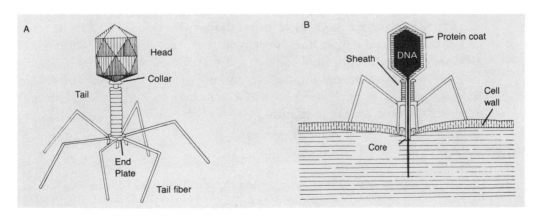

phages are *temperate bacteriophages*; their viral genome does not take over the host cell. The temperate phage DNA is injected into the bacterium, but causes no damage to the cell. Then, each time the host cell divides, the viral genome also replicates and is passed to each daughter cell. Thus, each daughter cell is infected with the phage DNA.

The relationship between the phage and its host cell is called *lysogeny*. The infected bacteria are said to be *lysogenic bacteria*; and the phages that infect them are *temperate phages*, which inject the latent phage genome (DNA) into the host cell. This latent viral genome is a *prophage*.

In some cases, under appropriate environmental conditions (heat, UV light, certain chemicals), the prophage may be stimulated to produce new complete phages and lyse the bacterial cell. This involves a process called *induction* of the lytic cycle.

Viruses and Genetic Changes

Much research in genetics has been accomplished using bacteria and bacteriophages. Some pathogens are identified by the specific bacteriophages that infect them. When bacteria are injected with the genetic material from a bacteriophage, the genetic constitution of those bacteria is changed by the addition of the phage DNA. This process is called *lysogenic conversion*. An example of such a conversion is the pathogenic diphtheria bacterium, which is pathogenic only when the phage genes are present. Evidently, the genes that enable diphtheria bacteria (*Corynebacterium diphtheriae*) to produce a lethal toxin are injected with the phage DNA. Other genetic changes produced in bacteria by bacteriophages are discussed in Chapter 4.

Viroids and Prions

Although viruses are very small, nonliving infectious agents, viroids and prions are even smaller and less complex, infectious agents. *Viroids* consist of circular, single-stranded RNA that can infect the nucleus of a plant cell. They are transmitted between plants by mechanical means (birds, insects) or via pollen. It is believed that they cause more than 10 plant diseases, such as potato spindle-tuber disease, chrysanthemum stunt disease, and exocortosis of citrus trees.

Prions are proteinaceous infectious particles that may cause nervous system diseases in livestock and humans, such as scrapie in sheep and goats and kuru and Creutzfeldt-Jakob disease in humans.

Summary

As you recognize the differences between the various types of microorganisms, you can understand why organisms are classified into kingdoms, phyla, orders, classes, families, genera, and species. You will also learn many of the characteristics used to describe each of these types of organisms and why some appear to be more primitive than others. A study of the various types of cells, especially the unicellular microorganisms, helps you to understand why it is believed that the microbes were probably the first kinds of cells on earth. Moreover, you discover how certain chemotherapeutic drugs, including antibiotics, work to destroy or inhibit certain pathogens but do not kill the patient.

This survey of the types of microorganisms emphasizes the characteristics that enable them to carry on beneficial ecological functions. Without these various types of microbes, the earth would not be habitable.

Study Outline

I.   Cells: eucaryotes and procaryotes
   A.   Cell theory: Hooke, Schleiden, Schwann, and Virchow
   B.   The cell: the fundamental living unit of life
     1.   Obtains food and metabolizes it
     2.   Reproduces itself
     3.   Responds to the environment
   C.   Eucaryotic cells: animal, plant, fungi, algae, and protozoa
     1.   Cell membrane
     2.   Nucleus
       a.   Nuclear membrane
       b.   Chromosomes
       c.   Nucleolus
       d.   Nucleoplasm
     3.   Cytoplasm
       a.   Endoplasmic reticulum, ribosomes
       b.   Golgi apparatus
       c.   Lysosomes
       d.   Mitochondria
       e.   Centrioles
       f.   Chloroplasts in plants
     4.   Cell wall
   D.   Procaryotic cells: bacteria and cyanobacteria
     1.   Nucleoid

     2.   Cytoplasm
     3.   Cytoplasmic particles
     4.   Cell membrane
       a. Mesosomes
     5.   Bacterial Cell Wall
     6.   Capsules
     7.   Flagella
     8.   Fimbriae, pili
     9.   Endospores
   E.   Differences between procaryotes and eucaryotes
II. Microbial classification
III. Bacteria
   A.   Characteristics
     1.   Morphology (grouping)
     2.   Staining characteristics
     3.   Motility
     4.   Colony characteristics
     5.   Nutritional requirements
     6.   Biochemical activities
     7.   Pathogenicity
   B.   Rudimentary forms of bacteria
     1.   Rickettsias
     2.   Chlamydias
     3.   Mycoplasmas
IV. Protozoa
   A.   Classified by means of locomotion
     1.   Cilia
     2.   Flagella

Problems and Questions

1.   Which microbes are eucaryotic cells?
2.   Which microorganisms are procaryotes?
3.   What function do the mitochondria and mesosomes have in common?
4.   Where does protein synthesis occur in eucaryotic cells and in procaryotic cells?
5.   Which microorganisms do not have a nuclear membrane?
6.   List five differences between eucaryotic animal cells and procaryotic bacterial cells.
7.   What is the difference between bacterial flagella and protozoan flagella?
8.   Describe peritrichous, amphitrichous, lophotrichous, and monotrichous flagellation in bacteria.
9.   Describe a symbiotic relationship of a parasitic protozoan.
10.   What is the role of fungi in recycling nutrients?
11.   What are the differences between protozoa and green algae?
12.   List five properties of viruses that distinguish them from other living cells.
13.   Describe the lytic and lysogenic cycles of viruses.

Self Test

After you have read Chapter 2, examined the objectives, studied the new words, reviewed the study outline, and answered the questions at the end of the chapter, complete the following self test.

Matching Exercises

Complete each statement from the list of words provided with each section.

Descriptive Terms

amphitrichous   diplococci   procaryotes
axial filaments   eucaryotes   spirilla
bacilli   lophotrichous   staphylococci
cocci   monotrichous   streptobacilli
diplobacilli   peritrichous   streptococci

1. The cyanobacteria and bacteria are _procaryotes_.
2. Bacteria with flagella on both ends are _amphitrichous_.
3. The rods or elongated bacteria are _bacilli_.
4. Some spirochetes have two flagellalike fibrils attached at each end, called _axial filaments_.
5. Fungi, protozoa, green algae, plants, and animal cells are _eucaryotes_.
6. Bacteria that have a tuft of flagella are _lophotrichous_.
7. The coiled or curved bacteria are known as _spirilla_.
8. Cocci that are found in pairs are _diplococci_.
9. Cells that have no true nuclear membrane are _procaryotes_.
10. Plant cells have cellulose cell walls, and animal cells have no cell wall, but both are _eucaryotes_.
11. The spherical or round bacteria have the shape of _cocci_.
12. Salmonella organisms are motile because they have flagella covering their surfaces; they are _peritrichous_.
13. Cells that have invaginations of the cell membrane, called mesosomes, for cellular respiration are _procaryotes_.
14. Cocci that appear as grapelike clusters on a stained smear are _staphylococci_.
15. Cells that have one naked chromosome composed of DNA are _procaryotes_.
16. Bacilli that usually appear in pairs are _diplobacilli_.

17. Some bacteria that live in the intestine have only one flagellum; they
    are _monotrichous_.
18. Bacilli that form long chains are _Streptobacilli_.
19. Bacteria that have a very complex cell wall are classified as
    procaryotes.
20. Cells that have membrane-bound organelles, such as mitochondria,
    endoplasmic reticulum, and Golgi bodies are _eucaryotes_.
21. Cocci that form many chains are _Streptococci_.

Characteristics of Microorganisms

algae   viruses   chlamydias
protozoa   rickettsias   *Escherichia coli*
fungi   mycoplasmas

1. Most of the saprophytic organisms, which live on decaying organic
   materials, are _fungi_.
2. All the organisms in this group are photosynthetic; they are
   algae.
3. The single-celled animals that are classified by their means of
   locomotion are _protozoa_.
4. The group that contains both eucaryotic and procaryotic organisms is
   the _algae_.
5. The bacteria that must obtain their energy (ATP) from their host cells
   are _chlamydias_.
6. The bacteria that have little or no cell wall, but are free-living, are
   mycoplasmas.
7. The bacteria that are normally found as a part of the normal flora of
   the human intestine are _Escherichia coli_.
8. The bacteria that must be transmitted from person to person by
   arthropod vectors such as fleas, lice, and ticks are _rickettsias_.
9. The smallest microorganisms, which consist mainly of the genetic
   material and a protein coat, are called _viruses_.

Diseases and Microorganisms

Match the following diseases with the type of microorganisms that cause them,
using the following words:

virus   mycobacteria   streptococci
chlamydias   protozoa   staphylococci
rickettsias   fungi   spirilla
mycoplasmas   spirochete   curved rods

1. "Strep" sore throat _Streptococci_
2. Typhus _rickettsias_
3. "Cold sores" _viruses_
4. Boils, wound infections _Staphlococci_
5. Atypical pneumonia, sinusitis _mycoplasmas_
6. Cholera _curved rod_
7. Rabies _virus_
8. Syphilis _spirochete_
9. Smallpox _virus_
10. Tuberculosis _mycobacteria_
11. Poliomyelitis _virus_
12. Lymphogranuloma venereum _chlamydias_
13. Influenza _virus_

True or False (T or F)

___T___   1. Microorganisms, with the exception of viruses, exhibit the properties found in all living systems.
___T___   2. Mitochondria are the powerhouses that generate energy for eucaryotic cells.
___F___   3. The chromosomes of procaryotic cells consist of histone proteins and DNA.
___T___   4. Lysosomes contain lysozyme to aid in the digestion of dead or dying cells and bacteria.
___F___   5. Nuclei of cyanobacteria have a well-defined nuclear membrane.
___T___   6. Bacterial flagella are structurally like protozoan flagella and cilia.
___F___   7. Viruses contain both DNA and RNA.
___T___   8. An icosahedron is a 20-sided figure.
___T___   9. Bacteriophages are viruses that infect bacteria.
___T___ 10. Most fungi reproduce sexually and asexually.
___F___ 11. Pathogenic rickettsias differ from viruses in that they require living cells for growth and reproduction.
___T___ 12. Molds differ from bacteria in that they are multicellular and reproduce by spores.
___T___ 13. During the cyst stage protozoa resemble bacterial spores because they have thick walls, are dormant, and resist drying.
___F___ 14. Bacteria reproduce by budding, and yeasts reproduce by transverse fission.
___T___ 15. Vibrio organisms (like _Vibrio cholerae_) are curved rod-shaped bacteria.
___F___ 16. PPLO, like the L-forms, have a rigid cell wall.
___T___ 17. Rickettsial diseases are usually transmitted by an arthropod vector.

Multiple Choice

1. The semipermeable structure
   controlling the entry and exit of
   materials between the cell and its
   environment is the
   a. cell wall
   b. protoplast
   c. cytoplasm
   d. plasma membrane
2. Procaryotic cells reproduce by
   a. gamete production
   b. budding
   c. mitosis
   d. binary fission
3. Centrioles are
   a. cylindrical organelles
   b. involved in cell division
   c. found in eucaryotes
   d. structurally similar to cilia and
      flagella
   e. all of the above
4. The group of bacteria that lack
   rigid cell walls and take on
   irregular shapes is
   a. rickettsia
   b. chlamydia
   c. clostridium
   d. mycoplasma
5. Sporulation in bacteria is a
   a. means of reproduction
   b. degeneration of organelles
   c. means of survival
   d. development of a cell wall

6. Lysogenic bacteria may be induced
   to enter a lytic cycle by exposure to
   a. ultraviolet light
   b. sunlight
   c. heat
   d. certain chemicals
   e. all of the above
7. Gram-positive bacteria stain
   a. purple
   b. red
   c. blue
   d. green
8. Rickettsias are the causative agent in
   a. vaginitis
   b. Rocky Mountain spotted fever
   c. trichomoniasis
   d. typhoid fever
9. Infections of the male and female
   genital tracts may be caused by
   Trichomonas vaginatis, which is a
   a. protozoin
   b. virus
   c. yeast
   d. fungus
10. During the lysogenic cycle, the virus
    a. lyses the host cell
    b. is latent in the cell
    c. has not yet infected the cell
    d. induces the production of
       more viruses

Chapter 3

Introduction to Chemistry of Life

Objectives

After studying this chapter, you should be able to

1. Differentiate among elements, atoms, molecules, and compounds
2. Describe an acid-base reaction
3. Discuss the importance of water in biochemical reactions
4. List the characteristics of monosaccharides, disaccharides, and polysaccharides
5. Describe four main types of biochemical molecules
6. Distinguish between organic and inorganic compounds
7. Discuss the structure of carbohydrates, fats, proteins, and nucleic acids and their breakdown products
8. Describe the role of enzymes in metabolism
9. Discuss how DNA directs cellular activities

New Words

Acid (a'-sid). Any substance that when in an aqueous solution results in sufficient hydrogen ions to produce a pH above 0 but below 7.0

Adenosine triphosphate (ATP) (a-den'-o-sin tri-fos'-fate). High-energy organic molecule

Atom (at'-um). Smallest unit of an element

Bases (base'-es). Substances with sufficient hydroxide ions in solution to produce a pH above 7.0 but below 14

Carbohydrates (car-boh-high'-drates). Organic compounds containing carbon, hydrogen, and oxygen in a ratio of $1:2:1$

Compound (com'-pound). Chemical substance containing more than one kind of atom

Deoxyribonucleic acid (DNA) (dee-ox'-ee-rye'-boh-new-clay'-ick). Genetic macromolecule in chromosomes

Disaccharide (die'-sack'-car-ride). A carbohydrate consisting of two sugar units

Electrolyte (ee-lect'-troh-light). A substance that exists as ions in a water solution

Element (el'-e-ment). General name given to a substance composed of identical atoms

Enzyme (en'-zime). A protein molecule that catalyzes (stimulates) the occurrence of biochemical reactions

Glycogen (gly'-ko-jen). A polysaccharide stored by animal cells

Hydrocarbons (high'-droh-car-buns). Organic compounds consisting of only hydrogen and carbon atoms.

Hydrolysis (high-drol'-e-sis). Reaction in which a compound is broken apart by the addition of water

Ion (i'-on). A positively or negatively charged atom or group of atoms

Inorganic (in-or-gan'-ick). Chemical compounds not classified as organic

Lipids (li'-pids). Organic compounds containing carbon, hydrogen, and oxygen that are insoluble in water but soluble in fat solvents

Metabolite (met-tab'-boh-light). Substance that furnishes energy and building blocks for the vital processes of a cell

Monosaccharide (mon-oh-sack'-car-ride). A carbohydrate consisting of one sugar unit

Nucleic acids (new-clay'-ick). Polymers of DNA and RNA that carry the genetic information of a cell and direct protein synthesis

Nucleotides (new'-clee-o-tides). Basic subunits of the nucleic acids, each consisting of a purine or pyrimidine combined with a ribose sugar and a phosphate group.

Organic (or-gan'-ic). Chemical compounds with a carbon base

Polymer (pol'-e-mer). Long-chain molecule consisting of repeated subunits

Polysaccharide (pol-ee-sack'-car-ride). Carbohydrate consisting of many sugar units

Protein (pro'-teen). Macromolecule consisting of one or more polypeptide chains of amino acids

Purine (pure'-een). A nucleic acid base; adenine or guanine

Pyrimidine (pi-rim-i-dean). A nucleic acid base; thymine, cytosine, or uracil

Ribonucleic acid (RNA) (rye'-boh-new-clay'-ick). Nucleic acid necessary for protein synthesis; transcribed from DNA

Replication (rep-li-kay'-shun). Duplication of DNA or chromosomes

Salt. Any solid ionic compound that forms ions other than hydrogen and hydroxide in solution

Solute (so'-lute). The substance dissolved in a solution

Solution (so-loo'-shun). A homogenous molecular mixture, usually a solid dissolved in water

Solvent (sol'-vent). The liquid in which another substance dissolves

Substrate (sub'-strāt). The material that an enzyme or microbe acts upon

Transcription (trans-cript'-shun). Process involved in transcribing the genetic message from DNA to RNA.

Translation (trans-lay'-shun). Process of translating the message carried by mRNA to synthesize proteins in the cell

The various ways microorganisms function and survive in their environment depend on the chemical makeup of the microorganisms. To understand microbial cells and how they work, one must have a basic knowledge of the chemistry of atoms, molecules, and macromolecules (large and complex molecules). As explained in Chapter 2, even procaryotic cells consist of very large macromolecules of DNA, RNA, proteins, lipids, polysaccharides as well as many combinations of these macromolecules that combine to make up the capsule, cell wall, cell membrane, mesosomes, cytoplasm, and nuclear material. These macromolecules can be broken down into smaller units, or molecules, of nucleotides, amino acids, glycerol, fatty acids, and monosaccharides, or simple sugars. Each of these molecules, in turn, may be broken down into *inorganic* molecules of water, carbon dioxide, ammonia, sulfides, and phosphates, and finally into the atoms of carbon, hydrogen, oxygen, nitrogen, sulfur, and phosphorus. Basic inorganic chemistry is introduced in this chapter and is followed by a discussion of the organic chemistry and biochemistry of the major macromolecules found in living cells. Organic chemistry is the study of compounds containing carbon; biochemistry is the chemistry of living cells; inorganic chemistry includes all other reactions.

Only when all of these units are in place and working together properly can the cell function like a well-managed industrial plant. As in industry, the cell must have the appropriate structures and parts, the regulatory molecules (enzymes) to control its activities, the fuel (nutrients or light) to provide energy, and raw materials (nutrients) for manufacturing end products.

Basic Chemistry

Atoms, Molecules, Elements, Compounds

All substances, whether gas, liquid, or solid, have certain fundamental characteristics in common. If one could break down any substance into its smallest elemental units, it would be composed of *atoms*. Although it is difficult to observe atomic structure, atoms are known to consist of a mass of positively charged protons, noncharged (or neutral) neutrons, tiny negatively charged electrons, and other even smaller subparticles. An atom has equal numbers of electrons and protons; thus it has a total charge that is zero. When an atom loses or gains electrons it becomes a negatively or positively charged *ion* (e.g., Na^+, Cl^-). The protons and neutrons are found in a central nucleus, and the electrons float around the nucleus, like negatively charged satellites attracted to a positively charged planet.

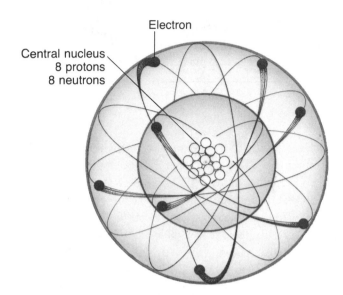

Central nucleus
8 protons
8 neutrons

Electron

Figure 3–1. Representation of an oxygen atom. Eight protons and eight neutrons are tightly bound in the central nucleus, around which the eight electrons revolve. (Rosdahl CB: Textbook of Basic Nursing, 4th ed. Philadelphia, JB Lippincott).

Figure 3–1 illustrates an oxygen atom. When a multitude of atoms with identical numbers of electrons and protons and the same chemical properties exist together, the substance is known as an *element*, for example, carbon (C), hydrogen (H), oxygen (O), nitrogen (N), sulfur (S).

The atoms of each element have their own special weight (or mass) called *atomic weight*, which is the total mass of the number of protons and neutrons each of which is assigned a value of 1. Electrons are negligible in weight. The atomic weight of a specific element is an average of the weights of all isotopes of that element as they occur in nature. *Isotopes* are atoms of the same element, with identical chemical characteristics but with different atomic weights. They differ in weight because they have various numbers of neutrons within the atoms. For example, carbon-12 has six protons and six neutrons for an atomic weight of 12, whereas carbon-14 has six protons and eight neutrons for an atomic weight of 14; both are isotopes of the element carbon. Elements are also identified by a number that indicates the number of positive charges, or protons, in the nucleus. This is called the *atomic number*. Thus the atomic number of carbon is 6. Atomic weights and atomic numbers can be found in a periodic table of the elements in any chemistry book; some atomic weights and numbers are shown in Table 3–1.

Two or more atoms of the same or different elements that combine into a single stable unit form a *molecule*; examples include carbon dioxide (CO_2), water (H_2O), or sulfur dioxide (SO_2). When many molecules exist together in a substance that can be seen or weighed, the substance is called a *compound, e.g.,* carbon dioxide gas (CO_2). Although there are only 106 known elements, the number of compounds that are known is already in the millions, and new ones are being created and discovered each year. The component parts of living cells and systems are

Table 3-1. The First 20 Elements

Element	Symbol	Atomic Number	Atomic Weight
Hydrogen	H	1	1
Helium	He	2	4
Lithium	Li	3	6.9
Beryllium	Be	4	9
Boron	B	5	10.8
Carbon	C	6	12
Nitrogen	N	7	14
Oxygen	O	8	16
Fluorine	F	9	19
Neon	Ne	10	20.1
Sodium	Na	11	23
Magnesium	Mg	12	24.3
Aluminum	Al	13	27
Silicon	Si	14	28.1
Phosphorus	P	15	31
Sulfur	S	16	32.1
Chlorine	Cl	17	35.5
Argon	Ar	18	40
Potassium	K	19	39.1
Calcium	Ca	20	40.1

composed of many macromolecules that interact to produce and maintain life. You will learn about many of these macromolecules, such as the polysaccharides, structural proteins, regulatory enzymes, and DNA, although many of the most complex still remain to be fully identified.

Chemical Bonding

In general, atoms form molecules by gaining or losing electrons (forming ionic bonds) or by sharing electrons (forming covalent bonds). An *ionic bond* holds together molecules, such as sodium chloride (NaCl, common table salt) and many others, that ionize in water. When sodium chloride dissolves in water, the sodium atom (Na) loses a negative electron and assumes a positive charge, thus becoming a positive ion (Na^+) in the water. Likewise, the chlorine atom (Cl) accepts one electron from the donor sodium atom (Na) to become a chloride ion (Cl^-). The ionic bonds between sodium and chlorine atoms are easily broken; however, they re-form in the water because the unlike charges are attracted to each other. They may temporarily form NaCl molecules, and then dissociate into ions again (Fig.

3–2). Positively charged ions are called *cations*; and negatively charged ions are *anions*.

Other molecules are held together by covalent bonds. A *covalent bond* is formed by atoms sharing one or more pairs of electrons. In Figure 3–3, the methane (CH_4) molecule has hydrogen atoms that each share two electrons with the carbon atom (Fig. 3–3). This is a much stronger bond than an ionic bond; thus, the molecule is much more stable. Carbon compounds are especially good examples of covalent bonding. All of organic chemistry is based on the stable covalently bonded carbon molecules and how they react with other molecules. Biochemistry, the chemistry of living cells and systems, is a study of the large macromolecules composed of covalently bonded carbon, hydrogen, oxygen, nitrogen, phosphorus, and sulfur atoms. The loosely bound electrons on the surface of the macromolecules enable them to react and bind with other molecules in living organisms. Peptide bonds, which hold amino acids together in a protein, and glycosidic bonds, which bind the sugar groups of polysaccharides together, are also covalent bonds.

Hydrogen bonding occurs when a hydrogen atom that is covalently bonded to an oxygen or nitrogen atom is attracted to another oxygen or nitrogen atom on a different molecule or group, as seen in the α-helix of DNA and protein structure.

Importance of Water in Living Cells and Systems

Water is the most abundant molecule in living cells; it is absolutely essential for the functioning of living cells. The water molecule, consisting of two hydrogen atoms on one side of an oxygen atom, gives the molecule *polarity*, that is, a water molecule has positive and negative areas (Fig. 3–4). This characteristic makes water an ideal solvent, or suspending medium, for other ionic or charged molecules. The hydrogen bonding (i.e., the attraction between water molecules) is called *polar bonding*.

This polarity of water molecules accounts for four major characteristics that make it an essential part of living cells.

1. Water is an excellent solvent (a liquid in which molecules of one or more other chemicals, called the solutes, are dissolved, thus forming a solution). Nutrients and waste materials may move in and out of a cell, crossing the cell membrane, because they are dissolved in water.
2. Its polarity makes the molecules adhere, producing surface tension and capillary action, hence, water can move within and among cells and tissues.
3. It also serves as an excellent buffer against heat changes to protect the cell from fluctuation in temperature, because it can absorb and hold large amounts of heat.
4. Water enters into *hydrolysis* reactions (digestion of large macromolecules like cellulose by breaking apart the molecular units) and *dehydration* reactions (in which the macromolecules are synthesized with the removal of a water molecule).

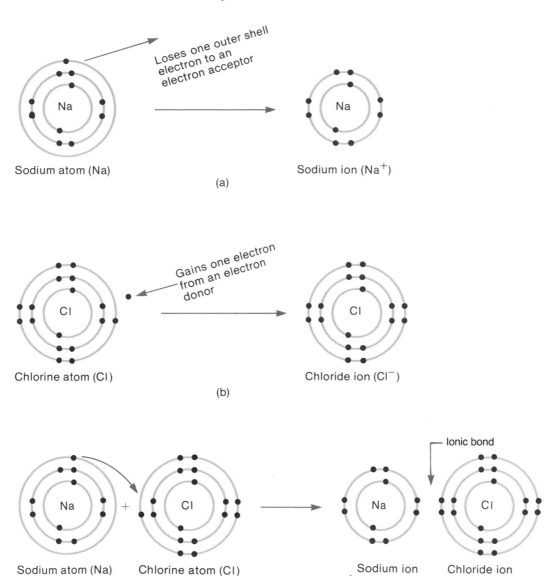

Figure 3–2. Ionic bond formation. (*A*) A sodium atom loses an electron to become a positively charged sodium ion (Na$^+$). (*B*) A chlorine atom gains an electron to become a negatively charged chloride ion (Cl$^-$). (*C*) The positive sodium ion is attracted to the negative chloride ion to form the sodium chloride molecule, which is held together by a weak ionic bond.

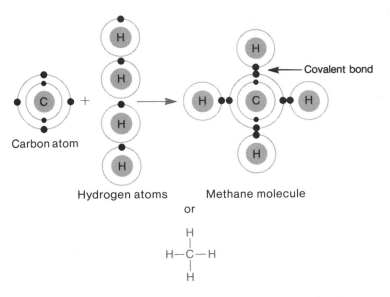

Carbon atom

Hydrogen atoms   Methane molecule

Covalent bond

or

H
|
H—C—H
|
H

Figure 3–3. Covalent bond formation. The methane molecule with four hydrogen atoms sharing electrons with a carbon atom, forming four covalent bonds.

Solutions, Acids, Bases, Salts, pH

Solutions of various types result from the mixing of elements with elements, elements with compounds, or compounds with compounds. It is these homogeneous (evenly distributed throughout) mixtures, that form almost all existing substances. The most common solutions are those in which a compound is dissolved in the solvent water. Other solvents, such as alcohol, are more commonly used with organic compounds. There are two types of compounds that have characteristics that set them apart from all others; these are acids and bases. One interesting feature of these two groups is that any acid will react with any base, almost without exception. This certain reactivity is not true for other classes of compounds. Also, it is relatively easy to measure the acidity or alkalinity of solutions of acids and bases.

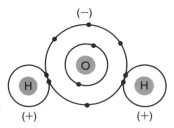

Figure 3–4. A water molecule, showing two hydrogen atoms covalently bonded to an oxygen atom. The arrangement gives the molecule a more positive charge near the hydrogen protons and a negative charge near the oxygen electrons, thus providing an attraction between water molecules (polar bonding).

Table 3 – 2. A Few Common Acids and Their Formulas

Acid	Formula	Location or Use
Hydrochloric acid	HCl	Acid in stomach
Sulfuric acid	H_2SO_4	Industrial mineral acid and battery acid
Boric acid	H_3BO_3	Eye wash
Nitric acid	HNO_3	Industrial oxidizing acid
Acetic acid	$HC_2H_3O_2$	Acid in vinegar
Formic acid	$HCHO_2$	Acid in some insect bites
Carbonic acid	H_2CO_3	Acid in carbonated drinks

Acids The sour taste of lemons, grapefruit, and vinegar is a familiar sensation. Acids can be recognized by this sour taste. However, this is *not* a safe method of identification because they may be poisonous or very destructive to human tissues. Acids are identified by a more reliable, safer technique using chemical indicators or dyes that exhibit a distinct color in an acid solution. Some common acids are shown in Table 3 – 2.

All acids behave in a similar way because they all share a common feature: the ability to produce hydrogen ions when in solution. An acid molecule has at least one hydrogen atom. As an illustration, consider hydrogen chloride or hydrochloric acid, which has the formula HCl. Hydrochloric acid in pure form is a gas, but when bubbled into water, it releases a hydrogen ion (H^+), by donating an electron to form the chloride ion (Cl^-). The result is a cation (the positively charged hydrogen ion) and an anion (the negatively charged chloride ion), as illustrated in the reaction equation (Fig. 3 – 5).

Note that the HCl is an electrolyte; that is, it is a substance with charged particles that can conduct electricity. All acids produce hydrogen ions, which are the particles that contribute to the sour taste of acids and also affect the color of indicators. Indicator dyes are acidic or basic compounds that have distinctive color when in acidic or basic solutions.

Figure 3 – 5. The ionization of hydrochloric acid in water.

$$HCl \quad + \quad H_2O \quad \longrightarrow \quad H^+ \; + \; Cl^- \quad + \quad H_2O$$

Hydrogen chloride molecule + Water molecule   Hydrogen ion + Chloride ion + Water molecule

Table 3–3.   Some Common Bases

Base	Formula	Location or Use
Sodium hydroxide	NaOH	Caustic soda
Potassium hydroxide	KOH	Caustic potash
Ammonium hydroxide	NH_4OH	Household cleaners
Calcium hydroxide	$Ca(OH)_2$	Limewater
Magnesium hydroxide	$Mg(OH)_2$	Antacid drug

Bases   If you have had the misfortune to taste soap, you know the bitter taste of bases. However, due to their potentially toxic nature, this is not a wise method to use for identification of a base. These substances have a hydroxide ion (OH^-) as their common feature. When dissolved in water, they release the hydroxide ion and a cation, and become electrolytes. Table 3–3 lists some common bases. Notice the hydroxide ion in their formulas.

As mentioned before, all acids will react with all bases. When they react they form one common product, water (H_2O). To illustrate, three reactions between different acids and bases are listed in Fig. 3–6.

Acid-base reactions can be summarized by a general statement: *An acid plus a base produces a salt and water.*

Salts   Salts are another general class of electrolytic compounds. Chemical formulas are often written in a manner to assist in determining whether a substance is acid, base, or salt. For example, acids are written with H at the left, as in HCl and H_2SO_4. Bases have an OH at the right, such as NaOH and $Mg(OH)_2$. The formulas for salts have neither an H at the left nor an OH at the right. Sodium chloride, NaCl, and sodium hydrogen carbonate, $NaHCO_3$, are examples.

It is important for all living creatures, including microorganisms, to have and maintain the appropriate acid, base, and salt balance to metabolize and function properly. When a nutrient medium is prepared for growing microbial cells in the laboratory, the correct acid-base-salt balance is as important as the availability of the necessary nutrients.

pH   pH is a measure of acidity. Naturally, acids are "acidic," and bases are "basic" or "alkaline" in nature. The pH scale used to indicate acidity or alkalinity ranges from 0 to 14, with 7 as the neutral point (Fig. 3–7). Pure water has a pH of

$$HCl + NaOH \longrightarrow NaCl + H_2O$$
$$H_2SO_4 + Mg(OH)_2 \longrightarrow MgSO_4 + 2\ H_2O$$
$$H_2CO_3 + NaOH \longrightarrow NaHCO_3 + H_2O$$

Figure 3–6. General equation: "acid" + "base" $\longrightarrow$ "salt" + "water."

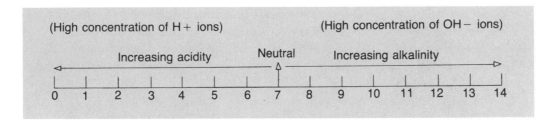

Figure 3-7. The pH scale is derived by using a complex mathematical formula to determine the free hydrogen ion (H^+) concentration. (Rosdahl CB: Textbook of Basic Nursing, 4th ed. Philadelphia, JB Lippincott)

7. If an acid is added to the water, the pH decreases to between 0 and 7. Adding a base to water gives a pH between 7 and 14. Table 3-4 lists some common substances and the pH for each.

The pH of a substance can be measured with a pH meter, with indicator solutions, or with chemically treated papers that turn a definite color within certain pH ranges. These papers are called indicator papers. In the human body the pH of various fluids (blood, lymph) must remain within very narrow ranges to keep the delicately balanced metabolic process working properly; as with microbial cells, if the pH varies too far from optimum, metabolism is disrupted and death may result.

Organic Chemistry

Organic chemistry is that branch of the science of chemistry that deals primarily with the element carbon and its covalent bonds. This definition makes organic chemistry a broad and important branch of the science of chemistry.

Carbon Bonds

In our current understanding of life, carbon is the primary requisite for all living systems. The element carbon exists in three forms: diamond, graphite, and carbon

Table 3-4. The pH of Some Common Substances

Substance	pH
Household ammonia cleaner	11.9
Blood (human)	7.35-7.45
Pure H_2O	7
Milk	6.9
Black coffee	5
Orange juice	2.9
Gastric juice (stomach acid)	1.5

or carbon black. These three forms have dramatically different physical properties, and it is difficult to believe that they are truly the same element. In addition to these unique physical differences, carbon has a valence of 4, which means that its atoms bond to four other atoms. For convenience, the carbon atom is illustrated in this text with the symbol C and four bonds:

$$-\overset{|}{\underset{|}{C}}-$$

The uniqueness of carbon lies in the ability of its atoms to bond to each other to form a "multitude" of compounds. The variety of carbon compounds increases still more when atoms of other elements also attach in different ways to the carbon atom.

When two carbon atoms bond together there are three types of resulting covalent bonds: *single bonds*, *double bonds*, and *triple bonds*. Each line represents a bond between the carbon atoms, which is formed from a pair of shared electrons.

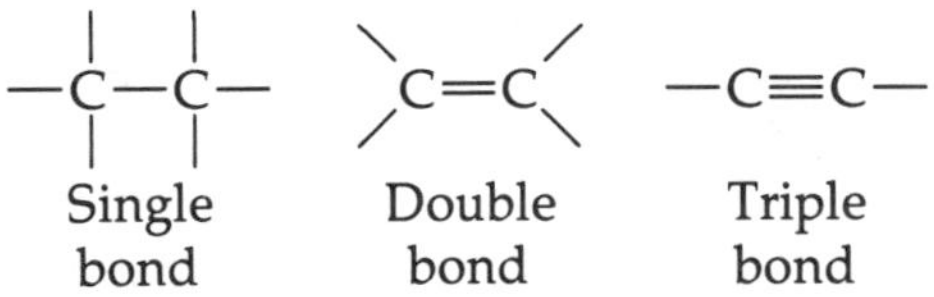

$$-\overset{|}{\underset{|}{C}}-\overset{|}{\underset{|}{C}}- \qquad \overset{\diagdown}{\diagup}C=C\overset{\diagup}{\diagdown} \qquad -C\equiv C-$$

Single   Double   Triple
bond   bond   bond

When atoms of other elements attach to additional available bonds of the carbon atoms, stable compounds are formed. For example, if hydrogens are bonded to the available bonds, compounds called *hydrocarbons* are formed. Just a few of the many hydrocarbon compounds are shown in Figure 3–8.

When more than two carbons are linked together, longer molecules are formed. A series of many carbon atoms bonded together is logically called a *chain*. The long-chain hydrocarbons are usually liquid or solid; the short-chain hydrocarbons, such as the ones in Figure 3–8, are gases.

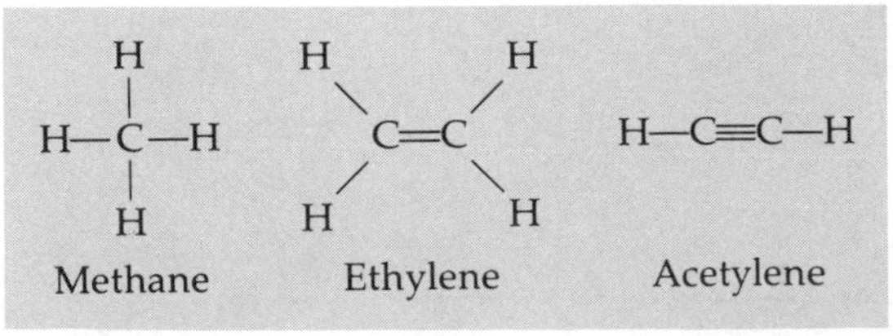

Figure 3–8. Simple hydrocarbons.

$$H-\overset{\overset{\displaystyle H}{|}}{\underset{\underset{\displaystyle H}{|}}{C}}-H \qquad \overset{\displaystyle H}{\diagdown}C=C\overset{\displaystyle H}{\diagup}$$

Methane   Ethylene $H-C\equiv C-H$ Acetylene

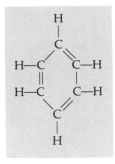

Figure 3–9. The benzene ring.

Cyclic Compounds

Carbon atoms may link to carbon atoms to close the chain, forming ring or cyclic compounds. An example is benzene, which has six carbons and six hydrogens bonded, as shown in Figure 3–9.

Biochemistry

Biochemistry is the study of living matter and its biochemical changes or metabolism. The large biochemical molecules, called macromolecules, are present in every cell in animals, plants, and microorganisms. These macromolecules are of many different types and are classified as carbohydrates, lipids, proteins, and nucleic acids. The vitamins, enzymes, hormones, and high-energy molecules, such as adenosine triphosphate (ATP), are also included among these biochemicals.

Humans obtain their nutrients from the foods they eat. The carbohydrates, fats, nucleic acids, and proteins contained in these foods are digested, and their components are absorbed by the blood and carried to every cell in the body. In the body cells, the components from the food biochemicals are absorbed and rearranged. In this way, the proper compounds necessary for cell structure and function are synthesized. Microorganisms also absorb their essential nutrients into the cell by various means to be described in Chapter 4. These nutrients are then used in metabolic reactions as sources of energy and as building blocks for enzymes and structural macromolecules as well as for genetic materials.

Carbohydrates

Carbohydrates are composed of carbon (C), hydrogen (H), and oxygen (O) in the ratio of $1:2:1$, or simply CH_2O.

Monosaccharides   The simplest carbohydrates are sugars; the smallest molecule of sugar is the monosaccharide (Gr. *mono* = one; *sakcharon* = sugar). The most important monosaccharide in nature is *glucose* ($C_6H_{12}O_6$), which may occur in the chain or alpha or beta ring configurations, as shown in Figure 3–10.

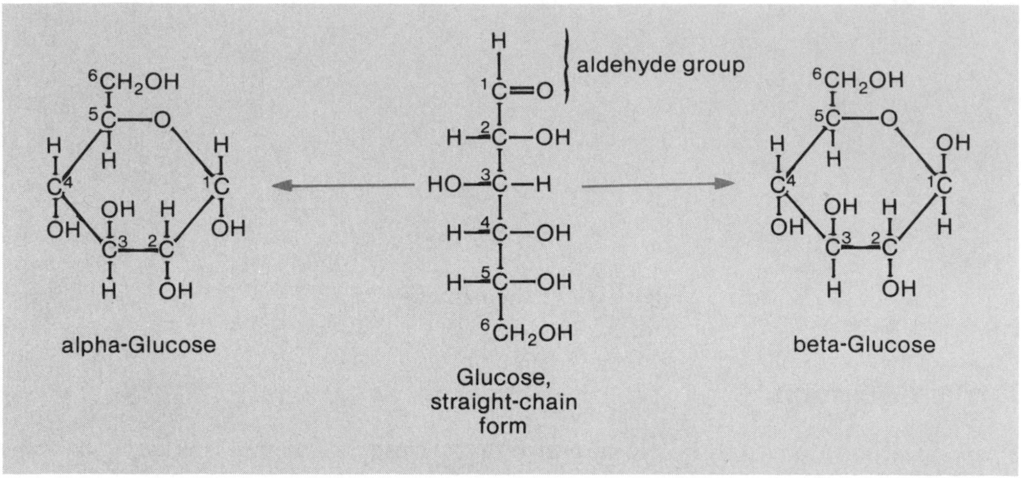

Figure 3–10. Glucose. The straight-chain and α and β forms may all exist in equilibrium in solution.

The main source of energy for body cells, glucose (dextrose), is found in most sweet fruits and in blood sugar. The glucose carried in the blood to the cells is oxidized to produce the high-energy molecule ATP with its high-energy phosphate bonds. This ATP molecule is the main source of energy used to drive most metabolic reactions. Other monosaccharides, with the aldehyde group on the first carbon, are galactose and ribose (a five-carbon sugar). An important monosaccharide that has a ketone group on the second carbon is *fructose* (Fig. 3–11). Fructose, the sweetest of the monosaccharides, is found in fruits and honey.

Disaccharides   Disaccharides are sugars that result from the combination of two monosaccharides. Sucrose (or table sugar) is a sweet *disaccharide* made up of a glucose molecule and a fructose molecule (Fig. 3–12).

Disaccharides react with water in a process called hydrolysis. This causes them to break down into two monosaccharides:

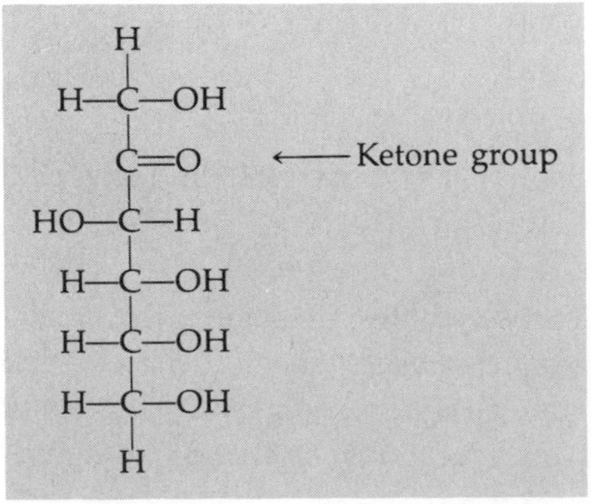

Figure 3–11. Fructose in straight-chain form. (Fructose may also exist in the ring form as shown in Figure 3–12.)

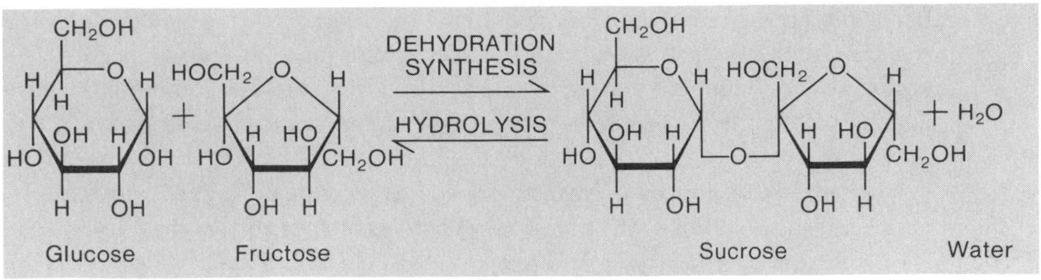

Figure 3–12. The dehydration synthesis and hydrolysis of sucrose.

$$\text{disaccharides} \rightleftharpoons 2 \text{ monosaccharides}$$
$$\text{maltose} + H_2O \rightleftharpoons \text{glucose} + \text{glucose}$$
$$\text{lactose} + H_2O \rightleftharpoons \text{glucose} + \text{galactose}$$
$$\text{sucrose} + H_2O \rightleftharpoons \text{glucose} + \text{fructose}$$

Maltose is the sugar in malt. Lactose is the sugar found in milk. Sucrose comes from sugar cane, sugar beets, and maple sugar. The synthesis of disaccharides from two monosaccharides with the removal of water is called *dehydration synthesis* (see Fig. 3–12).

Polysaccharides   Polysaccharides, such as starch, cellulose, and glycogen, are essentially made up of hundreds of repetitive glucose units, that is, they consist of long chains of the monosaccharide, glucose, which are held together by glycosidic bonds. They are *polymers*, which means they consist of many similar subunits. These large polysaccharide molecules are made of many monosaccharide molecules. Some of these molecules are so large that they are insoluble in water. In the presence of the proper enzymes or acids, polysaccharides may be hydrolyzed or broken down into disaccharides and then finally into monosaccharides (Fig. 3–13).

Polysaccharides serve two main functions. One is to store energy that can be

Figure 3–13. The hydrolysis of starch.

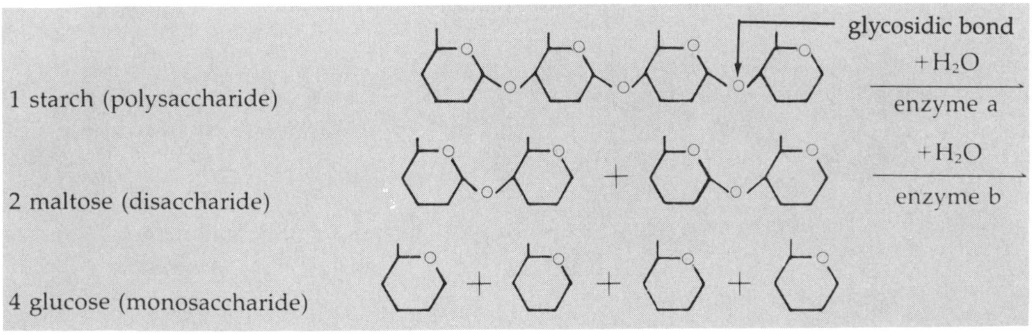

1 starch (polysaccharide)

2 maltose (disaccharide)

4 glucose (monosaccharide)

used when the external food supply is low. The common storage molecule in animals is *glycogen*, which is found in the liver and in muscles. In plants, glucose is stored as *starch* and is found in potatoes and other vegetables and seeds. Some algae store starch; and bacteria contain glycogen granules as a reserve nutrient supply.

The other function of polysaccharides is to provide a "tough" molecule for structural support and protection. Many bacteria secrete polysaccharide capsules for protection against drying and phagocytosis. Plant and algae cells have cellulose cell walls to provide support and shape, as well as protection against the environment.

Cellulose is insoluble in water and indigestible for humans and most animals. Some protozoa, fungi, and bacteria have enzymes that will break the β-glycosidic bonds linking the glucose units in cellulose. These are the microorganisms (saprophytes) that are able to disintegrate dead plants in the soil and that live in the digestive organs of herbivores (plant eaters). Starch and glycogen are easily digested by animals because they have the digestive enzyme to hydrolyze the α-glycosidic bonds that link the glucose units into long, helical or branched polymers (Fig. 3–14).

Fibers of cellulose extracted from certain plants are used to make paper, cotton, linen, and rope. These fibers are relatively rigid, strong, and insoluble because they consist of 100 to 200 parallel strands of cellulose.

When polysaccharides are combined with other chemical groups (amines, lipids, and amino acids), extremely complex macromolecules are formed that serve specific purposes. Glucosamine and galactosamine (amine derivatives of glucose and galactose, respectively) are important constituents of the supporting polysaccharides in connective tissue fibers, cartilage, and chitin. Chitin is the main component of the hard outer covering of insects, spiders, crabs, and fungi. The main portion of the rigid cell wall of bacteria consists of aminosugars and short polypeptide chains that combine to form the peptidoglycan layer.

Figure 3–14. The difference between cellulose and starch.

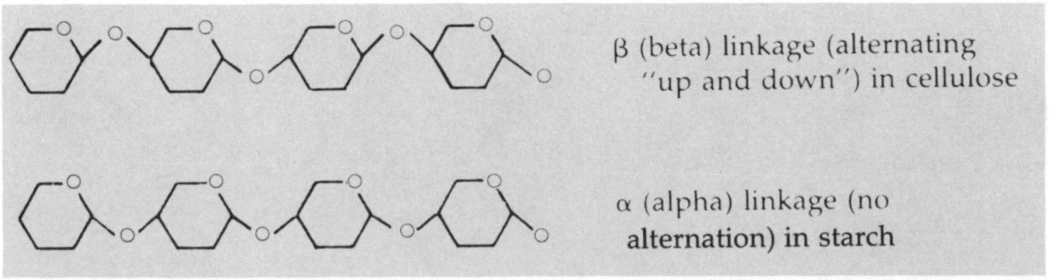

β (beta) linkage (alternating "up and down") in cellulose

α (alpha) linkage (no alternation) in starch

Lipids

Lipids are a class of biochemical compounds consisting mainly of fats and oils. Most of them are insoluble in water but soluble in fat solvents such as ether, chloroform, and benzene. Lipids are essential constituents of almost all living cells. They may be classified into the following categories:

1. Simple lipids (contain C, H, O)
   a. Fats and oils (butter, vegetable oils)
   b. Waxes (beeswax, lanolin)
2. Compound lipids (contain C, H, O, N, and P)
   a. Phospholipids (in cell membranes)
   b. Glycolipids (in nerve cells)
3. Derived lipids (contain C, H, O)
   a. Steroids (sex hormones, cholesterol)
   b. Fat-soluble vitamins A, D, E, K

The simple lipids (*fats* and *oils*) consist of one molecule of glycerol and three fatty acid molecules joined together by the removal of three molecules of water (dehydration synthesis), which produces a triglyceride fat or oil (Fig. 3–15).

If the hydrocarbon side chains have no double bonds between carbons, it is called a *saturated fatty acid* because every carbon atom is saturated with hydrogen. When there are double bonds between the carbons (C=C), it is an *unsaturated fatty acid*. Sources of unsaturated fats are peanut, olive, corn, soybean, and cottonseed oils. Fats are liquids or low-melting solids at room temperature, depending on the relative composition of the fatty acids. Unsaturated fatty acids with short carbon chains are usually liquids. Many people are on low-saturated fat diets to help prevent lipid cholesterol deposits in their hearts and arteries.

Figure 3–15. The synthesis of a fat.

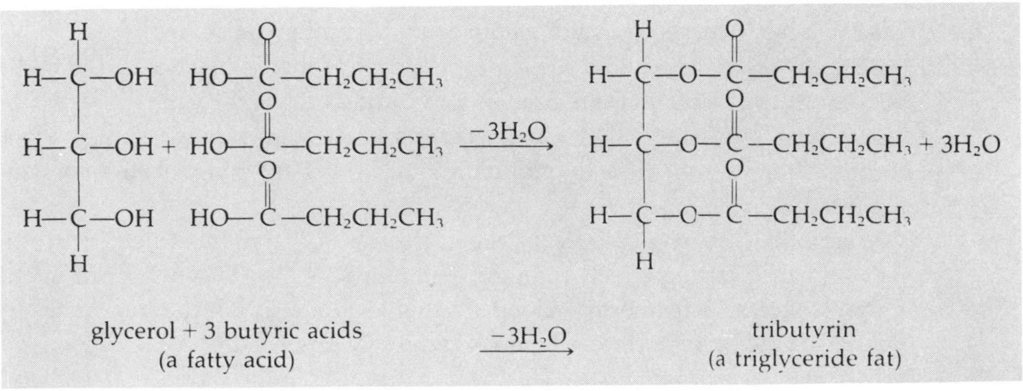

glycerol + 3 butyric acids $-3H_2O$ tributyrin
(a fatty acid) $\longrightarrow$ (a triglyceride fat)

A nutritious human diet should include at least the two essential fatty acids that the body cannot synthesize. These are linoleic acid ($C_{17}H_{31}COOH$), from fish liver oils and vegetable oils, and arachidonic acid ($C_{19}H_{31}COOH$) from egg yolk, liver, kidney tissues, and fish liver oils. However, different fatty acids are produced by and are necessary for the growth of bacteria and other microorganisms, depending on the species of the organism.

Saponification is the hydrolysis of a fat into glycerol (glycerin) and its three fatty acids. When NaOH or KOH (strong alkalis) are used to hydrolyze fats, the results are sodium or potassium salts of the fatty acids, which are soaps. Detergents, bile salts, and fat-digestive enzymes also saponify fats.

Waxes   Waxes are chemically different from fats because they are long-chain or complex alcohols, other than glycerol, with fatty acids attached. Waxes are semisolid substances that serve as a protective coating on the surfaces of leaves, stems, fruits, insects, and some bacteria.

Compound Lipids   Compound lipids include the phospholipids of cell membranes and the glycolipids of nerve and brain cells. Even when an organism is starving, the amount of these nonfat lipids in the cells does not vary.

Derived Lipids   Derived lipids are classified as lipids because they are also soluble in fat solvents. These complex molecules of four interlocking carbon rings are called steroids. Many steroid anti-inflammatory medications are produced by fungi and bacteria and are used in the treatment of arthritis and cancer patients. Other examples of steroids include cholesterol, male and female hormones, adrenal cortex hormones, and vitamin D. Vitamin A, E, and K are *not* steroids but are fat-soluble vitamins.

Cholesterol is a necessary body metabolite. It is found in most eucaryotic membranes and in nervous tissues and aids in fatty acid adsorption. It is also essential for the production of sex hormones, vitamin D, and adrenal cortex hormones. However, an excess of cholesterol may be deposited in either the arteries, causing heart disease, or in the gallbladder, becoming gallstones.

Vitamin D helps maintain the calcium and phosphorus balance in the body. Good sources of vitamin D are fish oils and fortified foods. Vitamin A can be obtained from liver, eggs, butter, cheese, carrots, and green leafy vegetables; a lack of this vitamin can lead to night blindness or hardening of the mucous membranes.

Vitamin E (from plant oils, leafy vegetables, and eggs) reduces sterility in animals and the wasting effects of aging. Vitamin K, which is synthesized in the body, is necessary for normal blood clotting. Some colon bacteria (specifically *Escherichia coli*) also secrete vitamin K, which is absorbed into the blood.

Proteins

Proteins are among the most essential chemicals in all living cells. Some are the structural components of membranes, cells, and tissues, whereas others are enzymes and hormones that chemically control the metabolic balance within both the cell and the individual organism. All proteins are polymers of amino acids; however, they vary widely in the number of amino acids present and in the sequence of amino acids, as well as in their size, configuration, and functions.

Proteins are synthesized by plants, algae, and bacteria from carbon dioxide, water, nitrates, and sulfates, through the process called photosynthesis. In this process, the chemicals combine with the aid of the sun's energy. Humans can synthesize proteins, but they must ingest eight essential amino acids to synthesize the other amino acids necessary in the building of proteins. Nonphotosynthetic microorganisms also must absorb their essential amino acids that are not synthesized or stored in living cells. All the amino acids (ingested and synthesized) must be present during the protein synthesis process in the cells. Any excess can be used to produce energy or eliminated with the soluble wastes.

Amino Acid Structure   There are 20 different amino acids. Each is composed of carbon, hydrogen, oxygen, and nitrogen; three of the amino acids also have sulfur atoms in the molecule. The general formula for amino acids is shown in Figure 3–16. In this figure, the "R" group represents any of the 20 groups that may be substituted into that position to build the various amino acids. For instance, —H in place of the —R represents glycine, and —CH_3 in that position results in a structural formula representing alanine.

The thousands of different proteins in the body are composed of a great variety of amino acids in various arrangements and amounts. The number of proteins that can be synthesized is virtually unlimited. They are not limited by the number of different amino acids, just as the number of words in the written language is not limited by the number of letters in the alphabet. The actual number of proteins produced by an organism and the amino acid sequence of those proteins are determined by the particular genes present on the chromosomes.

Figure 3–16. The basic structure of amino acids.

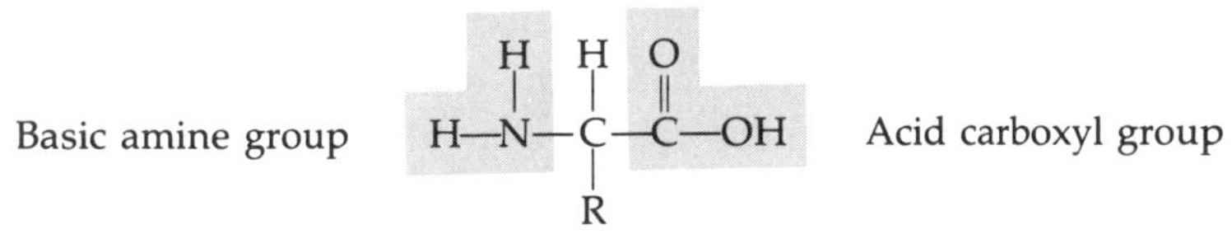

$$\text{Basic amine group} \quad \underset{\displaystyle R}{H-N-\overset{\displaystyle H}{\underset{|}{C}}-\overset{\displaystyle O}{C}-OH} \quad \text{Acid carboxyl group}$$

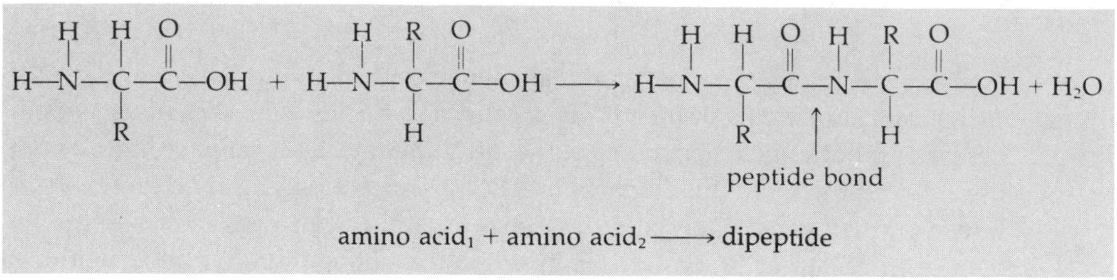

Figure 3–17. The formation of a dipeptide (R = any amino acid side-chain group).

Protein Structure   When water is removed, by dehydration synthesis, the amino acids are linked together by a peptide bond as shown in Figure 3–17. A *dipeptide* is formed by bonding two amino acids; three amino acids form a *tripeptide*. A long chain or polymer of amino acids is referred to as a *polypeptide*. Polypeptides are said to have *primary protein structure*, a sequence of amino acids in a chain (Fig. 3–18). Some fibrous proteins are made of strands of polypeptides bonded to each other by hydrogen bonds and wound together into a helix. Collagen, found in connective tissue, scars, and tendons is another fibrous protein, consisting of three polypeptides in a triple helix, forming a very strong structure.

Most polypeptide chains naturally twist into spirals or helices as a result of the charged side chains protruding from the carbon-nitrogen backbone of the molecule. This helical configuration is referred to as *secondary protein structure* and is found in fibrous proteins such as the keratin fibers of hair, nails, and skin, and the microtubules and microfilaments of cells.

Because a long coil can become entwined by folding back on itself, a polypeptide helix may become globular (see Fig. 3–18). In some areas the helix is retained, but other areas curve randomly. This globular, *tertiary protein structure* is stabilized, not only by hydrogen bonding but also by disulfide bond cross-links between two sulfur groups (S—S). This three-dimensional configuration is characteristic of enzymes, which work by fitting on and into specific molecules (see the next section).

When two or more polypeptide chains are bonded together by hydrogen and disulfide bonds, the resulting structure is referred to as *quaternary protein structure* (see Fig. 3–18). For instance, hemoglobin consists of four globular myoglobins. The size, shape, and configuration of a protein is specific for the function it must perform. If the amino acid sequence and, thus, the configuration of hemoglobin in red blood cells is not perfect, the red blood cells may become distorted and assume a sickle shape (as in sickle cell anemia). In this state they are unable to carry oxygen, which is necessary for cellular metabolism. Myoglobin, the oxygen-binding protein found in skeletal muscles, was the first protein to have its primary, secondary, and tertiary structure defined.

Ser—Tyr—Ser—Met—Glu—His—Phe—Arg—Trp—Gly—Lys—Pro—Val—Gly—Lys

A

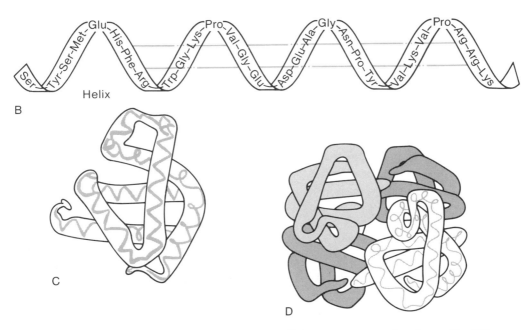

B

Helix

C

D

Figure 3–18. Basic protein structure. (A) Primary sequence of amino acids. (B) Secondary helix. (C) Tertiary globular structure. (D) Quarternary structure with four polypeptide chains.

Enzymes *Enzymes* are protein molecules produced by living cells as "ordered" by the DNA or genes on the chromosomes. Enzymes are essential as catalysts in the biochemical reactions of metabolism; in other words, they speed up these reactions. Almost every reaction in the cell requires the presence of a specific enzyme. All enzymes are proteins; many consist of protein only, whereas others require a nonprotein *cofactor*, such as metal ions (Ca^{2+}, Fe^{2+}, Mg^{2+}, Cu^{2+}) or organic compounds such as vitamin C. Although enzymes influence the direction of the reaction and increase its rate of reaction, they do not provide the energy needed to activate the reaction.

Enzymes are usually named by adding the ending *-ase* to the word indicating the compound or types of compounds on which an enzyme exerts its effect. For example, proteases, carbohdrases, and lipases are enzymes specific for proteins, carbohydrates, and lipids, respectively.

Poisons and toxins usually cause damage to the body by interfering with the action of certain necessary enzymes. For example, cyanide poison binds to the iron and copper ions in the cytochrome systems of the mitochondria of cells. As a result, the cells cannot use oxygen to synthesize ATP, which is essential for energy production, and they soon die.

Proteins, including enzymes, may be denatured by heat or certain chemicals. In a denatured protein, the bonds that hold the molecule in a tertiary structure are broken. With the bonds broken, the protein is no longer functional. Enzymes are also discussed in Chapter 4.

Nucleic Acids

The fourth major group of macromolecules in living cells are the nucleic acids: deoxyribonucleic acid (DNA) and ribonucleic acid (RNA). DNA is the macromolecule that makes up the major portion of the chromosomes. Its important task is to carry the genetic information for each cell of an organism. The information from the DNA must be carried to the rest of the cell for the cell to function properly; this is accomplished by RNA. Thus, RNA is found not only in the nucleus but in the cytoplasm as well.

Function Nucleic acids have two very important functions. First, the nucleic acids determine precisely all the proteins that are synthesized, and those protein enzymes that are synthesized control the metabolism of the organism. DNA's second role is to act as the genetic "molecular blueprint of life." The genetic information must be passed from one generation to the next, from each parent cell to each daughter cell via the DNA.

Structure In addition to carbon, hydrogen, oxygen, and nitrogen, DNA and RNA contain the element phosphorus, whereas the proteins (described previously) contain sulfur. The building blocks of these nucleic acid polymers are the *nucleotides*. These are more complex monomers (single molecular units that can be repeated to form a polymer) than the amino acids, which are the building blocks of proteins. The nucleotides consist of three subunits: a nitrogen-containing base, a five-carbon sugar, and a phosphate group joined together, as shown in Figure 3–19.

Figure 3–19. Two nucleotides consisting of a nitrogen base, a five-carbon sugar, and a phosphate group.

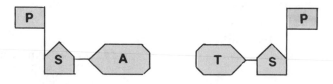

As previously stated, there are two kinds of nucleic acids in cells: DNA and RNA. DNA contains deoxyribose as its five-carbon sugar (a pentose), whereas RNA contains the sugar ribose. There are three types of RNA, which are named for the function they serve: messenger RNA (mRNA), ribosomal RNA (rRNA), and transfer RNA (tRNA). The five most important nitrogen-containing bases are adenine (A), guanine (G), thymine (T), cytosine (C), and uracil (U). Thymine occurs in DNA and uracil in RNA. The other bases occur in both DNA and RNA.

The nucleotides join between their sugar and phosphate groups to form very long polymers, 100,000 or more monomers long, as shown in Figure 3–20.

DNA Structure   In 1953, James Watson and Francis Crick proposed a double-stranded helical structure for DNA to indicate how it could copy (replicate) itself exactly to pass the genetic information to each daughter cell. For a double-stranded DNA to form, the bases must bond together. It was found that adenine always bonds with thymine (with two hydrogen bonds) and guanine with cytosine (with three hydrogen bonds) because of the size and bonding attraction between the molecules. The bonding forces of the double-stranded polymer cause it to assume the shape of a double α-helix, which is similar to a right-handed spiral staircase (Fig. 3–21).

Replication   When a cell is preparing to divide, all of the DNA molecules in the chromosomes of that cell must duplicate, thereby ensuring that the same genetic information is passed to both daughter cells. This process is called DNA replication. It occurs by the separation of the DNA strands and the building of complementary strands by the addition of the correct nucleotides, as indicated in Figure 3–22. The duplicated DNA of the chromosomes can then be separated during or-

Figure 3–20. One small section of a nucleic acid polymer.

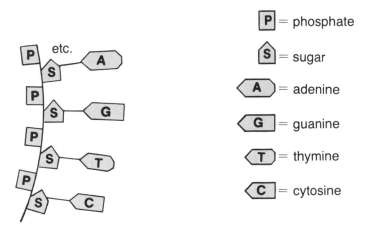

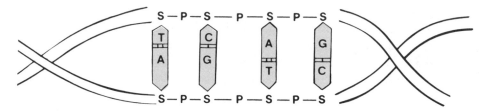

Figure 3–21. The DNA double helix.

dinary cell division so that the same number of chromosomes, the same genes, and the same amount of DNA as in the parent cell are found in each daughter cell (except during meiosis, the reduction division to produce egg and sperm cells).

Protein Synthesis   In a normally functioning living cell, the DNA of the chromosomes controls all the metabolic activities. It accomplishes this by directing the synthesis of the protein enzymes that regulate the chemical reactions occurring in metabolism.

The translation and interpretation of the information carried by the DNA molecule to produce the proper proteins is a complex procedure. It is the sequence of the four nitrogen-containing bases (A, T, C, and G) that carries the code for the amino acid sequences of the protein to be synthesized in the cytoplasm of the cell. A diagrammatic representation of this process is shown in Figure 3–23.

You should remember that the *chromosomes*, which are located in the nuclear region of the cell, consist of many *genes* that carry the genetic information for the inherited traits of the organism. Each gene consists of several *cistrons*, which are the portions of the chromosomal DNA that code for *one* particular protein or enzyme.

Figure 3–22. Replication of DNA before cell division.

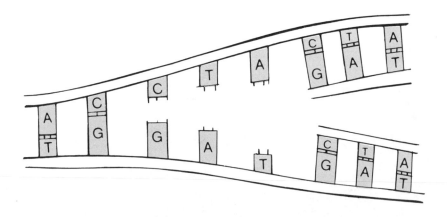

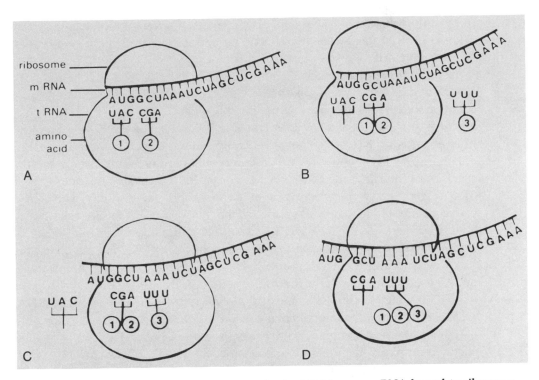

Figure 3-23. Outline of protein synthesis. (A) Messenger RNA bound to ribosome. Amino acids 1 and 2 are bonded to their transfer RNAs. The t-RNA-amino acid 1 is bound to the peptidyl binding site. The t-RNA-amino acid 2 is bound to the amino acid binding site. (B) Amino acid 1 is released from its t-RNA and is joined to amino acid 2 through a peptide bond. (C) The ribosome moves along the m-RNA, and t-RNA 1 leaves the peptidyl binding site. The t-RNA 2 with the attached dipeptide moves to the peptidyl site and t-RNA amino acid 3 binds to the amino acid binding site. (D) Amino acid 2 is bonded to amino acid 3 as in step B. The process repeats until the protein is completed.

When a cell is stimulated (by need) to produce a particular protein, such as insulin, the DNA of the appropriate cistron is activated to unwind temporarily from its helical configuration. This unwinding exposes the bases, which then attract the bases of free nucleotides, and a *messenger RNA* (mRNA) begins to build on one strand, the activated strand, of the opened DNA. Thus, the DNA has served as a *template*, or pattern, and has coded for a complementary mirror image of its structure in the RNA. This procedure is called *transcription* because the message from the DNA is transcribed onto the mRNA. After the mRNA has been synthesized over the length of the cistron, it is freed from the active DNA strand to carry the message to the cytoplasm and direct the synthesis of that particular protein, which is insulin in this case.

In eucaryotes, the freed mRNA passes through the pores of the nuclear membrane into the cytoplasm, and takes its position on the protein "assembly line";

that is, the ribosomes containing ribosomal RNA (rRNA), which attract the mRNA. The ribosomes usually reside on the endoplasmic reticulum membranes in eucaryotic cells.

In procaryotes, the ribosomes may attach to the mRNA as it is being transcribed at the DNA genome, because no nuclear membrane is present; thus transcription and translation may occur simultaneously.

The base sequence of the mRNA is read or interpreted by the rRNA in groups of three bases, called *codons*. The sequence of a codon's three bases is the code that determines which amino acid goes in that position in the protein being synthesized. The amino acids must be transferred or carried by an activated *transfer RNA* (tRNA) from the cytoplasmic matrix to the site of protein assembly. The three-base sequence of the codon determines which tRNA brings its specific amino acid to the ribosome, because the RNA has an *anticodon*, three-base sequence, which is complementary to, or attracted to, the codon of the mRNA. For example, the tRNA with the anticodon base sequence UUU carries the amino acid lysine to the mRNA codon AAA. Similarly, the mRNA codon CCG codes for the tRNA anticodon GGC, which carries the amino acid proline at the opposite end of the tRNA molecule. This information system is called the *genetic code*. A chart can be prepared to show which sequence of three bases in the DNA codes for a particular codon in mRNA, which calls a particular anticodon on the tRNA carrying a specific amino acid.

The process of translating the message carried by the mRNA and decoded by the rRNA, which calls the particular tRNAs to bring the amino acids to be bound together in the proper sequence to make a specific protein (*e.g.*, insulin), is called *translation*. This process is summarized in Figure 3–23. It should be noted that the living cell is constantly producing mRNA in its nucleus, which directs the synthesis of all the proteins, including metabolic enzymes necessary for the normal functions of that specific type of cell. Also, the mRNA and tRNA are short-lived nucleic acids that may be reused many times, then destroyed and resynthesized in the nucleus. The rRNA is made in the dense portion of the nucleus called the nucleolus; the ribosomes last longer in the cell than the mRNA.

As the tRNA molecules attach to mRNA while it is sliding over the ribosomes, they bring the correct activated amino acids into contact with each other so that peptide bonds are made and a polypeptide is formed. As the polypeptide grows and becomes a protein, it folds into the unique shape determined by the amino acid sequence. This characteristic shape allows the protein to perform its specific function. If one DNA cistron base is out of sequence, the amino acid sequence will not be correct and the protein configuration will not allow the protein to function properly. For instance, some diabetics may not produce insulin properly because a mutation in the DNA of their chromosomes caused a rearrangement of the bases in the cistron that codes for insulin. DNA errors are the basis for most genetic and inherited diseases, such as phenylketonuria (PKU), sickle cell anemia, cerebral palsy, cystic fibrosis, cleft lip, clubfoot, extra fingers, albinism, and many other birth defects. Likewise, nonpathogenic microbes may mutate to become pathogens, and pathogens may lose the ability to cause disease by mutation, or a change in the DNA sequence.

The new science of genetic engineering attempts to repair the genetic damage in some diseases. As yet, the morality of manipulation of human genes has not been resolved by society. However, many genetically changed microbes are able to produce substances, such as human insulin, interferon, growth hormones, new pharmaceutical agents, and vaccines, that will have a substantial effect on the medical treatment of humans.

Summary

To understand how a cell lives, metabolizes, and reproduces, one must comprehend some of the chemical aspects and reactions involved. In this chapter, a brief introduction to atoms and molecules and how they combine by ionic, covalent, and polar bonds was given. The importance of water, hydrolytic reactions, and acid-base reactions was discussed. The structure, function, characteristics, and breakdown products of carbohydrates, lipids, proteins, and nucleic acids were emphasized so that the functions of enzymes and metabolic reactions may be better understood.

Study Outline

I. Basic chemistry
  A. Atoms, molecules, elements, compounds
  B. Chemical bonding
  C. Importance of water
  D. Solutions, acids, bases, salts, pH
II. Basic organic chemistry
  A. Carbon bonds
  B. Cyclic compounds

III. Biochemistry
  A. Carbohydrates
  B. Lipids
  C. Proteins
    1. Enzymes
  D. Nucleic acids
    1. DNA, RNA
    2. RNA
    3. Protein synthesis

Problems and Questions

1. Describe the relationship between electrolyte, solvent, solute, and solution.
2. Differentiate between acids and bases, and give some examples of each.
3. If a nutrient growth medium is too acidic or too basic, might a bacterial culture die? Why?
4. Why is it possible for humans to digest starch but not cellulose and chitin? Which microorganisms can digest cellulose?
5. Is the peptidoglycan layer of bacterial cell wall a polymer? If so, provide reasons to support this claim.

6. Are the fat-soluble vitamins lipids? Why? Where would lipids be found in bacterial cells?
7. What are the differences between structural proteins and enzyme proteins in a cell? Describe the primary, secondary, tertiary, and quaternary structure of proteins. How does an enzyme function?
8. Draw a hypothetical bacterium and indicate the types of macromolecules found in its various parts.
9. Explain the chemical characteristics of polymers, carbohydrates, polysaccharides, sugars, cellulose, starch, lipids, proteins, fats, waxes, enzymes, peptides, and nucleic acids.
10. Differentiate between DNA, mRNA, rRNA, and tRNA. Which four bases are found in DNA? In RNA?

Self Test

After you have read Chapter 3, examined the objectives, studied the new words, reviewed the study outline, and answered the questions at the end of the chapter, complete the following self test.

Matching Exercises

Complete each statement from the list of words provided with each section.

Basic Chemistry

neutrons	covalent	molecule
electrons	ionic	hydrolysis
atoms	polar	dehydration synthesis
ions	isotope	metabolism

1. Matter is composed of fundamental units called _____.
2. Charged atoms that have gained or lost electrons are _____.
3. Isotopes of an element differ in the number of _____.
4. When electrons are actually transferred from one atom to another _____ bonds form.
5. When atoms share electrons rather than transferring them, _____ compounds form.
6. _____ involves the breakdown of large organic molecules into their subunits through the process of _____, and the synthesis of large organic molecules by dehydrolysis or _____.

Biochemistry

primary   monosaccharides   RNA
secondary   enzymes   glycerol
tertiary   substrate   glucose
polysaccharides   DNA   proteins
nucleotides

1. A fat molecule is composed of three fatty acid molecules and one _____ molecule.
2. The order, or sequence, of amino acids in a protein molecule constitutes its _____ structure.
3. _____ is the genetic material of living systems, the subunits of which are called _____.
4. Glycogen, starch, and cellulose are examples of _____.
5. Most metabolic reactions are made possible through the action of _____, or organic catalysts.
6. The substance acted on by an enzyme is called a/an _____.

Match the chemicals in Column I with an appropriate group in Column II. An answer from Column II may be used more than once.

Column I
____ 1. Cholesterol
____ 2. Triglyceride
____ 3. Hemoglobin
____ 4. Glucose
____ 5. DNA
____ 6. Sucrose
____ 7. Glycerol and fatty acids
____ 8. RNA
____ 9. Phospholipid
____ 10. Cellulose

Column II
a. Lipid
b. Carbohydrate
c. Nucleic acid
d. Peptide
e. Protein

True or False (T or F)

____ 1. In general DNA molecules are double-stranded.
____ 2. RNA contains the base cytosine instead of guanine.
____ 3. Transcription occurs in the nuclear area, whereas translation occurs on the ribosome.
____ 4. In DNA, the molecule guanine normally pairs with cytosine.
____ 5. Lipids are generally insoluble inorganic solvents.

____ 6. Steroids are a form of lipid.
____ 7. The chief polysaccharide of animals is starch.
____ 8. Uracil is common nitrogenous base of DNA.
____ 9. The chemical bond linking amino acids to one another is a
         disulfide bond.

Multiple Choice

1. The four major organic
    macromolecular groups include
    a. carbohydrates, sugars, starch,
        cellulose
    b. amino acids, proteins,
        enzymes, peptides
    c. lipids, proteins, nucleic acids,
        carbohydrates
    d. carbohydrates, lipids,
        vitamins, proteins

2. Proteins are polymers of
    a. sugars
    b. enzymes
    c. amino acids
    d. glycerol and fatty acids
    e. nucleotides

3. DNA is a polymer of
    a. deoxyribose
    b. phosphate
    c. organic bases
    d. nucleotides
    e. peptides

4. RNA is a polymer of
    a. triglycerides
    b. carbohydrates
    c. peptides
    d. nucleotides
    e. amino acids

5. Which of the following is *not* a
    true difference between DNA and
    RNA?
    a. DNA is a double helix and
        RNA is a single helix.

    b. DNA contains deoxyribose
        sugar and RNA contains
        ribose sugar.
    c. DNA contains thymine and
        RNA contains uracil.
    d. DNA is synthesized in the
        nuclear area and RNA is
        synthesized on the ribosome.
    e. All of these are differences
        between DNA and RNA.

6. Which of the following is an
    example of a lipid?
    a. Glycogen
    b. Amide
    c. Starch
    d. Cholesterol
    e. Deoxyribose

7. Which of the following is *not* an
    example of a complex
    polysaccharide?
    a. Cellulose
    b. Glucosamine
    c. Glycogen
    d. Starch
    e. None of these

8. Which of the following
    components is *not* found in DNA?
    a. Thymine
    b. Cytosine
    c. Uracil
    d. Guanine
    e. Adenine

9. The term "peptide bonds" is associated with which compound?
   a. Carbohydrates
   b. Fats
   c. Phospholipids
   d. Proteins
   e. Nucleic acids

10. Digestion is equivalent to
    a. hydrolysis
    b. dehydration synthesis
    c. metabolism
    d. nutrition
    e. dehydrolysis

11. A charged atom that has achieved structural stability through the gain or loss of electrons is called a/an
    a. isotope
    b. isomer
    c. ion
    d. radical
    e. molecule

12. The notation C=O indicates that a carbon atom and an oxygen atom share how many electrons?
    a. One
    b. Two
    c. Three
    d. Four
    e. Five

13. Isotopes of an element differ in the number of
    a. protons
    b. neutrons
    c. electrons

14. The chloride ion carries a net charge of -1 because it has more
    a. protons than neutrons
    b. electrons than protons
    c. neutrons than electrons
    d. protons than electrons
    e. neutrons than protons

15. Lipids are commonly found, along with proteins, as part of the
    a. plasma membrane
    b. cell walls
    c. ribosomes
    d. nuclei
    e. solutions

16. DNA:
    a. exists in the cell as a double helix
    b. uses its message for the synthesis of specific proteins
    c. carries messages that control the activities of the cell
    d. all of the above
    e. none of the above

Chapter 4

Physiology of Microorganisms

Objectives

After studying this chapter, you should be able to

1. List the nutritional types of bacteria
2. Discuss how the nutritional types fit into the biosphere
3. State the meaning of autotroph, heterotroph, chemotroph, and phototroph
4. Define producers, consumers, and decomposers
5. Describe and give an example of catabolism, anabolism, respiration, and photosynthesis
6. List six uses for energy in the cell
7. Draw and label the bacterial growth curve
8. List the reasons bacteria die during the death phase
9. Describe the bacterial chromosome
10. List and describe five ways by which the genetic constitution of bacteria can be changed

New Words

Anabolism (an-ab'-boh-lizm). Metabolic reactions that result in the biosynthesis of complex cellular materials

Autotrophs (awe'-toe-trophs). Organisms that obtain carbon from inorganic sources, as from carbon dioxide

Catabolism (ca-tab'-boh-lizm). Metabolic reactions that break down organic materials into simple molecules

Catalyst (cat'-ah-list). A chemical agent that speeds up a reaction

Catalyze (cat'-ah-lyz). To speed up a reaction

Chemolithotrophs (key-moe-lith'-oh-trofs). Organisms that use a chemical source of energy and an inorganic source of nutrients

Chemoorganotrophs (key-moe-or-gan'-oh-trofs). Organisms that use a chemical source of energy and an organic source of nutrients

Chemotrophs (key'-moe-trofs). Organisms that obtain their energy from chemical sources

Corynebacterium diphtheriae (co-ri'-knee-back-tear-ee-um dif-theer'-ee-ee). Species of bacteria that causes diphtheria

Escherichia coli (es-ur-eek'-ee-uh co'-lie). A normal intestinal bacterium

Filamentous (fil-uh-men'-tus). Having many threads or filaments

Gene (jean). A portion of a chromosome, carrying genetic information for one polypeptide

Glycolysis (gly-col'-eh-sis). The anaerobic breakdown of glucose to pyruvic acid or lactic acid with the production of energy

Heterotrophs (het'-ter-oh-trofs). Organisms that obtain carbon from organic sources

Logarithm (log'-uh-re-them). Mathematically, the power to which a number must be raised to produce a given number

Metabolism (muh-tab'-boh-lizm). The sum of all the chemical reactions in living cells

Mutagenic (mew-tuh-jen'-ick). Producing mutations or genetic changes in organisms

Mutation (mew-tay'-shun). An inheritable change in a gene

Mutant (mew'-tant). An organism that has survived mutation

Mycobacterium tuberculosis (my-co-back-tear'-ee-um tu-bur-cue-low'-sis). Species of bacteria that causes tuberculosis

Photolithotrophs (foe-toe-lith'-oh-trofs). Organisms that use light for energy and inorganic chemicals for nutrients

Photoorganotrophs (foe-toe-or-gan'-oh-trofs). Organisms that use light for energy and organic chemicals for nutrients

Phototrophs (foe'-toe-trofs). Organisms that use light as their source of energy

Protoplasm (pro'-toe-plaz-um). The substance inside a cell

Protoplast (pro'-toe-plast). A bacterial cell with no cell wall

Pseudomonas (sue-doe-moan'-us). A genus of soil bacillus; may cause wound or lung infections

Saprophyte (sap'-row-fight). Organism that obtains its nutrients from dead, decaying organic matter

Staphylococci (staff-ill-oh-coc'-sigh). Cocci occuring in clusters; some may cause "staph" infections

Streptococci (strep-toe-coc'-sigh). Cocci in chains; some may cause "strep" infections

Vibrio cholerae (vib'-ree-oh col'-lar-ree). A species of bacteria that causes cholera

Microorganisms are perhaps the best organisms to use in our study of the basic metabolic processes of life. Species of bacteria can be found that represent each of the nutritional types of organisms on earth. We can learn much about ourselves by studying the nutritional needs of bacteria, their metabolic cycles, and why under certain conditions they grow or die. The population growth cycles of bacteria illustrate the growth phases of any population of a species of organism including humans.

Each tiny single-celled bacterium strives to produce more cells like itself, and it often does so at a rate that is alarming, as long as water and the nutrient supply are available. Under favorable conditions, in 24 hours, the offspring of a single *Escherichia coli* bacterium would outnumber the entire human population on the earth!

Bacteria are easy to find, grow, and maintain in the laboratory. Their morphology, their nutritional needs, and some of their metabolic reactions are easily observable; thus, when these normal characteristics change in a pure culture, the resultant mutant (a genetically changed organism) can be quickly identified. Because some bacteria, molds, and viruses produce generation after generation so rapidly and easily, they have been used extensively in genetic studies. In fact, most of the genetic knowledge of today was and is being obtained from the study of these microorganisms.

Nutrition

The study of bacterial nutrition and other phases of microbial physiology helps one to understand the vital chemical processes of every living cell, including those of the human body.

Nutritional Requirements

All living protoplasm consists of six major chemical elements: carbon, hydrogen, oxygen, nitrogen, phosphorus, and sulfur. Other elements usually necessary in lesser amounts include sodium, potassium, chlorine, magnesium, calcium, iron, iodine, and some trace elements. The combinations of all of these elements make up the vital macromolecules of life, including carbohydrates, fats, proteins, and nucleic acids (DNA and RNA).

Each organism must have a source of energy and nutrient chemicals to build the necessary cellular materials of life. Those materials that organisms cannot synthesize in building the macromolecules of protoplasm are termed *essential nutritional requirements*. These are the nutrients that must be continually supplied to every organism for it to live. Essential nutrients vary from species to species.

The majority of microbes are *aerobes*, which means that they grow best in an atmosphere that contains oxygen. *Anaerobes* are microbes that grow in the absence of oxygen. *Facultative* anaerobes can grow either with or without oxygen, whereas *obligate* anaerobes live only in the absence of oxygen.

Nutritional Types

Because microorganisms have evolved from the beginning of life on earth, there are microbes representing each of the nutritional types.

Heterotrophs are organisms that obtain carbon from organic materials. All animals, including humans, and most microorganisms, including the pathogens, are heterotrophic organisms. Even the saprophytic fungi and bacteria that live on dead, decaying animal and plant material are heterotrophs.

Autotrophs are organisms that use inorganic carbon dioxide (CO_2) as their basic carbon source. Plants, algae, and many bacteria are autotrophic organisms.

Heterotrophs and autotrophs may be further divided into *chemotrophs* and *phototrophs* according to their sources of energy. Chemotrophs are those organisms that use chemical substances as a source of energy, whereas phototrophs are those that use light for their energy source.

Descriptive terms have been developed to indicate both the sources of energy and the chemical nutrients for each type of microorganism by combining the words chemotroph and phototroph with terms indicating the sources of chemical nutrients. *Organo-* indicates the organic nutrients derived from living or dead material, such as carbohydrates, fats, proteins, and nucleic acids; *litho-* indicates inorganic sources of nutrients, such as water, carbon dioxide, nitrates, phosphates, and sulfates. Thus, the first part of the words *chemoorganotroph, chemolithotroph, photoorganotroph,* and *photolithotroph* indicates the source of energy, and the middle portion of the word identifies the source of nutrients for the living organism (*-troph*). Another group of terms often used instead of these four are, respectively, *chemoheterotroph, chemoautotroph, photoheterotroph,* and *photoautotroph.* These relationships are further explained in the following outline:

I.   Heterotrophic organisms (those using an organic carbon nutrient source)
  A. Chemoorganotrophs (chemoheterotrophs) are those chemotrophs that have a chemical source of energy and use organic materials as a source of nutrients. All animals, protozoa, fungi, and most bacteria fall into this subdivision.
  B. Photoorganotrophs (photoheterotrophs) include those phototrophs that use the ultraviolet rays of the sun as a source of energy and organic matter for nutrients. A few bacteria and a few types of algae are of this nutritional type.
II. Autotrophic organisms (those using an inorganic carbon nutrient source)
  A. Chemolithotrophs (chemoautotrophs) are chemotrophs that use inorganic chemicals such as iron, sulfur, water, carbon dioxide, nitrates, and phosphates as sources of energy and nutrients. This nutritional type includes only a few groups of bacteria—those that oxidize nitrogen, iron, sulfur, uranium, methane, and carbon monoxide—but they are very important in the environmental cycles of these compounds.

B. Photolithotrophs (photoautotrophs) are phototrophs that trap the sun's ultraviolet energy source and use inorganic materials, such as water, carbon dioxide, nitrates, and phosphates, as sources of food nutrients. Most plants, algae, and the photosynthetic bacteria are photolithotrophic organisms. They contribute energy to the ecosystem by trapping energy from the sun and using it to build organic compounds (carbohydrates, fats, nucleic acids, and proteins) from the inorganic materials in the soil, water, and air. In photosynthesis, oxygen also is released for respiration by animals.

The *ecosystem* consists of the interaction between the living organisms and the nonliving environment. The interrelationships among the different nutritional types are of prime importance in the functioning of the ecosystem. The photolithotrophs (plants) are the producers of food and oxygen for the chemoorganotrophs (animals). Dead plants and animals would clutter the earth as debris if the chemoorganotrophic saprophytic decomposers (fungi and bacteria) did not break down the dead organic matter into the inorganic compounds (carbon dioxide, nitrates, phosphates) of the soil and air so that they could be utilized and recycled by the photolithotrophs.

Enzymes, Metabolism, and Energy

Microorganisms are able to grow only if they obtain the proper raw materials for nutrients and for the manufacture of the enzymes necessary to promote metabolic reactions. These processes are similar to those in our own body cells. The term *metabolism* designates all chemical reactions that occur within any cell. These metabolic reactions are enhanced and regulated by enzymes.

Enzymes

Metabolic Enzymes

Enzymes are organic catalysts; that is, they are organic molecules that accelerate the rate of a biochemical reaction at certain temperatures without being used up in those reactions. These reactions would occur at the same temperature without enzymes but at a much slower rate. A *substrate* is a compound on which an enzyme exerts its effect. The enzyme must fit the combining site of the substrate, as a key fits a lock. Usually, an enzyme is specific, that is, it works on only one type of substrate, but occasionally it can attach to different substrates because the shapes of the combining sites on the substrate molecules are similar (Fig. 4–1).

All enzymes are protein molecules; the three-dimensional shape of the protein enables it to attach to one or more substrates to accelerate a very slow reaction, without causing the enzyme to change in the process. The enzyme continues to

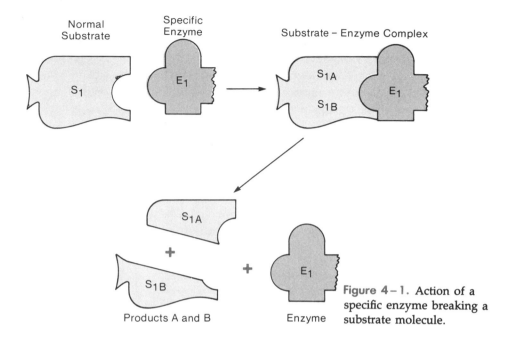

Figure 4–1. Action of a specific enzyme breaking a substrate molecule.

move from substrate molecule to substrate molecule at a rate of several hundred each second, producing a supply of the end product, as long as this particular end product is needed by the cell. However, enzymes do not last indefinitely; they finally degenerate and lose their activity. Therefore, the cell must synthesize and replace these important proteins. Because there are hundreds of metabolic reactions continually occurring in the cell, there must be thousands of enzymes available to control and direct the essential metabolic pathways. At any particular time, all of the required enzymes need not be present; this situation is controlled by the genes on the chromosomes and the needs of the cell, which are determined by the internal and external environment. Those enzymes found inside the cell are called *endoenzymes*, and those secreted outside the cell to perform extracellular functions are *exoenzymes*. The digestive enzymes within phagocytes are good examples of endoenzymes. Exoenzymes are the enzymes secreted by saprophytes, which are then able to digest materials outside the organism. These nutrients digested outside are then absorbed into the organism.

Some enzymes require *cofactors* to activate them to perform their intended functions because they normally exist in the cell in an inactive state. These cofactors are usually mineral ions such as magnesium, calcium, or iron. Other enzymes function only in the presence of a *coenzyme* that acts as a carrier of small chemical groups (such as H_2) that are removed from the substrate. These coenzymes are small organic vitamin-type molecules such as flavin-adenine dinucleotide (FAD) and nicotinamide-adenine dinucleotide (NAD). The activity of these coenzymes is easily recognized in the citric acid cycle for the production of energy from glucose; these oxidation-reduction reactions are discussed later in this chapter. Coenzymes, like enzymes, do not have to be present in large amounts because they are recycled through many reactions. However, the lack of certain vitamins from which the coenzymes are synthesized will halt all those reactions involving that particular coenzyme-enzyme complex.

Some enzymes may also be called hydrolases because they break down macromolecules by the addition of water in a process called *hydrolysis*. These hydrolytic processes enable saprophytes to break apart such complex materials as leather, wax, cork, wood, rubber, hair, some plastics, and even mechanical equipment. Some of the enzymes involved in the formation of large polymers, DNA, and RNA, are called polymerases. These polymerases are active each time the DNA of a cell is replicated and during the synthesis of RNA molecules.

Inhibition of Enzymes

Many factors affect the activity of enzymes (see Fig. 4–1). Any physical or chemical change may diminish or completely stop enzyme activity, because these protein molecules function properly only under optimum conditions. Optimum conditions for enzyme activity include a relatively limited range of pH (acidity) and temperature, and the appropriate concentration of enzyme and substrate. Extremes in heat and acidity can denature (or alter) enzymes by breaking the bonds responsible for their three-dimensional shape, resulting in the loss of enzymatic activity. This explains why bacteria grow best at certain temperatures and pH, characteristic for each species of organism.

Although the mineral ions, calcium, magnesium, and iron, enhance the activity of enzymes by serving as cofactors, other heavy metal ions such as lead, zinc, mercury, and arsenic usually act as poisons to the cell. These toxic ions inhibit enzyme activity by replacing the cofactors, or sometimes replacing only hydrogen, at the combining site of the enzyme, thus inhibiting normal metabolic processes. Some disinfectants containing mineral ions are effective in inhibiting the growth of bacteria by this means.

Sometimes, a similar substrate can be used as an inhibitor to deliberately interfere with a particular metabolic pathway. It binds with the enzyme; thus the end product is not produced. For example, a chemotherapeutic agent, such as a sulfonamide drug, may bind with certain enzymes to prevent essential metabolites from being formed and thereby inhibits the growth of a pathogen.

Cellular Metabolism

Because metabolism is the total of all the chemical reactions in the cell, it includes the production of energy and intermediate products (metabolites) as well as the end products. Furthermore, these reactions must proceed in many directions simultaneously, breaking down some materials to provide energy and raw materials for the synthesis of other compounds. Thus, most metabolic reactions fall into two categories: catabolism and anabolism. *Catabolism* is the metabolic degradation (breakdown) of organic compounds that results in the production of energy and smaller molecules. *Anabolism* refers to those biosynthetic processes that use energy for the synthesis of protoplasmic materials needed for growth, maintenance, and other cellular functions. In this manner, the cell works much like a factory. It gathers and produces raw materials to be used in the production of macromolecules for building, maintenance, and repair. It must also have fuel or energy available to run this metabolic machinery. This energy may be trapped from the rays of the sun (as in photosynthesis), or it may be produced by certain catabolic reactions. Then the energy is bound into high-energy bonds in special molecules, usually adenosine triphosphate (ATP). These high-energy molecules serve as the fuel, just as coal is used to fire the furnaces in the production of steel and other important alloys.

The most important high-energy compound found within the cell is ATP, but it is not the only one. It is found in all cells because it is used to transfer energy from energy-yielding molecules, like glucose, to an energy-using reaction. Thus, ATP is a temporary, intermediate molecule. If ATP is not used shortly after it is formed, it is soon hydrolyzed to adenosine diphosphate (ADP), a more stable molecule, and adenosine monophosphate (AMP) in catabolic reactions. ADP can also be used as an emergency energy source by the removal of another phosphate group to produce AMP (a catabolic reaction; Fig. 4–2). Both AMP and ADP bind with high-energy phosphate groups to produce ATP when the energy is removed from energy-yielding reactions.

Figure 4–2. Conversion of bond energy to cellular energy.

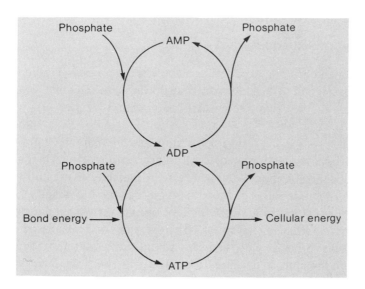

Although the metabolic pathways require the production of much energy, energy must also be available to the organism for growth, reproduction, sporulation, and movement. Some organisms even use energy for bioluminescence, such as the plankton that glow in the darkness of the ocean. Much energy of any system is lost in the form of heat.

Energy Metabolism

Chemical reactions are essentially energy transformation processes during which the energy that is stored in chemical bonds is transferred to other newly formed chemical bonds. The cellular mechanisms that release small amounts of energy as the cell needs it, usually involve a sequence of catabolic and anabolic reactions, many of which are oxidation-reduction reactions.

In oxidation-reduction reactions, electrons are transferred from one chemical to another. Whenever an atom, ion, or molecule loses one or more electrons (e^-) in a reaction, the process is called *oxidation*, and the molecule is said to be *oxidized*. The electrons lost do not float about at random but, since they are very reactive, attach immediately to another molecule. The resulting gain of one or more electrons by a molecule is called *reduction* and the molecule is said to be *reduced*. Within the cell, an oxidation reaction is always paired (or coupled) with a reduction reaction; thus the term *oxidation-reduction* or *"redox"* reaction.

Many biological oxidations are referred to as *dehydrogenations* because hydrogen ions (H^+) as well as electrons are removed. Concurrently, those H^+ must be picked up in a reduction reaction. Many good illustrations are found in the metabolism of glucose to form pyruvic acid and the concurrent synthesis of ATP and water (see the discussion of the citric acid cycle that follows).

Energy Production (Catabolism)

Cellular Respiration of Glucose

The complete catabolism of glucose takes place in three phases: (1) glycolysis, (2) the citric acid cycle, and (3) the electron-transport system. The first phase is anaerobic, whereas the last two require aerobic conditions (Fig. 4–3).

Glycolysis   Glycolysis is the term for the stepwise breakdown of glucose into pyruvic acid in the absence of oxygen. It is the basic set of reactions in the anaerobic phase of cellular respiration. Somewhere in the metabolism of almost all cells, glycolysis, or the degradation of glucose, takes place to produce small amounts of ATP. Heterotrophs can degrade starch and glycogen to provide glucose for these glycolytic reactions. Other sugars, such as fructose, can also be used in these reactions. Autotrophs synthesize glucose during photosynthesis so that they can derive energy from the glucose to drive other metabolic reactions. The amount of

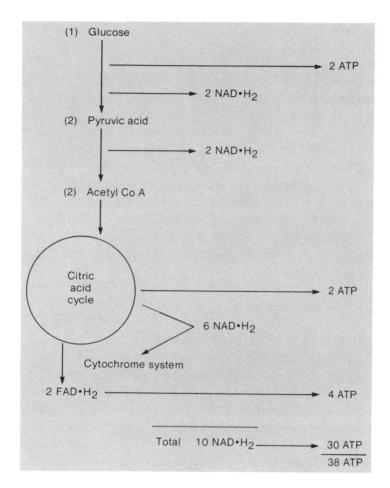

Figure 4–3. Summary tabulation of high-energy molecules produced by aerobic cellular respiration of one molecule of glucose.

energy (ATP) derived from a glucose molecule depends on how much oxygen is available to bond with the hydrogen atoms released during the aerobic phase of cellular respiration. It should be noted that the aerobes and facultative anaerobes are much more efficient in energy production than the obligate anaerobes because they have oxygen available to aid in the production of much more ATP.

Citric Acid Cycle and Electron Transport System   In the aerobic phases of cellular respiration, oxygen is used as the final hydrogen acceptor following a long series of molecular reactions controlled by specific enzymes. Aerobic microorganisms and facultative anaerobes use pyruvic acid to produce about nine times more energy than obligate anaerobes can produce by the fermentation of glucose and the other sugars. Even in the presence of oxygen, obligate anaerobes do not have the appropriate enzymes and coenzymes to catalyze this metabolic pathway.

The citric acid cycle is also known as the tricarboxylic acid cycle (TCA) and is often called the Krebs cycle after the scientist who defined this phase of aerobic cellular respiration. As indicated in Figure 4–3, the citric acid cycle involves a series of reactions, which are controlled by specific enzymes, that yield the end products carbon dioxide and hydrogen atoms. These activated hydrogen atoms are temporarily bound to NAD and FAD and are transferred to the electron transport system, where the cytochromes aid in the oxidative phosphorylation of ADP to ATP, and the hydrogen bonds with the oxygen to form water (cellular water).

The complete process of cellular respiration of one molecule of glucose yields 38 ATP molecules. Two ATP molecules are gained from the glycolysis phase and two from the citric acid cycle; the other 34 result form oxidative phosphorylation in the electron transport system. The chemical equation representing this highly efficient catabolic reaction is

$$C_6H_{12}O_6 + 6\ O_2 + 38\ ADP + 38\ ⓟ \rightarrow 6\ H_2O + CO_2 + 38\ ATP$$

where ⓟ indicates activated phosphate groups.

Although the metabolic pathway and amount of energy that can be produced from cellular respiration of glucose has been shown as an illustration, one must be aware that there are many variations to this pathway depending on the individual organism and its available nutrient and energy resources. Some bacteria degrade glucose to pyruvic acid by other metabolic pathways. Also, glycerol, fatty acids from lipids, and amino acids from protein digestion may be fed into the citric acid cycle to produce energy for the cell when necessary, that is, when there are insufficient carbohydrates available (Fig. 4–4).

Anaerobic Fermentation

When the hydrogen atoms released from the breakdown of sugars are bound to organic molecules instead of oxygen, the glycolytic process is referred to as *fermentation*. Pyruvic acid usually accepts the hydrogen atoms to produce lactic acid or ethanol (ethyl alcohol), but other end products may be formed. The products produced depend on the species of the organism and on the sugar used as the source of carbohydrate. In human muscle cells, the lack of oxygen during extreme exertion results in pyruvic acid's being converted to lactic acid. This compound, existing in the muscle tissue, is the cause of the soreness that develops in exhausted muscles. There are some bacteria (*Lactobacillus* and *Streptococcus*) that also produce lactic acid during the fermentation process. These organisms are found in the mouth where the presence of lactic acid can promote tooth decay,

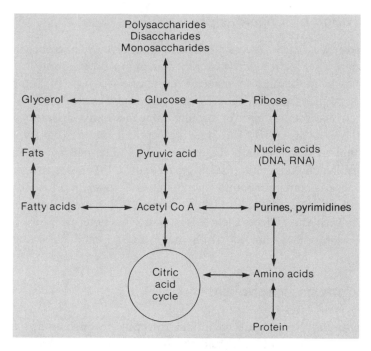

Figure 4–4. Other nutrients entering and exiting from the metabolism of glucose.

and their presence in milk causes the normal souring of milk into curd and whey. The yeasts, *Saccharomyces*, can ferment grain and fruit sugars into ethanol, the alcohol found in beer, wines, and liquors. Acetic acid bacteria (*Acetobacter*) are able to oxidize ethanol to acetic acid and spoil the beer and wine by changing them to vinegar. These and other various end products of fermentation have many industrial applications.

Aerobic Oxidation by Chemolithotrophs

Certain autotrophs, the chemolithotrophs, are able to perform respiration reactions by oxidizing hydrogen (H_2) to water (H_2O), carbon (C) and carbon monoxide (CO) to carbon dioxide (CO_2), ammonia (NH_3) and nitrite ions (NO_2^-) to nitrate ions (NO_3^-), hydrogen sulfide (H_2S) and free sulfur (S) to sulfates (SO_4^{2-}), and iron to iron oxides. As one can imagine, these microorganisms (usually soil and water bacteria) are very important in recycling the elements and some compounds into forms more usable by plants and other microorganisms. They also must be acknowledged as major factors in the destruction of iron parts of machinery, since they also promote rust.

Anaerobic Respiration by Chemotrophs

Oxidation-reduction reactions occur, biologically, in certain anaerobes in the absence of oxygen. The electron donor usually is an organic compound such as glucose, but it may be inorganic iron or sulfur compounds (as used by *Thiobacillus*). Inorganic compounds (nitrates, sulfates, and carbonates) serve as the final electron (hydrogen) acceptors in place of oxygen. Some facultative anaerobes convert nitrates (NO_3^-) to nitrites (NO_2^-) and free atmospheric nitrogen gas (N_2). Others reduce carbonates (CO_3^{2-}) to carbon dioxide (CO_2) and to methane (CH_4). Some obligate anaerobes convert sulfate (SO_4^{2-}) to free sulfur (S) or to hydrogen sulfide gas (H_2S). These bacteria are found in the soil, sea water, marine mud, fresh water, acid mine waters, sewage, and sulfur springs. Obviously, they are unable to produce as much as ATP from their energy sources as heterotrophic organisms because their nutrients do not contain as much bound chemical energy.

Metabolic Biosynthesis (Anabolism)

Energy Conversion   In general, chemoheterotrophs produce energy from organic compounds by fermentation, anaerobic respiration, and aerobic respiration, as previously discussed. However, all of the phototrophs (algae, cyanobacteria, photosynthetic bacteria, and plants) must derive their energy from light, usually the sun, by *photosynthesis*. This process provides energy to the greatest mass of organisms, not only all of the photosynthetic organisms but heterotrophs as well, because the heterotrophs consume phototrophs.

Energy Use   The biosynthesis of organic compounds requiring the use of energy is called *anabolism*, or an anabolic reaction. In living cells this biosynthetic metabolism may be one of two types: *photosynthesis* by photolithotrophs or photoorganotrophs, or *chemosynthesis* by chemolithotrophs or chemoorganotrophs.

In photosynthesis, light energy is converted to chemical bond energy to be used to synthesize organic biochemicals. Those phototrophic organisms using inorganic raw materials (CO_2, H_2O, H_2S, S) for biosynthesis are the photolithotrophs (photoautotrophs). Those phototrophs using small organic molecules, such as acids and alcohols, to build carbohydrates, fats, proteins, nucleic acids, and other important biochemicals are the photoorganotrophs (photoheterotrophs).

Photosynthesis   The goal of photosynthetic processes is to trap and convert the radiant energy of light into chemical bond energy in ATP and carbohydrates, particularly glucose, which can then be converted into more molecules of ATP via the respiratory pathways. The general overall photosynthesis reaction is

$$6\ CO_2 + 12\ H_2O \xrightarrow[\text{ATP}]{\text{light}} (CH_2O)_6 + 6\ O_2 + 6\ H_2O + ADP + \circledP$$

Notice that this reaction is almost the reverse of the oxidative respiration reaction, and it is nature's way of balancing substrates in the environment.

The photosynthetic process may be considered as two major reactions, the light phase and the dark phase. During the *light phase*, chlorophyll or other photosynthetic pigments absorb light and are activated by the radiant energy to release electrons into a series of reactions resulting in the formation of ATP. Simultaneously, hydrogen from H_2O is bound to the coenzyme NADP as NADP · H_2, releasing oxygen. In the *dark phase* of photosynthesis, ATP, NADP · H_2, and CO_2 are combined to synthesize carbohydrates, usually in the form of glucose and starch. These compounds can then be used in the glycolytic production of ATP or for maintenance and growth of the organism.

Photosynthesis does not necessarily require the presence of oxygen; in other words, it can take place anaerobically, as occurs in the purple and green bacteria (obligate anaerobic photoautotrophs). These bacteria do not use H_2O but instead use H_2 or H_2S gas or other hydrogen donor molecules produced by other bacteria in soil or mud. The overall reaction of anaerobic bacterial photosynthesis then becomes

$$6 \ CO_2 + 12 \ H_2S \xrightarrow{\text{light}} (CH_2O)_6 + 6 \ H_2O + 12 \ S$$

or

$$6 \ CO_2 + 12 \ H_2 \xrightarrow{\text{light}} (CH_2O)_6 + 6 \ H_2O$$

The bacterial photosynthetic pigments use shorter wavelengths of light, which penetrate deep within a pond or into mud where it appears to be dark.

In the absence of light, some photolithotrophic organisms may survive anaerobically by the fermentation process alone. Other phototrophic bacteria also have a limited ability to use simple organic molecules in photosynthetic reactions; thus, they become photoorganotrophic organisms under certain conditions. A few species of cyanobacteria have also been found to exist as facultative phototrophs and facultative autotrophs, meaning that in certain environments they become photoheterotrophs. In other words, they have backup metabolic systems.

Chemosynthesis   The chemosynthetic process involves a chemical source of energy and raw materials to synthesize the necessary metabolites and macromolecules for growth and functioning of the organisms. These chemotrophic organisms may be either autotrophs or heterotrophs.

The chemoautotrophs are the same chemolithotrophic bacteria, previously discussed, that obtain energy by aerobic oxidation of inorganic compounds or by anaerobic respiration of inorganic substances. These are the only organisms that do not depend on the radiant energy from the sun. They are considered among the most primitive bacteria and are frequently found near volcanoes deep within the ocean.

The chemoorganotrophs have been defined as those organisms that derive both their energy and nutrients from organic materials. Most bacteria, as well as protozoa, fungi, and all animals belong to this group. Although they vary greatly in the details of their metabolism, they all use carbohydrates, lipids, and proteins to synthesize their own carbohydrates, lipids, proteins, nucleic acids, and high-energy molecules such as ATP. These metabolic pathways may be carried on with or without oxygen by aerobic or anaerobic respiration, fermentation, and other biodegradation and biosynthetic reactions.

Microbial Growth

Bacterial growth is represented by an increase in the number of organisms rather than in their size. When each bacterial cell reaches its optimum size, it divides by binary fission (*bi* equals two) into two daughter cells. Binary fission means that each bacterium simply splits into two similar cells. These in turn divide, and as a result, a viable, healthy colony of cells is maintained as long as the nutrient supply, water, and space allow. This process continues until the waste products from cells build up to a toxic level or until the nutrients are depleted. The actual division of staphylococci by binary fission is shown in the electron micrograph in Figure 4–5.

The growth of microorganisms in nature (*in vivo*) as well as in the laboratory (*in vitro*) is greatly influenced by temperature, *p*H (acidity), moisture content, available nutrients, and the character of other organisms present. Therefore, the number of bacteria in nature fluctuates unpredictably because these factors vary with the seasons, rainfall, temperature, and time of day.

In the laboratory, however, a pure culture of a single species of bacteria can usually be grown if the appropriate growth medium and environmental conditions are provided. The temperature, *p*H, and amount of oxygen are quite easily controlled to provide optimum conditions for growth. Then the appropriate nutrients must be provided in the growth medium. Some bacteria are so fastidious (having complex nutritional requirements) that they will not grow outside of living cells; thus, they must be cultured in living animals, egg embryos or tissue cultures.

Culture Media

Basically, there are two types of media for culturing bacteria: (1) a chemically defined synthetic medium and (2) a rich, natural, complex medium containing digested extracts from meats, fish, and plants providing the necessary nutrients, vitamins, and minerals. These media can be used in liquid or broth form, which is available in tubes, or they may be solidified by the addition of agar and poured into tubes or petri dishes so that the bacteria can be grown within or on the surface of the agar.

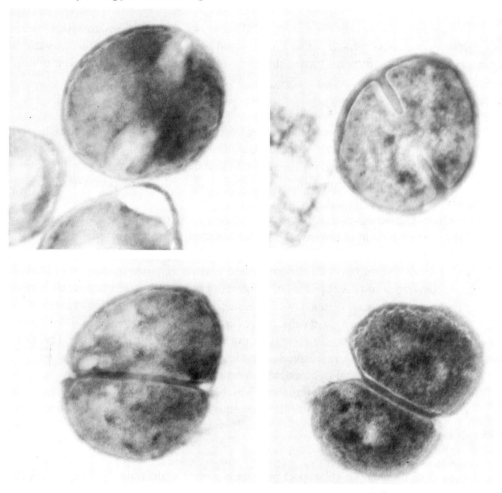

Figure 4–5. Binary fission of staphylococci (original magnification ×30,000). (Photograph courtesy Ray Rupel)

An *enriched medium* is a broth or solid medium containing a rich supply of special nutrients that promotes the growth of a particular fastidious organism while not promoting growth of other microorganisms that might be present. Thus, the desired species grows best and predominates in the culture, and a pure culture could easily be obtained from a mixed specimen. A good example of this is Thayer-Martin agar for the growth of *Neisseria* species.

A *differential medium* is used to grow several species of bacteria, but each bacteria grown has a distinctive appearance. Eosin methylene blue (EMB) agar is frequently used to separate and identify gram-negative organisms in fecal specimens.

A *selective medium* has added inhibitors that discourage the growth of certain organisms without inhibiting the growth of the one sought. For example, mannitol salt agar encourages the growth of staphylococci but inhibits growth of other gram-positive bacteria. It is also a differential agar because the colonies of various species of *Staphylococcus* have a different appearance on mannitol salt medium.

Population Counts

Once the desired species of bacteria has been separated from other organisms in a specimen, it can be grown as a pure culture under the best possible conditions. The changes in an isolated bacterial population over an extended period follows a definite predictable pattern that can be shown by plotting the population growth curve on a graph (Fig. 4–6).

Often microbiologists need to know the rate of bacterial growth and how many bacteria are present at any one time. This information is particularly important in determining the degree of bacterial contamination in drinking water, milk, and other food. The number can be determined by counting the total number of bacterial cells, living and dead, in 1 ml of solution, or by counting only the viable (or living) bacteria present. A total count is easier and faster but it differs because it includes both living and dead cells; however, if the 1-ml sample is taken when the microorganisms are growing and dividing rapidly in the growth phase, few dead cells are found. In many hospitals, electronic cell counters are incorporated into the autoanalyzers used in blood, urine, and spinal fluid analysis. Many research laboratories use spectrophotometers, which determine the number of organisms present by measuring the turbidity (cloudiness) of the solution due to the number

Figure 4–6. Population growth curve of living organisms. The logarithm of the number of bacteria per milliliter of medium is plotted against time. (*A*) Lag phase. (*B*) Logarithmic growth phase. (*C*) Stationary phase. (*D*) Death phase.

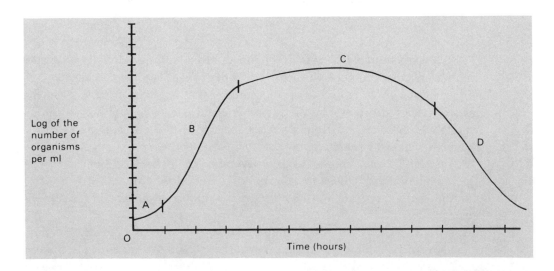

of organisms. Chemical analyses of nitrogen or carbon content also can be used to determine the number of bacteria present by chemically destroying them.

The *viable plate count* is usually the most accurate method for determining the number of living bacteria in a milliliter of liquid, which may be milk, water, diluted food, or broth. In this procedure, as shown in Figure 4–7, 1 ml of solution is

Figure 4–7. The viable plate count technique. One milliliter of the original culture is successively diluted and cultured on agar plates.

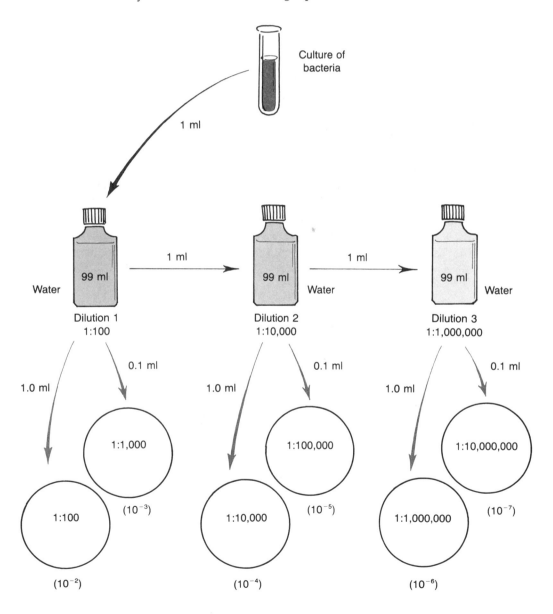

diluted to 100 ml three times in sequence, and samples are taken from each dilution. Then 0.1-ml and/or 1-ml samples are grown on nutrient agar. The number of colonies observed growing on the nutrient agar plates the following day indicates the number of viable bacteria present at that particular dilution. This number multiplied by the dilution factor indicates the number of living bacteria in the original culture at the time the sample was taken. For example, if 220 colonies were counted on an agar plate grown from a 1-ml sample from the second dilution bottle (1 : 10,000 dilution), there were $220 \times 10,000 = 2,200,000$ bacteria in 1 ml of the original material at the time the dilutions were made and cultured. Practically, it is easier to culture only 0.1 ml of each dilution, while increasing the dilution factor by 10, as shown in Figure 4–7. For the count to be statistically significant and most accurately representative of the number of living microorganisms in the solution, the number used in the calculations should be taken from the agar plate that has between 30 and 300 colonies.

A similar technique has been developed to count viruses. The diluted viruses are grown on a "lawn" of bacteria or a layer of tissue culture cells. Each cell lysed by a virus causes a clear zone (plaque) in the culture of cells following incubation. Thus, the number of plaques represents the number of viruses in 1 ml of the diluted solution. This number must then be multiplied by the dilution factor.

A method of approximating the number and type of bacteria in urine involves streaking a known volume of urine from a calibrated inoculation loop onto various appropriate differential media. The color and number of colonies enables a microbiologist to determine the presence of large numbers of certain bacteria that often cause urinary infections, including species of *Staphylococcus*, *Streptococcus*, and particularly *Escherichia coli* (*E. coli*) as well as other coliforms.

Population Growth Curve

The population growth curve for any particular species of bacteria may be determined by growing the organism in pure culture (a culture of only one organism) at a constant temperature. The graph in Figure 4–6 is constructed by plotting the logarithm of the number of bacteria against the incubation time.

The first stage of the growth curve is the *lag phase* (see *A* in Fig. 4–6), during which the bacteria absorb nutrients, synthesize enzymes, and prepare for reproduction. In the *logarithmic growth phase* (exponential growth phase; *B* in Fig. 4–6), the bacteria multiply so rapidly that the population number doubles during each generation time. The generation time, which is the time between the formation of a new bacterium and its division into two daughter cells, varies with the species of bacteria. The growth rate is the greatest during the logarithmic growth phase. *E. coli* from the intestine, *Vibrio cholerae* (which causes cholera), *Staphylococcus*, and *Streptococcus* all have a generation time of about 20 minutes, whereas *Pseudomonas*, from the soil, may divide every 10 minutes, and *Mycobacterium tuberculosis* may divide only once in 18 hours. The logarithmic growth phase is always brief unless the rapidly dividing culture is maintained by constant addition of nutrients and oxygen and frequent removal of the waste products and excess microorganisms. Many industrial and research procedures depend on the maintenance of an essential species of microorganism. These are continuously cultured in a controlled environment called a *chemostat* (Fig. 4–8), which regulates the supply of nutrients and the removal of waste products and excess microorganisms. Chemostats are used in industries where yeast is grown to produce beer and wine, where fungi and bacteria are cultivated to produce antibiotics, where *E. coli* are grown for genetic research, and in any other process needing a constant source of microorganisms.

As the nutrients and oxygen in the culture tube are used up and waste products from the metabolizing bacteria build up and change the *p*H of the culture medium, the rate of division slows, such that the number of bacteria dividing equals the number dying. The result is the *stationary phase* (*C* in Fig. 4–6). It is during this phase that the culture reaches its greatest population density.

As overcrowding occurs, the toxic waste products increase and the nutrient supply decreases. The microorganisms then die at a rapid rate; this is the *death* or *decline phase* (*D* in Fig. 4–6). The culture may die completely or a few microorganisms may continue to survive for months. If the bacterial species is a sporeformer, it will form spores to survive beyond this phase. When the cells are observed in old cultures of bacteria in the death phase, some of them look different

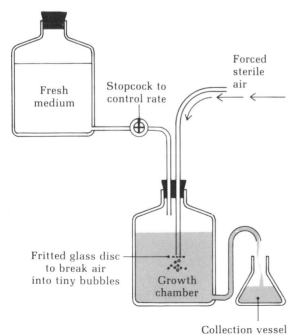

Figure 4–8. Chemostat used for continuous cultures. Rate of growth can be controlled either by controlling the rate at which new medium enters the growth chamber or by limiting a required growth factor in the medium. (Volk WA, et al.: Essentials of Medical Microbiology, 4th ed. Philadelphia, JB Lippincott, 1991)

Fresh medium

Stopcock to control rate

Forced sterile air

Fritted glass disc to break air into tiny bubbles

Growth chamber

Collection vessel

from the healthy organisms seen in the growth phase. As a result of the unfavorable conditions, morphological changes in the cells may appear. Some cells undergo involution and assume a variety of shapes, becoming long, multinucleated, filamentous rods, or branching or globular forms that are difficult to identify. Some develop without a cell wall (protoplasts) and others take an L shape because they have very little cell wall (L-forms). When these involuted forms are inoculated into a fresh nutrient medium, they usually revert to the original shape of the healthy bacteria.

A population growth curve may be plotted for all organisms, including humans. At present, the human population is in the logarithmic growth phase with a generation time of 35 years. No population of organisms is known to continue in this phase forever without careful control of the food supply, numbers of individuals, and proper disposal of waste products. Eventually, the forces of nature (food shortages, epidemics, wars, toxic waste products) will probably cause the world population to stabilize in the stationary growth phase and, hopefully, this stationary phase will not proceed beyond to the terminal death phase.

Bacterial Genetics

The nucleoid region of bacteria usually consists of only one DNA type of chromosome with no protein on the outside as is found in eucaryotic chromosomes. This chromosome is a circular strand of genes linked together. Genes are the fundamental units of heredity that carry the information needed for the special characteristics of each different species of bacteria. Thus, the genes direct all functions of the cell, providing it with its own particular traits and individuality. Because there is only one chromosome that replicates just before cell division, identical traits of a species are passed from the parent bacterium to the daughter cells after binary fission has occurred.

The DNA of any gene on the chromosome is subject to accidental alteration, which changes the trait controlled by that gene. If the change in the gene alters or deletes (eliminates) a trait in such a way that the cell does not die or become incapable of division, the altered trait is transmitted to the daughter cells of each succeeding generation. A change in the characteristics of a cell caused by a change in the DNA molecule (genetic alteration) that is transmissible to the offspring is called a *mutation*. A lethal mutation is one that causes the cell to die because an essential functional gene is missing. It may perhaps be one that codes for an essential enzyme. Spontaneous mutations usually occur about once in every 10 million cell divisions. The mutation rate can be increased by exposing the cells to physical or chemical agents that affect the DNA molecule. These agents are called *mutagens*. In the research laboratory, x-rays, ultraviolet light, and radioactive substances, as well as certain chemical agents, are used to induce more frequent mutations (Fig. 4–9). These mutants are used in genetic and medical research and in the development of vaccines. The types of mutagenic changes frequently ob-

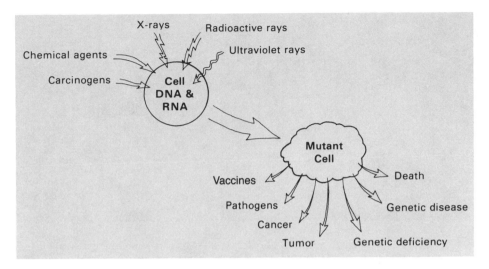

Figure 4–9. Agents that may cause mutagenic changes.

served in bacteria involve color, colony appearance, cell shape, biochemical activities, nutritional needs, antigenic sites, virulence, pathogenicity, and drug resistance. The nonpathogenic living virus vaccines, such as the Sabin vaccine for polio, are examples of laboratory-induced mutations of pathogenic microorganisms.

Changes in Bacterial Genetic Constitution

There are at least four ways, other than mutation, that the genetic composition of bacteria can be changed: lysogenic conversion, transduction, transformation, and conjugation. These types of gene transfers result in extra genetic material in the recipient cell. If this extra bit of DNA remains in the cytoplasm of the cell, it is called a *plasmid* (Fig. 4–10). Some plasmids contain many extra chromosomal genes, others only a few, but the cell is changed by the addition of these genetic components. Plasmids can replicate themselves simultaneously with chromosomal DNA replication or at various other times. When a plasmid becomes incorporated into the chromosome, it is referred to as an episome. Some plasmid genes can be expressed as extrachromosomal genes, but others must become chromosomal episomes before the genes become functional.

Lysogenic Conversion

The genetic change or lysogenic conversion occurs when a temperate bacteriophage (bacterial virus) infects a bacterium changing it to a *lysogenic* bacterium (i.e., a bacterium that has the potential to be lysed by the viral genes) (Fig. 4–11)

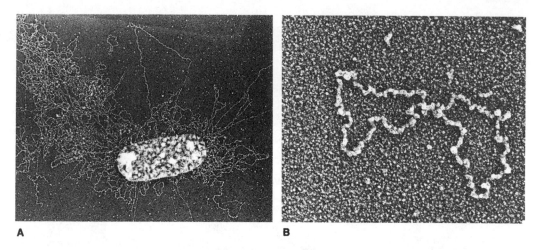

A   **B**

Figure 4–10. (*A*) Disrupted cell of *Escherichia coli*; the DNA has spilled out and a plasmid can be found slightly to the left of top center. (*B*) Enlargement of a plasmid (about 1 μm from side to side). (Volk WA, et al.: Essentials of Medical Microbiology, 4th ed. Philadelphia, JB Lippincott, 1991)

by injecting its DNA into the cytoplasm of the bacterium. This plasmid, consisting of viral genes, can be called a *prophage* because it contains the genes to make new bacteriophages under certain circumstances (see the discussion of bacteria and bacteriophages in Chapter 2). The number of genes in the bacterium is thus increased by the number of genes injected by the phage. For example, the diphtheria bacterium (*Corynebacterium diphtheriae*) is pathogenic only when it has been infected by a bacteriophage that enables it to produce the toxin that causes diphtheria.

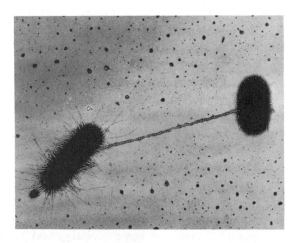

Figure 4–11. Initiation of conjugating in *Escherichia coli*. The donor cell (with numerous short pili) is connected to the recipient bacterium by an F pilus, as described in the text (original magnification ×3,000). (Anderson TF: Cold Spring Harbor Symp Quant Biol 18:197)

Transduction

Transduction means "to carry across." Some cellular genetic material may be carried across from one bacterial cell to another by a bacterial virus. This phenomenon may occur when a temperate bacteriophage infects a bacterial cell by injecting its DNA into the bacterium (in other words via lysogenic conversion). The viral DNA (prophage) then combines with the bacterial chromosome. If a stimulating chemical, heat, or ultraviolet light activates the prophage, it begins to produce new viruses by the production of phage DNA and proteins. Because the viral DNA has actually been a part of the bacterial chromosome, as the entire chromosome disintegrates, small pieces of bacterial DNA may remain attached to the maturing phage DNA. During the assembly of the virus particles, one or more bacterial genes may be incorporated into some of the mature bacteriophages. When all the phages are freed by cell lysis, they proceed to infect other cells, injecting bacterial genetic material as well as viral genes. Thus, cellular genes that are attached to the phage DNA are carried to new cells by the virus.

There are two types of transduction: *specialized* and *generalized*. The explanation in the previous paragraph describes *specialized transduction* in which the infecting phage integrates into the bacterial chromosome or a plasmid. As the virus genome breaks away to replicate and produce more viruses, it carries a few identifiable bacterial genes with it to the newly infected cell. In this way genetic capabilities involving the fermentation of certain sugars, antibiotic resistance, and other phenotypic characteristics can be transduced to other bacteria. This process has been shown in the laboratory to occur among species of *Bacillus*, *Pseudomonas*, *Haemophilus*, *Salmonella*, and *Escherichia*, and it is assumed to occur in nature.

In *generalized transduction*, the bacteriophage is a virulent lytic phage that does not incorporate into the bacterial genome or plasmid. Rather, it picks up fragments of bacterial DNA during the assembly of new virus particles and carries these genes to other cells that the new viruses infect. This generalized transduction has been observed in species of *Streptococcus*, *Staphylococcus*, and *Salmonella*, and in *Vibrio cholerae*.

Only small segments of DNA are transferred from cell to cell by transduction compared with the amount that can be transferred by transformation and conjugation.

Transformation

In the transformation process, a recipient bacterial cell is genetically transformed by the addition of DNA fragments from another strain of bacteria with at least one different observable characteristic. The first experiments in transformation

Insight: *Salmonella* Infections

Salmonellosis caused by various *Salmonella* species is the most frequently reported foodborne gastroenteritis in the United States. Foods containing poultry or other meats, eggs, or dairy products are the usual vehicles for transmitting the *Salmonella* from the meat, eggs, and feces of infected animals (usually poultry) and contaminated soil to humans. Poor personal hygiene of foodhandlers and improper food preparation may inoculate these organisms into other foods. If these contaminated foods are then improperly stored and served at room temperature, large numbers of people may be exposed to the organisms, especially at salad and food bars in restaurants and grocery stores.

In 1991, the news media indicated that some cantalopes were infected with *Salmonella* organisms, causing the American public to become alarmed; when they ceased to buy cantalopes, the melon farmers suffered great losses. In actuality, the melons from Texas and Mexico probably had *Salmonella* in the contaminated dirt on the surface of the melons.

The pathogens may be introduced from the unwashed skins onto the prepared food by food preparers. Cutting an unwashed melon through a contaminated rind may lead to the contamination of the edible parts via the cutting knife, dirty rinds, or hands. Excessive storage and serving time at room temperature may then permit bacterial growth before the food is eaten. Food freshly prepared and eaten immediately will not cause gastroenteritis, because the *Salmonella* do not have time to proliferate. Large numbers of *Salmonella* are necessary to cause the infection. The actual disease symptoms are induced by the endotoxins present in the cell wall of the pathogens.

To reduce the risk of salmonellosis from dirty melons, the FDA recommends that both produce retailers and consumers thoroughly clean melons with potable water before cutting them. (Some large producers also dip washed melons in a chlorine solution.) Prepare cut melons using clean hands and sanitized utensils and surfaces; store cut melons at a temperature below 45°F (7°C) until served or sold; and limit the display of cut melons to less than 4 hours if they are not refrigerated.

To decrease the risk for *Salmonella* food poisoning, it is important to (1) wash all fruits and vegetables before they are handled and consumed; (2) properly cook all poultry, eggs, and meats; and (3) use pasteurized milk and eggs in uncooked foods.

(From MMWR, Aug. 12, 1991, Vol. 40, #32.)

proved that DNA is, indeed, the genetic material. When a DNA extract from encapsulated pathogenic *Streptococcus pneumoniae* type 1 was added to a growing culture of nonencapsulated, nonpathogenic *S. pneumoniae* type 2, the resulting culture showed the presence of living encapsulated *S. pneumoniae* type 2 because some of the type 1 DNA was incorporated into the dividing type 2 DNA. Thus, the nonencapsulated streptococci must have been transformed by the genes coding for capsule that were incorporated into the cells. Although this type of genetic recombination is not widespread, it has been demonstrated in several genera including *Bacillus, Escherichia, Haemophilus, Pseudomonas,* and *Neisseria.* Transformations have even been shown to occur between two different species (*Staphylococcus,* and *Streptococcus*).

Large DNA molecules from a donor cell can only penetrate the cell wall and cell membrane of a *competent* recipient cell, that is, one capable of receiving the DNA molecule. Recipient bacteria usually become competent during the late logarithmic growth phase when the cell secretes a protein competence factor that increases its permeability to DNA.

Some competent bacterial cells have incorporated DNA fragments from certain animal viruses (*e.g.,* cowpox), retaining the latent virus genes for long periods. This knowledge may have some importance in the study of viruses that remain latent in humans for many years before they finally cause disease, as may be the case in Parkinson's disease. These human virus genes may hide in the normal flora bacteria until they are released to cause disease.

Conjugation

Conjugation occurs when two bacteria attach to each other, usually by a pilus bridge, and some genetic material is transferred from the donor cell to the recipient. Many biologists compare this transfer of genetic material to the sexual process in animals, labeling the donor "male" and the recipient "female." This type of genetic recombination occurs mostly among the species and among some genera of the enteric bacteria, but it has been reported within species of *Pseudomonas* and *Streptococcus* as well. In electron micrographs, microbiologists have noted sex pili that are larger than other pili. The donor sex pilus attaches to the recipient cell, which is usually nonpiliated, to form the pilus bridge. Genetic material from a plasmid or from the chromosomes is then transferred across the pilus bridge from donor to recipient cell (Fig. 4–12, Conjugation). Although many genes may be transferred by conjugation, the ones most frequently noted include those coding for antibiotic resistance, colicin (a protein that kills certain enteric bacteria), and the fertility factor (F^+, HFr^+). Bacteria with the F^+ or HFr^+ genes have the ability to produce pili, including sex pili; therefore, those bacteria may become donor cells. If the fertility factor is on a plasmid, it is an F^+ gene; whereas, if it is incorporated within the chromosome, it is referred to as the HFr^+ gene. A complete copy of the plasmid (with F^+) usually moves to the recipient (F^-) cell; thus, it usually becomes F^+. However, the recipient (F^-) cell usually receives only a portion of the chromosome from an HFr^+ cell, not including the HFr^+ gene; thus, the recipient remains HFr^- in that circumstance, does not produce pili, and cannot become a donor cell.

Transduction, transformation, and conjugation are excellent tools for mapping bacterial chromosomes and for studying bacterial and viral genetics. Although each of them is frequently used in the laboratory, it is believed that they occur in natural environments under certain circumstances.

Genetic Engineering

An array of techniques has been developed to transfer eucaryotic genes, particularly human genes, into other easily cultured cells to facilitate the large-scale production of important proteins. Bacteria, yeasts, human leukocytes, macrophages, and fibroblasts have been used as manufacturing plants for proteins, such as the human growth hormone, insulin, and interferon. In the near future, perhaps the genes themselves will be implanted into people with genetic deficiencies. This work is not conducted without some risk to mankind. The greatest fear is that genes introduced into bacteria may produce yet unknown toxins or diseases that cause harm to or even destroy the human race. With this in mind, extreme care and caution is exercised during genetic manipulation experiments.

Many industrial and medical benefits may be derived from genetic engineering (or genetic recombination) research. There is a potential for incorporating nitrogen-fixing capabilities into more of the soil microorganisms, for making animal proteins for food and medicines, for increasing the production of antibiotics, for synthesizing important enzymes and hormones for treatment of inherited diseases, and for making portions of viruses and bacterial pathogens to be used as vaccines. Such vaccines would contain only part of the pathogen (for instance, the capsid of the smallpox virus) to which the person would form protective antibodies in the absence of complete virulent pathogens.

Summary

This discussion of the physiology of microorganisms includes a discussion of the microbes' nutrient and energy sources that enable them to maintain the metabolic cycles of living organisms. These metabolic reactions are those involved in respiration, photosynthesis, catabolism, and anabolism.

When the organism has all the nutrients and energy it needs to maintain itself, it can then reproduce sexually or asexually. The growth curve represents the growth and downfall of any population of organisms.

As you learn about bacterial genetics and the ways that bacteria can be changed by the addition of genetic material, try to envision how many ways human body cells could be changed by similar procedures. These techniques open up a new field called genetic engineering.

Study Outline

I. Nutrition
   A. Nutritional requirements
      1. Six major elements
      2. Other elements necessary
   B. Nutritional types
      1. Heterotrophic organisms
         a. Chemoorganotrophs
         b. Photoorganotrophs
      2. Autotrophic organisms
         a. Chemolithotrophs
         b. Photolithotrophs

II. Metabolic Enzymes
   A. Factors affecting enzyme activity
      1. Substrate, enzyme, specificity
      2. Optimum conditions
      3. Cofactors, coenzymes
   B. Naming of enzymes
      1. Endoenzymes, exoenzymes
      2. Substrate types
      3. Reaction types
   C. Inhibition of enzymes
      1. Change optimum conditions
      2. Mineral ions
      3. Similar substrates

III. Cellular metabolism
   A. Catabolism and anabolism
   B. Energy production (catabolism)
      1. Cellular respiration of glucose
      2. Fermentation
      3. Aerobic oxidation by chemolithotrophs
      4. Anaerobic respiration by chemotrophs
   C. Metabolic biosynthesis (anabolism)
      1. Energy conversion
         a. Photosynthesis
         b. Chemosynthesis

IV. Microbial growth
   A. Factors that influence growth
   B. Culture media
   C. Techniques for determining the number of bacteria per milliliter
   D. Population growth curve

V. Bacterial genetics
   A. Chromosomes, genes, and DNA
   B. Changes in bacterial genetic constitution
      1. Mutations
      2. Lysogenic conversion
      3. Transduction
      4. Transformation
      5. Conjugation
   C. Genetic engineering

Problems and Questions

1. What factors influence the growth of microorganisms in nature?
2. What factors are kept constant to produce a population growth curve in the laboratory?
3. What factors contribute to the death of a pure culture of bacteria in a tube of nutrient broth?
4. What are the major elements found in living cells? What other elements are also necessary for the metabolic functions of the cell?
5. Compare (a) heterotrophs and autotrophs; (b) chemotrophs and phototrophs; (c) chemoorganotrophs and chemolithotrophs; (d) photoorganotrophs and photolithotrophs.
6. Why are saprophytic decomposers necessary for ecological balance?
7. Describe catabolism, anabolism, respiration, fermentation, and photosynthesis.
8. Describe five ways by which the genetic constitution of bacteria may be altered.
9. What is a plasmid? an episome?
10. Describe the process of genetic engineering and give an example.

Self Test

After you have read Chapter 4, examined the objectives, studied the new words and answered the questions at the end of the chapter, complete the following self test.

Matching Exercises

Complete each statement from the list of words provided with each section.

Nutritional Types

heterotrophs	phototrophs	chemolithotrophs
autotrophs	chemoorganotrophs	photolithotrophs
chemotrophs	photoorganotrophs	

1. Organisms that use light as a source of energy are _____.
2. Organisms that get their energy from a chemical source are _____.

3. Organisms that use an organic carbon source of nutrients are
   _____.

4. Organisms that use an inorganic source of carbon for nutrients are
   _____.

5. Organisms that use a chemical source of energy and an organic source
   of nutrients are _____.

6. Organisms that use a chemical source of energy and an inorganic
   source of nutrients are _____.

7. Those organisms that use light as a source of energy and use an
   organic source of nutrients are _____.

8. Organisms that use light as a source of energy and use an inorganic
   source of nutrients are _____.

9. Algae are which nutritional type? _____

10. Plants are which nutritional type? _____

11. Animals are which nutritional type? _____

12. Fungi and protozoa are which nutritional type? _____

Metabolic Reactions

catabolism   photosynthesis   fermentation
anabolism   aerobic respiration

1. The metabolic process by which plants and algae use light and carbon
   dioxide, water, and other inorganic compounds to build their
   carbohydrates, fats, and proteins is called _____.

2. The process in which simple molecules are used to build complex ones
   is _____.

3. The process in which complex macromolecules are broken down into
   simple molecules is _____.

4. A chemical reaction in which oxygen participates with carbohydrates to
   yield energy and carbon dioxide is _____.

5. An anaerobic respiration reaction that yields energy is
   _____.

6. The breakdown and recycling of red blood cells in the liver is an
   example of _____.

7. The synthesis of enzymes within a cell is an example of
   _____.

8. The production of alcoholic beverages from grain is an example of
   _____.

Growth Curve

lag phase   logarithmic growth phase
death phase   stationary phase

1. The organisms absorb nutrients, synthesize enzymes, and prepare to reproduce in the _____.
2. More organisms are dying than are reproducing in the _____.
3. The organisms are all alive and reproducing rapidly in the _____.
4. The number of living bacteria remain about the same in the _____.
5. The healthiest stage of growth is the _____.
6. A chemostat keeps the organisms in the _____.
7. An industry that produces products from microorganisms maintains the microbes in the _____.
8. Sporulation of certain genera of bacteria occurs during the _____.

Bacterial Genetics

mutation   conjugation   transduction
mutagens   transformation   lysogenic conversion

1. When living cells absorb and incorporate DNA from the surrounding medium, they are changed; this process is called _____.
2. The spontaneous change in the arrangement of the DNA molecule within a living cell is called _____.
3. The process by which a nonpathogenic bacterium could be produced for use in a vaccine is called _____.
4. When a bacteriophage carries a bit of bacterial DNA from the cell it came from to another cell, the process is called _____.
5. When a temperate bacteriophage injects its own DNA into a bacterial cell, the process is called _____.
6. When two bacteria join by a pilus bridge and genetic material is transferred from one to another, the process is called _____.
7. Ultraviolet light, x-rays, and some chemicals are used to increase the rate of mutation; these agents are called _____.

True or False (T or F)

_____ 1. Inorganic ions are basic nutrients required by living cells.
_____ 2. A mutant is an organism that has survived mutation.
_____ 3. Sodium, hydrogen, oxygen, and phosphorus are the most necessary elements in living protoplasm.
_____ 4. The macromolecules of living cells include the carbohydrates, fats, proteins, and nucleic acids.
_____ 5. The saprophytic fungi can get energy from the sun by photosynthesis.
_____ 6. Autotrophs use carbon dioxide as a nutrient source.
_____ 7. Only a few groups of bacteria are chemoorganotrophs.
_____ 8. The process of photosynthesis releases oxygen into the air for use by animals.
_____ 9. In all living cells enzymes control the metabolism of the cell.
_____ 10. All enzymes are proteins.
_____ 11. All photosynthetic organisms must contain some form of photosynthetic pigment.

Multiple Choice

1. A characteristic that humans, fungi, and saprophytic bacteria have in common is that they
   a. can be facultative anaerobes
   b. obtain carbon atoms from organic materials
   c. use carbon dioxide as a basic carbon source
   d. obtain their energy from light
2. _In vitro_, a culture that contains only one organism is known as
   a. singular
   b. specific
   c. a pure culture
   d. chemostatic
3. Viable plate counts are used to determine
   a. the number of bacterial cells present
   b. the turbidity of the solution
   c. the toxic levels in the original solution
   d. the number of living bacteria present
4. The greatest number of living organisms are present during
   a. the lag phase
   b. the logarithmic growth phase
   c. the death phase
   d. the stationary phase
5. The largest number of adenosine triphosphate (ATP) molecules are produced in what part of cellular respiration?

   a. Citric acid cycle
   b. Glycolysis
   c. Electron transport system
   d. Krebs' cycle

6. In conjugation, the DNA transferred is
   a. viral
   b. defective
   c. bacterial
   d. piliated

7. Saprophytes digest organic materials outside the organism by means of
   a. endoenzymes
   b. cofactors
   c. coenzymes
   d. exoenzymes

8. The process of converting light energy to chemical bond energy is
   a. oxidation
   b. photosynthesis
   c. catabolism
   d. phosphorylation

9. Viral DNA is transferred in
   a. transduction
   b. conjugation
   c. lysogenic conversion
   d. transformation

10. The soreness in muscles after extreme exertion is due to
    a. the conversion of lactic acid to pyruvic acid
    b. excess oxidation
    c. the conversion of pyruvic acid to lactic acid
    d. the accumulation of phosphates

11. Transduction and transformation differ in that transduction
    a. involves DNA
    b. is restricted to pneumococci
    c. requires a phage
    d. is a sexual process

Chapter 5

Control of Microbial Growth

Objectives

After studying this chapter, you should be able to

1. List three reasons why microbial growth must be controlled
2. Define sterilization, disinfection, bactericidal agents, and bacteriostatic agents
3. Differentiate between sterilization, pasteurization, and lyophilization
4. Describe aseptic, antiseptic, and sterile techniques
5. List the factors that influence the growth of microbial life
6. Describe the following types of microorganisms: psychrophilic, mesophilic, thermophilic, halophilic, haloduric, alkaliphilic, acidophilic, and barophilic
7. List several factors that influence the effectiveness of antimicrobial methods
8. List the common *physical* antimicrobial methods
9. List the common *chemical* antimicrobial compounds
10. Describe the mode of action of sulfonamide drugs on bacteria
11. Describe the action of penicillin on bacteria
12. List four reasons why antibiotics should be used with caution

New Words

Antibiotic (an-tie-buy-ot'-tick). Substance produced by microorganisms that inhibits or destroys pathogens during the disease process

Antimicrobial (an-ti-my-kro'-be-al). An agent that kills microorganisms or suppresses their growth

Antiseptic (an-ti-sep'-tick). A chemical disinfectant that is safe to use on living tissues

Asepsis (a-sep'-sis). Absence of infectious microorganisms on living tissue

Bactericide (back-tear'-i-side). An agent that kills bacteria

Chemotherapy (key-mow-ther'-uh-pee). The treatment of diseases and infection using chemicals

Disinfectant (dis-in-feck'-tant). A chemical agent used to destroy pathogens on or within nonliving materials

Fungicide (fun'-juh-side). A substance that kills fungi

Germicide (germ'-uh-side). A substance that kills microorganisms

Haloduric (hey-low-dur'-ick). Surviving in a salty environment

Hypertonic (hi-per-tahn'-ick). Having a greater osmotic pressure outside the cell membrane than inside the cell

Hypotonic (hi-po-tahn'-ick). Having less osmotic pressure outside the cell membrane than inside the cell

Isotonic (i-so-tahn'-ick). Having the same osmotic pressure inside and outside a cell membrane

Lyophilization (lie-off-fil-eh-za'-shun). Preservation by freeze-drying

Mesophilic (mess-oh-fill'-ick). Thriving at 30° to 45°C (86° to 113°F)

Microbial (my-crow'-bee-al). Pertaining to microbes

Microbistasis (my-crow-bi-stay'-sis). The inhibition of growth and reproduction of microorganisms

Microbicide (my-crow'-bi-side). An agent that kills microbes

Osmotic pressure (oz-mah'-tick). The pressure exerted on the cell membrane by the solution inside and surrounding the cell

Pasteurization (pass-tur-uh-zay'-shun). A process by which heat is used to kill pathogens in foods

Plasmolysis (plaz-moll'-uh-sis). The shrinking of the cell membrane and cytoplasm from the cell wall, causing the cell to shrink

Plasmoptysis (plaz-mop'-ti-sis). Process in which water enters a cell through the cell wall, decreasing the osmotic pressure

Psychroduric (sigh-crow-dur'-ick). Ability to endure −20° to 5°C (−5° to 40°F)

Sporicidal (spor-uh-sigh'-dull). Killing spores

Thermoduric (ther-mow-dur'-ick). Ability to survive boiling

Thermophilic (ther-mow-fill'-ick). Abiliy to thrive at temperatures above 45°C (113°F)

Tuberculocidal (too-bur-cue-low-sigh'-doll). Killing the bacteria that cause tuberculosis (*Mycobacterium tuberculosis*)

Virucide (vi'-ruh-side). A substance that kills viruses

The factors or agents that influence the growth of microorganisms are subject to continual study. On the basis of these studies researchers learn how the beneficial microbes can be encouraged to grow while growth of the pathogenic ones can be controlled, inhibited, or destroyed. The control of certain microorganisms is important (1) for the prevention and control of infectious diseases in man, animals, and plants; (2) for the preservation of food; (3) to prevent contaminating microbes from interfering with certain industrial processes; and (4) to prevent contamination of pure culture research. Preventing the spread of infectious diseases and controlling infections require many different procedures. The source of infection can be controlled by (1) destroying or inhibiting disease-causing microbes; (2) checking the sources, routes, and vectors of transmission of disease agents; and (3) protecting the infected person from the consequences of disease by building up the body's defenses and administering appropriate chemotherapeutic drugs.

An *infectious disease* is any disease caused by the invasion and multiplication of pathogenic microorganisms in the body. Thus, an infection indicates the presence of pathogens in living tissues. *Contamination* means that pathogenic microorganisms are present on or in nonliving materials, such as bed linens, discharges from human or animal sources, or food and water.

Long before people were aware of the existence of microorganisms, they tried to prevent the spoilage of food and wines, the transmission of diseases, and the infection of wounds. They developed many primitive procedures and "cures" that were often more harmful than helpful to the recipient. Today we know that the avoidance, inhibition, and destruction of potentially pathogenic microorganisms is imperative to control diseases. It is essential that those who work in the health fields appreciate the importance of controlling microbes in patients' rooms, operating rooms, treatment rooms, and emergency rooms. They must be aware of proper aseptic procedures to be followed for dressing wounds, giving injections and respiratory treatments, and assisting physicians, dentists, and all other personnel who have the responsibility for patient care. Health care workers must be able to properly handle contaminated linen and wound dressings, bedside equipment, and laboratory specimens to avoid infecting themselves, the patients for whom they are providing care, or other patients.

Definition of Terms

Before we can discuss the methods used to destroy or inhibit microbes, a number of terms should be understood as they apply to microbiology.

Sterilization The complete destruction of all living organisms, including cells, viable spores, and viruses, is called sterilization. Sterilization of objects can be accomplished by heat, autoclaving (heat and steam or ethylene oxide under pressure), various chemicals (such as formaldehyde), and certain levels of radiation with ultraviolet or gamma rays. These procedures are discussed later in this chapter.

Disinfection *Disinfection* is the destruction or removal of infectious or harmful microorganisms from nonliving objects by physical or chemical methods. The heating process developed by Pasteur to disinfect beer and wines is called *pasteurization*. It is still used to eliminate pathogenic microorganisms from milk and beer. It should be remembered that pasteurization is not a sterilization procedure, because not all the microbes are destroyed. Chemical agents are also used to eliminate pathogenic agents. The chemicals used to disinfect inanimate objects, such as bedside equipment and operating rooms, are called *disinfectants*. An *antiseptic* is a solution used to disinfect the skin or other living tissues. Disinfectants are strong chemical substances and are more destructive to living tissues than antiseptics. *Sanitization* reduces microbial populations to levels considered safe by public health standards, such as those applied to restaurants.

Microbicidal Agents   The suffix *-cide* or *-cidal* refers to killing. Thus, a microbicidal agent is one that kills microbes. A *bactericidal agent* (bactericide) kills bacteria, but not necessarily endospores of bacteria. A disinfectant that kills fungi is a *fungicide*, and similarly, an agent that destroys viruses is a *virucide*. The general term *germicide* refers to any agent that destroys germs or harmful microorganisms; this agent might be used in sanitization procedures.

Microbistatic Agent   The suffix *-stasis* or *-static* means the inhibition or cessation of growth and reproduction of microorganisms. A *bacteriostatic agent* is one that inhibits the metabolism and reproduction of bacteria, causing them to degenerate and die or be destroyed. Important microbistatic agents and processes include desiccation (drying), freezing temperatures, concentrated sugar and salt solutions, and some chemotherapeutic drugs (including the antibiotics).

Asepsis   Because sepsis refers to the growth of infectious microbes on living tissues, *asepsis* means the absence of infectious microorganisms on living tissues. Thus, *aseptic technique* is a procedure designed to eliminate and exclude all infectious microbes by sterilization of equipment, disinfection of environment, and cleansing of the body tissues with antiseptics. The *antiseptic technique* was developed by Lister in 1867. He used dilute carbolic acid to cleanse surgical wounds and equipment and a carbolic acid aerosol to prevent harmful microorganisms from entering the surgical field or contaminating the patient.

Sterile Technique   When it is necessary to prevent *all* microorganisms from gaining entrance into a laboratory or onto a surgical field, sterile technique is followed. A chemical agent used in sterilization is referred to as a *sterilant*.

Factors Influencing Microbial Growth

There are many environmental factors that enhance or inhibit the growth of microorganisms, including temperature, moisture, osmotic pressure, pH, barometric pressure, gases, radiations, chemicals, and the presence of neighboring microbes. Many concepts involving these factors may be applied to our everyday lives as well as to laboratory and hospital situations.

Temperature

There is an optimum temperature at which an organism grows best, a minimum temperature at which it ceases to grow, and a maximum temperature at which it is destroyed. These temperature ranges differ greatly among organisms. Their rate of growth and metabolism is generally slower at low temperatures and faster at higher temperatures, with the effect of temperature changes varying according to the species of organism. Microbes that thrive at 20° to 40°C (68° to 104°F) are called *mesophiles*, a group that includes most of the species that grow on plants and animals and in soil and water. *Psychrophiles* are capable of growth at temperatures near the freezing point; they thrive in oceans, soil, and refrigerated foods at temperatures between 0° and 20°C (30° to 68°F). Microorganisms that grow at temperatures above 45°C (113°F) are called *thermophiles*. These heat-loving microbes may be found in hot springs, compost pits, and silage; because they thrive at high temperatures, boiling is not an effective means of killing them. Refer to Table 5–1 for the minimum and maximum temperature ranges of psychrophilic, mesophilic, and thermophilic bacteria.

Most pathogens and normal flora are mesophilic, because they grow best at normal body temperature, 37°C (98.6°F). Thus, most pathogens are easily destroyed by boiling. The exceptions are the spores from spore-forming bacteria, the mycobacteria with resistant cell walls, and those microbes that are encased in a protective coating of organic material, such as mucus, vomitus, pus, or feces.

Microorganisms that can survive or endure very cold temperatures and can be preserved in the frozen state are known as *psychroduric* organisms. The fecal material left by early arctic explorers contained psychroduric *Escherichia coli* that survived the arctic temperatures. Also, many microbes and endospores can survive boiling and are therefore called *thermoduric* organisms. These microbes cause much of the color observed in hot springs.

Moisture

Living organisms require water to continue their normal metabolic processes. However, some microorganisms can survive the complete drying process called

Table 5–1. Bacteria Named on the Basis of Temperature Tolerance

Group	Temperature Range (°C)		
	Minimum	*Optimum*	*Maximum*
Psychrophiles	−20 to 5	0 to 20	19 to 35
Mesophiles	10 to 15	20 to 40 35	35 to 47 55
Thermophiles	40 to 45	55 to 75 60	60 to 90 80

(handwritten annotations:) Psychrotrophs −5 to 35   20   35
Thermodurrs short hot exposure

desiccation. Such organisms are in a dormant or resting state after they have been dried; then, as soon as they are placed in a moist nutrient environment, they grow and reproduce normally.

Another method of inhibiting growth of microbes is by dehydration (or drying) of frozen organisms, a process often called *lyophilization*. The lyophilized materials are frozen in a vacuum, which is then sealed to maintain the inactive state. This freeze-drying method is widely used in industry to preserve foods, antibiotics, antisera, microorganisms, and other biological materials. It should be remembered that lyophilization cannot be used as a method to sterilize or kill microorganisms, but rather, it is used to prevent them from reproducing.

Osmotic Pressure

Osmotic pressure is that pressure exerted on the cell membrane by the solution inside and outside the cell (Fig. 5–1). When cells are suspended in a solution, the normal osmotic pressure inside the cell should equal the pressure of the solution outside the cell; thus the cell neither shrinks nor swells; the solution outside the cell is then said to be an *isotonic solution*. Red blood cells in serum and bacterial cells in a nutrient broth remain normal in size because these solutions are isotonic — the osmotic pressure is equalized. When red blood cells are suspended in a *hypotonic* (more dilute than normal) solution, they increase in size because the water moves across the cell membrane into the concentrated cytoplasm of the cell. Often the cell membrane ruptures; this is called *hemolysis*. When bacterial cells are placed in water (a hypotonic solution), more water enters the cell than leaves the cell, greatly increasing the fluid pressure inside the bacterial cell, because the rigid cell wall prevents an increase in size. This condition is referred to as *plasmoptysis* and is found in plants and bacteria, which have rigid cell walls. If red blood cells

Figure 5–1. Changes in osmotic pressure. No change in pressure occurs inside the cell in an isotonic solution; pressure is increased in a hypotonic solution; pressure is decreased in a hypertonic solution. Arrows indicate direction of water flow.

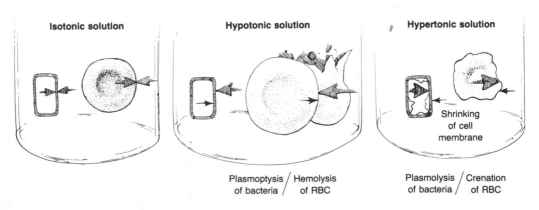

are suspended in a *hypertonic* (more concentrated than normal) salt or sugar solution, water is drawn from the cytoplasm of the cell to the surrounding solution, and the result is shrinking or *crenation* of the cell. When a bacterial cell is placed in a hypertonic solution, the cell membrane and cytoplasm shrinks away from the cell wall; this condition, *plasmolysis*, inhibits bacterial cell growth and metabolism. Refer to Figure 5–1 for a comparison of the differences of various solution concentrations on bacteria and human body cells.

Sugar solutions for jellies, and pickling brines (salt solutions) for meats, preserve these foods by inhibiting the growth of microorganisms. However, many types of molds and some types of bacteria can survive and even grow in a salty environment. Such organisms are known as *haloduric*, whereas those that thrive in concentrated salt water, such as the Great Salt Lake, are called *halophilic* (halo-, referring to salt, saltlike; and philos; Gr. for love), because they require an abundance of sodium ions.

*p*H

The term *p*H refers to the acidity or alkalinity of a solution (see Chapter 3). Most microorganisms prefer a neutral growth medium (about *p*H 7), but the *acidophilic* microbes, which can live in the stomach and in pickled foods, prefer a *p*H of 2 to 5. *Alkalophiles* prefer an alkaline environment, such as is found inside the intestine, that is about *p*H 9.

Barometric Pressure

Most bacteria are not affected by minor changes in pressure. They thrive at normal atmospheric pressure, and some, known as barophiles (baro-, referring to pressure), thrive deep in the ocean and in oil wells, where the atmospheric pressure is very high.

Autoclaves and home pressure cookers kill microbes by a combination of high pressure and high temperature. The increase in pressure raises the temperature above the temperature of boiling water. [At a pressure of 15 pounds per square inch (P.S.I.), the temperature of boiling water is 121°C.] However, home canning done without the use of a pressure cooker does not destroy the endospores of bacteria, notably *Clostridium botulinum*. Occasionally, the local newspapers report cases of food poisoning resulting from the release of *C. botulinum* endospores in improperly canned vegetables and meats.

Gases

The types of gases present and their concentrations determine which species of microbes are able to live in a particular environment. Most microbes are *aerobic*; that is, they grow best in an atmosphere containing oxygen. *Anaerobes* prefer to live without oxygen, usually in an atmosphere containing from 5 to 50% carbon dioxide from which the oxygen has been removed or a similar environment deep within the body tissues. *Obligate anaerobes* die when exposed to oxygen. For this reason, oxygen is sometimes forced into wound infections caused by anaerobes. For instance, wounds that may contain tetanus bacteria are lanced (opened) to expose them to the air. Another example is gas gangrene; this is a deep wound infection that is often treated by placing the patient in a hyperbaric (greatly increased pressure) oxygen chamber or in a room with high oxygen pressure, because the causative bacteria, *Clostridium perfringens,* cannot live in the presence of oxygen.

Antimicrobial Methods

The methods used to destroy or inhibit microbial life are either physical or chemical, and sometimes both types are used. The effectiveness of any antimicrobial procedure depends on (1) length of time it is applied, (2) temperature, (3) concentration, (4) nature and number of microbes and spores present (bioburden), and (5) presence of protective materials, such as the proteins in feces, blood, vomitus, and pus (Fig. 5–2).

Physical Antimicrobial Methods

The physical methods commonly used in hospitals, clinics, and laboratories to destroy or control pathogens are heat, pressure, drying, radiation, sonic disruption, and filtration.

Figure 5–2. The factors that determine the effectiveness of any antimicrobial procedure: time, temperature, concentration, presence of other microbes or spores, and presence of protein materials.

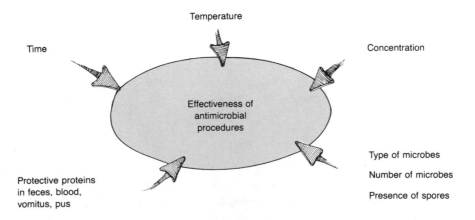

Heat   Heat is the most practical, efficient, and inexpensive method of disinfection and sterilization of those inanimate objects and materials that can withstand high temperatures. Because of these advantages, it is the means most frequently employed.

Two factors, *temperature* and *time*, determine the effectiveness of heat for sterilization. There is considerable variation from organism to organism in susceptibility to heat; pathogens usually are more susceptible than nonpathogens. Also, the higher the temperature, the shorter the time required to kill the organisms. The *thermal death point* of any specific species of microorganism is the lowest temperature that will kill all the organisms in a standardized pure culture within a specified period of time. The *thermal death time* is the length of time necessary to sterilize a pure culture at a specified temperature.

In practical applications of heat for sterilization, one must consider the material in which a mixture of organisms and their spores may be found. Pus, feces, vomitus, mucus, and blood contain proteins that serve as a protective coating to insulate the pathogens; when these discharges are present on bedding, bandages, surgical instruments, and syringes, very high heat is required to destroy the microorganisms and spores. In practice, the most effective procedure is to wash away the protein debris with strong soap, hot water, and a disinfectant and then sterilize the equipment with heat.

Heat applied in the presence of moisture, such as by boiling or steaming, is more effective than dry heat because moist heat causes the proteins to coagulate. Because cellular enzymes are proteins, they are also inactivated. This is exactly what happens when an egg is hard-boiled: the combination of heat and moisture causes the proteins to coagulate. Moist heat sterilization is faster than dry heat sterilization and can be done at a lower temperature; thus, it is less destructive to many materials that otherwise would be damaged by higher temperatures.

The vegetative forms of most pathogens are quite easily destroyed by boiling; however, bacterial endospores are particularly resistant to heat and drying. The autoclave, which combines heat and pressure, offers the most effective yet inexpensive means of destroying the spores. Two examples of sporeformers are *Clostridium tetani*, the causative agent of tetanus, and *C. botulinum*, which causes a food poisoning; they are usually found in contaminating dirt and dust. Botulism food poisoning is preventable by properly washing and pressure cooking (autoclaving) the food.

Certain viruses are remarkably resistant to heat. A case in point is the hepatitis virus, which is frequently transferred from one person to another by the reuse of contaminated syringes and needles that have not been adequately sterilized. It is recommended that all equipment used in the transfer of blood be sterilized in an autoclave at 121°C (250°F) for 20 minutes or boiled for 30 minutes or baked at 180°C (356°F) for 1 hour.

Dry heat   Dry heat baking in a thermostatically controlled oven provides effective sterilization for metals, glassware, some powders, oils, and waxes. These items must be baked at 160° to 165°C (320° to 329°F) for 2 hours or at 170° to 180°C (338° to 356°F) for 1 hour. An ordinary oven of the type found in most homes may be used if the temperature remains constant. The effectiveness of dry heat sterilization depends on how deeply the heat penetrates throughout the material, and the items to be baked must be placed so that the hot air circulates freely among them.

Incineration, or burning, is an effective means of destroying contaminated disposable materials. An incinerator must never be overloaded with moist or protein-laden materials, such as feces, vomitus, or pus, because the contaminating microorganisms within these moist substances may not be destroyed if the heat does not readily penetrate and burn them. Flaming the surface of heat-resistant material is an effective way to kill microorganisms on forceps and bacteriological loops and is a common laboratory procedure. Flaming is accomplished by holding the end of the loop or forceps in the yellow portion of a gas flame (Fig. 5–3).

Moist heat   As was stated, moist heat causes the cellular proteins (enzymes) in the microorganisms to become inactivated, and the cell dies. Boiling water and steam are favored in disinfection, because no expensive equipment is necessary and the required time is short. Most pathogens die after 10 minutes of steaming at 70°C (158°F); also, boiling for 10 to 30 minutes at 90° to 100°C (194° to 212°F), depending on the altitude, destroys most viable bacteria, fungi, and viruses. Clean articles made of metal and glass, such as syringes, needles, and simple instruments, may be disinfected by boiling for 30 minutes. However, this technique

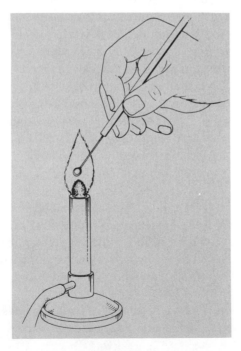

Figure 5–3. The technique for flaming the bacteriological loop.

is not always effective, because heat-resistant bacterial endospores, mycobacteria, and viruses may be present. As mentioned in Chapter 2, the endospores of the bacteria that cause anthrax, tetanus, gas gangrene, and botulism, as well as the hepatitis viruses, are notably heat resistant and often survive normal disinfection procedures.

An effective way to disinfect clothing, bedding, and dishes is to use hot water, above 60°C (140°F) with detergent or soap and to agitate the solution around the items. This combination of heat, mechanical action, and chemical inhibition is deadly to most pathogens.

Pressurized steam   An autoclave is a large pressure cooker that uses steam under pressure to completely destroy all microbial life. Pressure raises the temperature of the steam and shortens the time necessary to sterilize materials that can tolerate the high temperature and moisture. Autoclaving at a pressure of 15 p.s.i. at a temperature of 121.5°C (250°F) for 20 minutes kills viable microorganisms, viruses, and exposed bacterial endospores, if they are not hidden in pus, feces, vomitus, blood, or other protein substances. Some types of equipment and certain materials, such as rubber, which may be damaged by high temperatures, can be autoclaved at lower temperatures for longer periods. The timing must be carefully determined based on the contents and compactness of the load. All articles must be properly packaged and arranged within the autoclave to allow steam to penetrate each package (Fig. 5–4). Cans should be open, bottles covered loosely with foil or cotton, and instruments wrapped in cloths. Sealed containers should not be autoclaved.

Figure 5–4. Pressure-sensitive autoclave tape shows dark stripes after sterilization. (Volk WA, Wheeler MF: Basic Microbiology, 5th ed. Philadelphia, JB Lippincott, 1984)

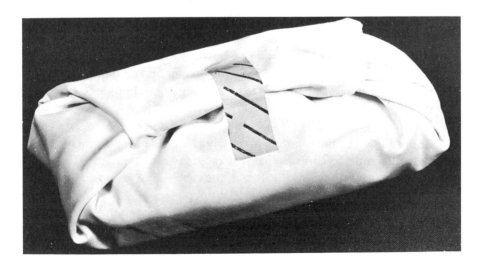

Cold Microorganisms are not killed by cold temperatures and freezing; their metabolic activities are slowed, greatly inhibiting their growth. Thus, freezing is a microbistatic method of preservation in which the microorganisms are in a state similar to suspended animation. When the temperature is raised above the freezing point, the metabolic reactions speed up and the organisms slowly begin to reproduce again. Refrigeration merely slows the growth of microorganisms; it does not altogether inhibit them. Many foods, biologic specimens, and bacterial cultures are preserved by rapid freezing to very low temperatures. It should be noted that slow freezing causes ice crystals to form within the cells and may rupture the cell walls of a few bacteria; hence, if it is important to preserve a pure culture of bacteria, such slow freezing should be avoided and rapid freezing should be performed, usually using liquid nitrogen.

Persons who are involved in the preparation and preservation of foods must be aware that thawing to room temperature allows bacterial spores to germinate and microorganisms to resume growth. Consequently, refreezing of thawed foods is an unsafe practice, because it preserves the millions of microbes and the food deteriorates quickly when it is rethawed. Also, if bacterial endospores of *C. botulinum* or *C. perfringens* were present, the viable bacteria would begin to produce toxins that would cause food poisoning.

Drying For many centuries, foods have been preserved by drying. When moisture and nutrients are lacking, many dried microorganisms remain viable, although they cannot reproduce. Foods, serums, toxins, antitoxins, antibiotics, and pure cultures of microorganisms are often preserved by lyophilization (discussed previously).

In the hospital or clinical environment, health care workers should keep in mind that dried viable pathogens may be lurking in dried matter, including blood, pus, fecal material, and dust that are found on floors, in bedding, on clothing, and in wound dressings. Should these dried materials be disturbed, such as by dry dusting, the microbes would be easily transmitted through the air or by contact. They would then grow rapidly if they settled in a suitable moist, warm nutrient environment such as a wound or a burn. Therefore, important precautions that must be observed include the following: wet mop and damp dust floors and furniture, roll the bed linens and towels carefully, and properly dispose of wound dressings.

Radiation The sun is not a particularly reliable disinfecting agent because it kills only those microorganisms that are exposed to direct sunlight. The rays of the sun include the long infrared (heat) rays, the visible light rays, and the shorter ultraviolet (UV) rays. The UV rays, which do not penetrate glass and building materials, are effective only in the air and on the surface of equipment. They do, however, penetrate cells and thus can cause damage to DNA. When this occurs, the genes may be so severely damaged that the cell dies (especially unicellular microorganisms) or is drastically changed.

In practice, the UV lamp is useful for reducing the number of microorganisms in the air. The UV lamp often is called a germicidal lamp. Its main component is a low-pressure mercury vapor tube. Such lamps are found in newborn nurseries, operating rooms, elevators, entryways, cafeterias, and classrooms, where they are incorporated into louvered ceiling fixtures designed to radiate across the top of the room without striking persons in the room. The sterility of an area may also be maintained by having a UV lamp placed in a hood or cabinet containing instruments, paper and cloth equipment, liquid, and other inanimate articles. Many biologic materials, such as serums, antiserums, toxins, and vaccines, are sterilized with UV rays.

Those whose work involves the use of UV lamps must be particularly careful not to expose their eyes or skin to the rays, because the rays can cause serious burns and cellular damage. Because UV rays do not penetrate cloth, metals, and glass, these materials may be used to protect persons working in a UV environment. It has been shown that skin cancer can be caused by excessive exposure to the UV rays of the sun; thus, extensive suntanning is harmful.

X-rays and gamma and beta rays of certain wavelengths from radioactive materials may be lethal or cause mutations in microorganisms and tissue cells, because they damage DNA and proteins within those cells. Work done in radiation research laboratories has demonstrated that these radiations can be used for the prevention of food spoilage, for preparation of organs for transplantation, for the sterilization of heat-sensitive surgical equipment, for the preparation of vaccines, and for the treatment of some chronic diseases such as cancer, all of which are very practical applications for laboratory research. When these radiations are used in the treatment of disease, care must be taken to focus the rays precisely on the specific area being treated to minimize damage to normal cells.

Ultrasonic Waves   In hospitals and clinics, ultrasonic waves are a frequently used means of cleaning and sterilizing delicate equipment. Ultrasonic cleaners consist of tanks filled with liquid solvent (usually water); the short sound waves are then passed through the liquid. The sound waves mechanically dislodge organic debris on instruments and glassware.

Glassware and other articles that have been cleansed in ultrasonic equipment must be washed to remove the dislodged particles and solvent and are then sterilized by another method before they are used.

Filtration   Filters of various pore sizes are used to filter or separate cells, larger viruses, bacteria, and certain other microorganisms from the liquids or gases in which they are suspended. The filtered solution (filtrate) is not necessarily sterile, because the small viruses may not be filtered out. The variety of filters is large and includes sintered glass (in which uniform particles of glass are fused), plastic films, unglazed porcelain, asbestos, diatomaceous earth, and cellulose membrane filters. Small quantities of liquid can be filtered through a syringe; large quantities require larger apparatuses.

A cotton plug in a test tube, flask, or pipette is a good filter for preventing the entry of microorganisms. Dry gauze and paper masks prevent the outward passage of microbes from the mouth and nose, at the same time protecting the wearer from inhaling airborne pathogens and foreign particles that could damage the lungs.

Chemical Antimicrobial Methods

Chemical disinfection means the use of chemical agents to inhibit the growth of microorganisms, either temporarily or permanently. The effectiveness of a chemical disinfectant depends on many factors: the concentration of the chemical; the time allowed for the chemical to work; the pH or acidity of the solution; the temperature; and the presence of proteins, blood, pus, feces, mucous secretions, and vomitus. Directions for the preparation and dilution of the disinfectant must be carefully followed, and the proper concentration, pH, and temperature must be maintained for the specified time period to ensure the best results. The items to be disinfected must first be washed to remove any material in which pathogens may be hidden. Although the washed article may then be clean, it is not safe to use until it has been properly disinfected. Health personnel need to understand an important limitation of chemical disinfection: many disinfectants that are effective against pathogens in the controlled conditions of the laboratory become ineffective in the actual hospital or clinical environment. Furthermore, the stronger and more effective antimicrobial chemical agents are of limited usefulness because of their destructiveness to human tissues and certain other substances.

Almost all bacteria in the vegetative growing state as well as fungi, protozoa, and most viruses are susceptible to many disinfectants, although the mycobacteria of tuberculosis and leprosy, the endospores of bacteria, fungal spores, and the hepatitis viruses are notably resistant. Therefore, chemical disinfection should never be attempted when it is possible to use proper physical sterilization techniques.

The disinfectant most effective for each situation must be carefully chosen. Chemical agents used to disinfect respiratory therapy equipment and thermometers must destroy all pathogenic bacteria, fungi, and viruses that may be found in sputum and saliva. One must be particularly aware of the oral and respiratory pathogens, including *Myobacterium tuberculosis*; *Pseudomonas* spp.; *Staphylococcus*; *Streptococcus*; and the various fungi that cause candidiasis, blastomycosis, coccidioidomycosis, and histoplasmosis, as well as all the respiratory viruses.

Because most disinfection methods do not destroy all bacterial endospores that are present, any instrument or dressing used in the treatment of an infected wound or of a disease caused by spore-formers must be autoclaved or incinerated. Gas gangrene, tetanus, and anthrax are examples of diseases caused by spore-formers that require the health worker to take such precautions. Formaldehyde and ethylene oxide, when properly used, are highly destructive to spores, mycobacteria, and viruses. Certain articles are heat sensitive and cannot be autoclaved or safely washed before disinfection; such articles are soaked for 24 hours in a strong detergent and disinfectant solution, washed, and then sterilized in the ethylene oxide gas autoclave. The use of disposable equipment whenever possible in these situations helps to protect the patient as well as the health care team members.

The effectiveness of a chemical agent depends to some extent on the physical characteristics of the article on which it is used. A smooth, hard surface is readily disinfected, whereas a rough, porous, or grooved surface is not. Thought must be given to selection of the most suitable germicide for cleaning patient rooms and all other areas where patients are treated.

The most effective antiseptic or disinfectant should be chosen for the specific purpose, environment, and pathogen or pathogens likely to be present. The characteristics of a good chemical antimicrobial agent are as follows:

1. It must kill pathogens within a reasonable time period and in specified concentrations.
2. It must be nontoxic to human tissues and noncorrosive and nondestructive to materials on which it is used.
3. It must be soluble in water and easy to apply. If a tincture (alcohol-water solution) is used, the concentration should be checked frequently. Evaporation of the alcohol solvent can cause a 1% solution to increase to a 10% solution, and at this concentration, it may cause tissue damage.
4. It should be inexpensive and easy to prepare for use with simple, specific directions.
5. It must be stable in the dissolved or solid form so that it can be shipped and stored for a reasonable period.
6. It should be stable to pH and temperature changes within reasonable limits.

Antisepsis

Most antimicrobial chemical agents are too irritating and destructive to be applied to the mucous membranes and the skin. Those that may be safely used on human tissues are called *antiseptics*. An antiseptic merely reduces the number of organisms on a surface but does not penetrate the pores and hair follicles to destroy microorganisms residing there. To remove organisms lodged in pores and folds of the skin, health personnel use an antiseptic soap and scrub with a brush. The surgeon wears sterile gloves on freshly scrubbed hands, and a mask and hood to cover face and hair, to prevent resident endogenous microflora from contaminating the surgical field. Also, an antiseptic is applied at the site of the surgical incision to destroy local microorganisms.

How Antimicrobial Chemicals Work

Injury of Cell Membranes   Soap and detergents are referred to as surfactants; this means that they are surface-active agents that help to disperse the bacteria, allowing them to more readily be rinsed away. These agents concentrate on the surface and thus reduce the surface tension; this characteristic makes them good wetting and dispersing agents. Some agents, such as Dial and Safeguard soaps, contain disinfectants, which also aid in killing bacteria. Certain concentrations of weak acids such as acetic acid and benzoic acids may also be used in disinfectant soaps.

Inactivation of Enzymes   Alcohols, such as ethyl and isopropyl, are good skin antiseptics at 70% solution. Ethyl alcohol has a low toxicity for humans, hence it is frequently used to disinfect clinical thermometers and other instruments. However, isopropyl alcohol causes severe gastrointestinal upset when taken internally, and methanol causes brain damage. Alcohols are turberculocidal (destructive of tuberculosis-causing organisms) but not sporicidal (destructive of spores).

The phenolics including phenol, carbolic acid, xylenols, orthophenylphenol, and cresol, are used as disinfectants in hospitals and laboratories. However, they are too irritating and toxic to be used on the skin. The commercial mixture of phenolics, Lysol, is an effective germicide, because it works in the presence of organic material, and remains active on hard surfaces for extended periods of time. These chemicals are tuberculocidal but not sporicidal.

The effectiveness of phenol was demonstrated by Joseph Lister in 1867, when it was used to reduce the incidence of infections following surgical procedures. The effectiveness of other disinfectants is compared to that of phenol using the *phenol coefficient test*. To perform this test, a series of dilutions of phenol and the experimental disinfectant are inoculated with the test bacteria, *Salmonella typhi* and *Staphylococcus aureus*, at 37°C. The highest dilutions that kill the bacteria after 10 minutes are used to calculate the phenol coefficient.

Salts of heavy metals such as mercury chloride (Merthiolate, Mercurochrome, Metaphen—generic names; thimerosal, merbromin, nitromersol, respectively) and silver nitrate (Argyrol, Protargol) are bacteriostatic antiseptics, but they are not sporicidal and are ineffective against many pathogens. Silver nitrate in low concentrations is used in the eyes of newborns to kill the gonococcus organism; this prevents gonorrheal infections, which could cause blindness.

Chemical oxidizing agents are useful disinfectants. Two of these are hydrogen peroxide and sodium perborate, which destroy bacteria and tissue debris and prevent anaerobic growth in damaged tissues. A third, potassium permanganate, is employed in weak solutions to treat urethral infections and fungal infections of the skin. Another agent in this group is ethylene oxide (Carboxide, Cryoxide, Oxygume), which is used as a sterilant in gas autoclaves to sterilize heat-sensitive materials. Although it is a good microbicide and sporicide, this gas must be used with great care, because it is inflammable and toxic to humans.

The elements and many compounds of chlorine, iodine, bromine, and fluorine are also useful disinfectants. For example, chlorine compounds (Clorox, Halozone, hypochlorites, Warexin) are used to disinfect water and sewage and for sanitation of dishes, floors, and plumbing fixtures. It has been found that the human immunodeficiency virus (HIV) otherwise known as acquired immunodeficiency virus (AIDS), can be destroyed on syringes and needles by soaking them in a Clorox (chlorine bleach) solution for 10 minutes. The iodine compounds, such as Wescodyne, Betadine, Isodine, and tincture of iodine, are effective skin antiseptics and disinfectants. These compounds can be dangerous, however; if an alcohol solution of iodine is left open to the air, allowing the alcohol to evaporate, the solution may become too concentrated, and an iodine burn may result if it is used on the skin. Most compounds of bromine and fluorine are too toxic at the effective concentrations to be used as antiseptics. All of these compounds are viricidal, bactericidal, and tubeculocidal; however, none are sporicidal.

Damage to the Genetic Material   The DNA of cells is inactivated by caustic compounds such as formalin. Formalin is a 37% aqueous solution of gaseous formaldehyde that inactivates proteins and nucleic acids. It is one of the few antimicrobial agents that are also sporicidal; however, it is so irritating to the skin and mucous membranes that it cannot be used on living tissues. Frequently, it is used to preserve tissue specimens.

Basic aniline dyes also inactivate nucleic acids. In this group are included gentian violet and crystal violet, which are useful in treatment of fungal skin infections (ringworm) and vaginal infections caused by yeasts (*Candida*) and grampositive bacteria, as well as intestinal infestations of roundworms. Pyridium is a dye classified in the same group. It is prescribed for urinary infections caused by gram-negative enteric organisms.

Chemotherapy

For thousands of years, people have been finding and using herbs and chemicals to cure diseases. Native witch doctors in Central and South America long ago discovered that the herb, ipecac, aided in the treatment of dysentery and that a quinine extract of cinchona bark was effective in treating malaria. During the 16th and 17th centuries, the alchemists of Europe searched for a way to cure smallpox, syphilis, and the many other diseases that were rampant during that period of history. Many mercury and arsenic chemicals that were used frequently caused more damage to the patient than to the pathogen.

Major Discoveries

The true beginning of modern chemotherapy was in the late 1800s when Paul Ehrlich began his search for chemicals that would destroy bacteria yet would not damage normal body cells. By 1909 he had tested and discarded more than 600 chemicals. Finally, in that year, he discovered an arsenic compound that proved effective against syphilis. Because this was the 606th compound Ehrlich had tried, he called it "compound 606." The technical name for it is arsphenamine and the trade name was salvarsan. Until the purification of penicillin in 1938, arsphenamine was used to treat syphilis. In 1928, Alexander Fleming noted that the waste products of a mold, *Penicillium notatum*, inhibited the growth of staphylococci on an agar plate. He also found that broth cultures of the mold not only were not toxic to his laboratory animals, but that they destroyed staphylococci and other bacteria. During World War II, two biochemists, Sir Howard Walter Florey and Ernst Boris Chain, purified penicillin and demonstrated its effectiveness in the treatment of various bacterial infections. By 1942, the American drug industry was able to produce sufficient penicillin for human use, and the search for other antibiotics began. In 1935, a chemist named Gerhard Domagk discovered that the red dye, Prontosil, was effective against streptococcal infections in mice. Further research demonstrated that Prontosil was degraded or broken down in the body into sulfanilamide, and that the sulfanilamide was the effective agent. For their outstanding contributions to scientific progress, these investigators, Ehrlich, Fleming, Florey, Chain, and Domagk, were all at various times Nobel Prize recipients.

Characteristics of Chemotherapeutic Agents

A *chemotherapeutic agent* or *antimicrobial drug* is any chemical used to treat infectious disease by inhibiting or killing pathogens *in vivo* (in the living animal). A chemotherapeutic substance that is derived from a living organism and that in small amounts kills or inhibits the growth of microorganisms is labeled an *antibiotic*; these substances are produced by molds, bacteria, and some plants. The term antibiotic was intended to distinguish between chemical therapeutic agents, such as sulfonamide drugs, and those that are extracted from secretions of living organisms, such as penicillin, streptomycin, and erythromycin; however, many of these drugs and their derivatives are now synthesized or manufactured in the laboratory.

The ideal chemotherapeutic agent should (1) kill or inhibit the growth of pathogens, (2) cause no damage to the host, (3) cause no allergic reaction in the host, (4) be stable when stored in solid or liquid form, (5) remain in specific tissues in the body long enough to be effective, and (6) kill the pathogens before they mutate and become resistant to it. However, almost all chemotherapeutic agents have some side-effects, produce allergic reactions, or permit development of resistant mutant pathogens.

How Chemotherapeutic Drugs Work

To be acceptable an antimicrobial drug must inhibit or destroy the pathogen without damaging the host. The agent does this by disrupting the pathogen's metabolism in an area that is slightly different from normal human metabolism; the following examples illustrate this action.

The sulfonamide drugs inhibit production of folic acid in those bacteria that require para-aminobenzoic acid (usually abbreviated PABA) to synthesize folic acid. The folic acid (a vitamin) is essential to these bacteria. Because the sulfonamide molecule is similar in shape to the PABA molecule, the bacteria attempt to metabolize the sulfonamide to produce folic acid (Fig. 5–5). However, the enzymes that convert the PABA to folic acid cannot produce folic acid from the sulfonamide molecule. Without the folic acid, the bacteria cannot produce some essential proteins and finally die. The sulfa drugs therefore are called *competitive inhibitors*, that is, by competing with an enzyme that metabolizes an essential nutrient, they inhibit the growth of the microorganisms. In other words, they are bacteriostatic. The cells of humans and animals do not synthesize folic acid from PABA (they get it from the food they eat), and consequently, they are unaffected by the sulfa drugs.

In most of the gram-positive bacteria, including the streptococci and staphylococci, penicillin, interferes with the synthesis of peptidoglycan required in the bacterial cell wall. Thus, by inhibiting cell wall synthesis, the penicillin destroys the bacteria. Why does penicillin not also destroy human cells? Human cells are eucaryotic cells and do not have a cell wall.

There are other chemotherapeutic drugs that have similar action; they inhibit a specific step that is essential to the microorganism's metabolism and thereby cause its destruction. Antibiotics are employed in this way against bacteria, and

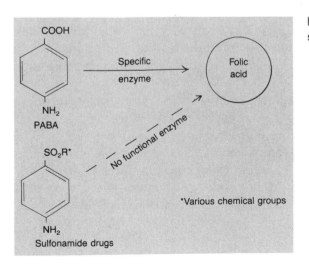

Figure 5–5. The effect of sulfonamide drugs.

they are highly effective. Some destroy gram-positive bacteria; some destroy gram-negative bacteria; those that are destructive to many gram-negative and gram-positive bacteria are called *broad-spectrum antibiotics*. Examples of broad-spectrum antibiotics are tetracycline, streptomycin, and ampicillin. Table 5–2 lists some of the antimicrobial drugs most frequently used against many common pathogens.

Antimicrobial drugs work well against bacterial pathogens because the bacteria (being procaryotic) have different cellular structures and metabolic pathways that can be disrupted by drugs that would not damage the host's (eucaryotic) cells. These antibacterial agents work in one of several ways.

1. To inhibit peptidoglycan cell wall synthesis, *e.g.*, penicillins, vancomycin, and cephalosporins
2. To act as competitive enzyme inhibitors to block the formation of essential metabolites; these "antimetabolites" include the sulfa drugs, trimethoprim, and ethambutol.
3. To inhibit protein synthesis by acting on 70S ribosomes, *e.g.*, tetracyclines, erythromycin, streptomycin, neomycin, and chloroamphenicol
4. To damage plasma membranes, such as polymyxin B
5. To inhibit nucleic acid synthesis, *e.g.*, rifamycin, nalidixic acid, and norfloxacin

It often happens that a single chemotherapeutic agent is not sufficient to destroy all the pathogens that develop during the course of a disease; thus, two or more drugs may be used simultaneously to prevent resistant mutant pathogens from emerging. In tuberculosis, for example, three drugs are routinely prescribed, and as many as twelve drugs may be required in resistant cases. Many urinary, respiratory, and gastrointestinal infections respond particularly well to a combination of trimethoprim and sulfamethoxazole; this combination is called co-trimoxazole.

It is much more difficult to use antimicrobial drugs against fungal and protozoal pathogens, because they are eucaryotic cells; thus, the drugs are much more toxic to the host. Antifungal agents work by (1) binding with cell membrane sterols, *e.g.*, nystatin and amphotericin B; (2) by interfering with sterol synthesis, *e.g.*, clotrimazole and micanazole; (3) by blocking mitosis or nucleic acid synthesis, *e.g.*, griseofulvin and 5-flucytosine. Antiprotozoal drugs are usually quite toxic and work (1) by interfering with DNA and RNA synthesis, *e.g.*, chloroquine, pentamidine, and quinacrine; or (2) by interfering with protozoan metabolism, *e.g.*, metronidazole.

Table 5 – 2.   Some Chemotherapeutic Agents Employed Against Important Pathogens

Pathogen	Disease	Chemotherapy or Treatment
Bacteria		
Bacillus anthracis	Anthrax	Penicillin, tetracyclines, erythromycin
Bordetella pertussis	Whooping cough	Erythromycin, ampicillin
Brucella abortus and B. melitensis	Brucellosis, undulant fever	Tetracyclines, streptomycin
Chlamydia trachomatis	Lymphogranuloma venereum	Sulfonamides, tetracyclines
Clostridium botulinum	Botulism (food poisoning)	(Antitoxin), penicillin, kanamycin
Clostridium perfringens	Gas gangrene, wound infections	(Antitoxin), penicillin, kanamycin
Clostridium tetani	Tetanus (lockjaw)	(Antitoxin), penicillin, kanamycin
Cornybacterium diphtheriae	Diphtheria	(Antitoxin), penicillin, erythromycin, cephalosporin
Escherichia coli	Urinary infections	Sulfonamides, gentamicin, cefazolin, nalidixic acid, norfloxacin, ampicillin
Francisella tularensis	Tularemia	Streptomycin, tetracyclines
Haemophilus ducreyi	Chancroid	Streptomycin, tetracyclines
Haemophilus influenzae	Meningitis, pneumonia	Ampicillin, streptomycin, tetracyclines, cefamandole
Klebsiella pneumoniae	Pneumonia	Colistin, cefazolin, gentamicin
Legionella pneumophilia	Legionellosis	Erythromycin, tetracycline
Mycobacterium leprae	Leprosy	Dapsone, tetracyclines, rifamide
Mycobacterium tuberculosis	Tuberculosis	Isoniazid, streptomycin, PAS, rifampin
Mycoplasma pneumoniae	Atypical pneumonia	Tetracyclines, erythromycin
Neisseria gonorrhoeae	Gonorrhea	Penicillin, tetracyclines, spectinomycin
Neisseria meningitidis	Nasopharangitis, meningitis	Penicillin, sulfonamides, ampicillin, tetracyclines, rifamide

continued

Table 5–2. Some Chemotherapeutic Agents Employed Against Important Pathogens (*Continued*)

Pathogen	Disease	Chemotherapy or Treatment
Proteus vulgaris and *P. morgani*	Gastroenteritis, urinary infections	Kanamycin, streptomycin, nalidixic acid
Pseudomonas aeruginosa	Respiratory and urogenital infections	Gentamicin, sulfonamides, mezlocillin, polymyxin
Rickettsia rickettsii	Rocky Mountain spotted fever	Tetracyclines, chloramphenicol
Salmonella typhi	Typhoid fever	Chloramphenicol, ampicillin, tetacyclines
Salmonella spp.	Gastroenteritis	Chloramphenicol, ampicillin, tetracyclines, co-trimoxazole
Shigella spp.	Shigellosis (bacillary dysentery)	Ampicillin, tetracyclines, sulfonamides, nalidixic acid
Staphylococcus aureus	Boils, carbuncles, pneumonia, septicemia	Bacitracin, erythromycin, gentamicin, vancomycin, cephalosporins
Streptococcus pyogenes	Strep throat, scarlet fever, rheumatic fever, septicemia	Penicillin, cephalosporin, erythromycin
Streptococcus pneumoniae	Pneumonia	Penicillin, cephalosporin, erythromycin
Treponema pallidum	Syphilis	Penicillin, erythromycin, tetracyclines
Vibrio cholerae	Cholera	Trimethoprim plus sulfamethoxazole
Yersinia pestis	Plague	Streptomycin, tetracyclines
Fungi		
Dermatophytes	Tineas	Nystatin, amphotericin B, griseofulvin
Candida	Mucosal candidiasis	Clotrimazole, micanazole, nystatin
Blastomyces		5-Flucytosine, amphotericin B
Histoplasma		5-Flucytosine, amphotericin B
Cryptococcus	Systemic mycosis	5-Flucytosine, amphotericin B
Coccidioides		5-Flucytosine, amphotericin B
Candida		Amphotericin B

Table 5–2. Some Chemotherapeutic Agents Employed Against Important Pathogens (*Continued*)

Pathogen	Disease	Chemotherapy or Treatment
Protozoa		
Trichomonas	Trichomoniasis	Metronidazole, griseofulvin
Giardia lamblia	Giardiasis	Metronidazole, quinacrine
Entamoeba histolytica	Amebiasis	Emetine, metronidazole
Toxoplasma	Toxoplasmosis	Clindamycin
Plasmodium spp.	Malaria	Clindamycin, chloroquine, pyrimethamine, sulfadiazine
Pneumocystis carinii	Pneumonia	Pentamidine, co-trimoxazole
Viruses		
Herpes spp.	Eye and lip herpes	Idoxuridine, acyclovir
	Genital herpes	Acyclovir
	Encephalitis	Vidarabine, acyclovir
Influenza A	Influenza	Amantidine, rimantadine
Human immunodeficiency virus (HIV)	AIDS	Azidothymidine (AZT), dideoxycytidine, ribavirin, suramin

Antiviral chemotherapeutic agents are particularly difficult to find and use because viruses are produced within the host's cells. A few have been found to be effective in certain conditions, and these work by interfering with the action of certain enzymes necessary for viral replication. These include amantadine and rimantadine, for influenza; acyclovir, for herpes; and azidothymidine (AZT, for acquired immunodeficiency syndrome AIDS). Some may interfere with DNA replication and RNA transcription; the action of others is unknown.

In cancer, in which the malignant cells are dividing more rapidly than the normal cells, chemical agents that inhibit DNA and RNA synthesis can be used, provided the dosage and total period of administration are carefully controlled. Cancer drugs interfere with normal DNA function in rapidly dividing cells, regardless of whether the cells are normal or malignant. Thus, the normal cells that are rapidly dividing, including skin cells, the erythroblasts that later become blood cells, and the sperm cells, are damaged along with the malignant cells. This is why blood cell counts are done frequently in cancer patients: the physician must be able to determine at what point the chemotherapy must be discontinued to avoid critical damage to the patient's normal cells.

Insight: AIDS Infections and AZT Therapy

From 1981 to 1990, 100,777 deaths due to AIDS infections were reported to the Centers for Disease Control (CDC); one third of these occurred in 1990.

An estimated 1 million people in the United States are infected with the human immunodeficiency virus (HIV), and 165,000–215,000 people will die of AIDS during the period from 1991–1993. The impact of HIV infections/AIDS on mortality rates through the decade into early 2,000 depends on present efforts to prevent and treat HIV infection.

AZT (azidothymidine or zidovudine) is being used extensively on HIV-infected adults who can afford the treatment, with positive results. Lower doses allow longer treatment periods with less toxic side effects. Recent clinical trials have indicated that AZT is even safe for infants infected perinatally. In many cases, the use of AZT delays the onset of AIDS symptoms among HIV-infected persons. It is still not the perfect drug. Other drugs, dideoxyinosine and dideoxycytosine (DDC), are being evaluated for use with or as a substitute for AZT. Combination therapy may prevent the development of drug resistance, which has already been detected. AZT therapy is not a cure; it appears to only prolong the life of HIV-infected patients 6 months to 1 year. There is no cure for the disease as yet. (Centers for Disease Control. Summary of notifiable diseases, United States, 1989. Morbidity and Mortality Weekly Report, 1991;40(3).)

Side Effects of Chemotherapeutic Agents

There are many reasons why chemotherapeutic drugs should not be used indiscriminately:

1. The microorganisms may mutate and become resistant to the antibiotic. Their metabolism may change, and they may produce an enzyme that can destroy the antibiotic or produce one that uses the antibiotic as a nutrient; or they may become impermeable to the antibiotic. To prevent these developments, several drugs, each of which has a different mode of action, often are administered simultaneously. If not properly treated, the drug-resistant pathogens may continue to flourish, causing a *superinfection*.

2. The patient may become allergic to the antibiotic. For example, penicillin G in low doses often sensitizes those who are prone to allergies; when these persons receive a second dose of penicillin at some later date, they may have a severe reaction known as anaphylactic shock, or they

may break out in hives. This reaction is described in more detail in Chapter 9.

3. Many chemotherapeutic drugs are toxic to humans, and some are so toxic they are administered only for serious diseases for which no other antibiotics are available. One such drug is chloramphenicol (Chloromycetin), which, if given in high doses for a long period, may cause a very severe type of anemia called aplastic anemia. Another is streptomycin, which can damage the auditory nerve and cause deafness.

4. With prolonged use, the broad-spectrum antibiotics may destroy the normal flora of the mouth, intestine, or vagina. The person no longer has the protection of the normal flora and, thus, becomes much more susceptible to infections caused by opportunists or secondary invaders. The result is a superinfection. An example of such an infection is diarrhea, which can result from prolonged antibiotic therapy owing to the loss of the normal protective microbes. This topic is discussed more fully in Chapter 6.

Therefore, chemotherapeutic drugs, including antibiotics, should be taken only when prescribed and only under a physician's supervision. Also, the proper dosage must be administered for the recommended period to prevent resistant organisms from gaining a foothold.

In recent years, scientific research has developed new antibiotics at such a rapid pace that many people, including some of the researchers, are beginning to fear that pathogens are becoming so resistant to antibiotics that the human race may be destroyed. Some problems already have arisen; a case in point is pneumonia. In the developed countries of the world, the types of pneumonia occurring at present are different from those that were seen 30 years ago, and sometimes they are highly resistant to treatment. Our hope is that antibiotics will be used with greater care and that effective vaccines may become available. We now have *H. influenzae* and a *Streptococcus pneumoniae* vaccine on the market to protect against some types of pneumonia, but not all. Also, resistant strains of gonococci, penicillinase-positive *Neisseria gonorrhoeae* (PPNG), have developed. We hope to soon see a vaccine against gonorrhea, syphilis, and acquired immunodeficiency syndrome. The difficulty then will be to convince the American public to take the vaccines to protect themselves against these pathogens.

Summary

It is important to learn how the growth of microorganisms can be inhibited or enhanced to prevent and control infectious diseases, prevent contamination of industrial processes, prevent spoilage of food and crops, and prevent contamination of pure culture research. Certain microbes are cultivated to produce vaccines, decompose decaying organic materials, and conduct research. Those people working in the health field must take special care not to transfer potentially pathogenic microbes from patient to patient, from themselves to patients, or from patients to themselves. Health care workers need to know the physical and chemical methods used to control pathogenic microorganisms and the conditions for the best use of these methods.

Study Outline

I. Control of growth of microorganisms
   A. Importance of controlling microbial growth
   B. Definitions
II. Factors influencing microbial growth
   A. Temperature
   B. Moisture
   C. Osmotic pressure
   D. pH (acidity)
   E. Barometric pressure
   F. Gases
III. Antimicrobial methods
   A. Physical methods
     1. Heat
     2. Cold
     3. Drying
     4. Radiations
     5. Ultrasonic waves
     6. Filtration
   B. Chemical methods
IV. Chemotherapy
   A. History
   B. Characteristics of a good chemotherapeutic agent
   C. How chemotherapeutic agents work
   D. Side effects of chemotherapy

Problems and Questions

1. Discuss why it is necessary to control microbial growth.
2. Give the definitions for sterilization, disinfection, pasteurization, and lyophilization.
3. What are the differences between sterile, aseptic, and antiseptic techniques? In what circumstances might each be used?
4. What are the characteristics of bacteria indicated by the following terms: psychrophilic, mesophilic, thermophilic, halophilic, haloduric, alkaliphilic, acidophilic?
5. What are the characteristics of a good antimicrobial agent?
6. List some effective physical and chemical means of controlling microbial growth.
7. How do chemotherapeutic agents destroy microbes without also killing the patient?
8. Discuss why antibiotics should be used discriminately.

Self Test

After you have read Chapter 5, examined the objectives, studied the key words, reviewed the study outline, and answered the questions at the end of the chapter, complete the following self test.

Matching Exercises

Complete each statement from the list of words provided with each section.

Terms

disinfection   sterilization   pasteurization
fungicidal agent   fungistatic agent   sepsis
asepsis   antiseptic technique   sterile technique
aseptic technique

1. A chemical that kills fungi is a _fungicidal agent_.
2. A chemical that inhibits the growth of the fungus that causes athlete's foot is a _fungistatic agent_.
3. The growth of infectious microorganisms in living tissues is _sepsis_.
4. The surgical technique of using disinfectants and antiseptics to cleanse the skin, instruments, and so on, is the _aseptic technique_
5. The lack of infectious microorganisms on living tissues is

   _____.
6. The surgical technique that eliminates and avoids pathogens is _sterile_ .
7. The process of opening a sterile packet without exposing the sterile equipment to any microorganisms is the _____.
8. A process during which all microorganisms are killed is called _sterilization_.
9. The process of destroying the harmful microorganisms from nonliving objects is called _sterilization_.
10. Heating milk to destroy the pathogens is called _pasteurization_.
11. To spray the base of the shower stall to kill the fungi growing there, one could use Lysol, a _fungicidal agent_.
12. When you apply iodine or Merthiolate to a cut or abrasion, you are using the _____ technique.
13. The microbes that spoil beer and wine can be destroyed by _pasteurization_.
14. Washing the tabletops with an antimicrobial agent is an example of _disinfection_.

Microbial Types

thermophiles   mesophiles   psychrophiles
halophiles   aerobes   acidophiles
alkalophiles   barophiles   obligate anaerobes
facultative anaerobes

1. Organisms that can thrive deep within the ocean, in a high barometric
   pressure, are _barophiles_.
2. Organisms that can live in the digestive tract or in the air are
   facultative anaerobes.
3. Microbes that die in the presence of oxygen are _obligate anaerobes_.
4. Microbes that thrive best in the air are considered _aerobes_.
5. The organisms that are not inhibited by chlorine or iodine disinfectants
   and tolerate a high salt concentration are called _____.
6. Those microbes that can live in the acid environment of the stomach
   are _acidophiles_.
7. Those microbes that prefer the basic environment of the intestine are
   alkalophiles.
8. The microbes found living in an iceberg are _psychrophiles_.
9. Those organisms that can live in hot springs are _thermophiles_.
10. Most pathogens are _mesophiles_ because they grow best at
    body temperature.
11. When you gargle with salt water most of the microbes are inhibited
    except the staphylococci, which are _____.
12. *Escherichia coli* and other enteric bacteria would be considered

    _____.

13. Pathogens of the genus *Clostridium* are all sporeformers, and they grow
    best in a closed wound or jar; they are therefore called
    obligate anaerobes.
14. The pathogen that causes botulism is one of the _____.

Physical Antimicrobial Methods

ultraviolet rays   x-rays   filtration
desiccation   autoclaving   sonic waves
osmotic pressure

1. Microorganisms of various sizes may be removed so that the remaining
   solution may be sterile by a process called _filtration_.

2. The use of concentrated salt and sugar solutions inhibits the growth of bacteria by changing the _osn atr pressure_.
3. An excellent method of cleaning and sterilizing delicate instruments, which also can be used to destroy the viruses that cause warts, is the use of _sonic waves_.
4. Rays that can be used to prepare organs for transplantation but that are lethal to human tissues as well as to pathogens are _ultraviolet rays x-rays_
5. The radiation used to keep certain areas sterile, such as cabinets containing sterile instruments and equipment, consists of _ultraviolet rays_.
6. When pressurized steam is used to kill microorganisms as well as spores, the process is called _autoclaving_.
7. When all the moisture is removed, microbes are inhibited by _desiccation_.
8. The rays of the sun that cause suntans and may cause skin cancer are the _ultraviolet rays_

Chemical Antimicrobial Methods

ethyl alcohol   isopropyl alcohol   detergent or soap
phenolics   hydrogen peroxide   mercury salts
formalin   ethylene oxide

1. The alcohol that is toxic when taken internally but is good for rubbing on the skin is _____.
2. The alcohol that is the best antiseptic, which may also be taken internally, is _____.
3. An oxidizing agent that is frequently used to cleanse wounds and remove pus is _____.
4. A solution that is sporicidal but is too caustic to use on living tissues is _____.
5. Lysol and carbolic acid are _____.
6. Merthiolate is one of the _____.
7. Before surgery, the doctor scrubs well with a _____ to destroy the surface bacteria on the skin.
8. A toxic, inflammable gas that is sporicidal and is used in gas autoclaves is _____.

Chemotherapy

antibiotic	penicillin	sulfanilamide
salvarsan	broad-spectrum	Prontosil
amphotericin B	antibiotics	

1. The first antibiotic, which was discovered by Fleming, purified by Florey and Chain, and isolated from a mold, is _____.
2. The antibiotics that are effective against many gram-positive and gram-negative pathogens are known as _____.
3. The drug that worked against *in vivo* streptococcal infections but was not effective *in vitro* was _____.
4. One drug that is effective against fungal infections is _____.
5. When Prontosil was broken apart, one half of the molecule was effective against gram-positive infections *in vitro*. This drug is

   _____.
6. A chemotherapeutic drug that is derived from a living organism (fungi, bacteria) is called an _____.
7. The chemotherapeutic agent that Ehrlich isolated after 605 unsuccessful attempts was _____.
8. The first chemotherapeutic drug found to be effective against syphilis was _____.
9. The chemotherapeutic drug used against syphilis today is

   _____.

True or False (T or F)

_____ 1. The sulfonamide drugs inhibit the production of the essential vitamin folic acid in all fungi.

_____ 2. Penicillin interferes with the synthesis of nuclei in bacteria.

_____ 3. Chemotherapeutic drugs work by inhibiting a specific essential step in the metabolism of a pathogen, which is different from the metabolism of a human cell.

_____ 4. Drugs that destroy viral infections generally also destroy host cells.

_____ 5. Drugs that destroy cancer cells affect all rapidly dividing cells.

_____ 6. Many pathogens can mutate to become resistant to chemotherapeutic drugs by changing their metabolic pathways.

_____ 7. The concentration of a disinfectant is not important; it will be effective at any concentration.

_____ 8. The mycobacteria that cause leprosy and tuberculosis are among the most resistant pathogens.

_____ 9. A rough, porous surface is more easily disinfected than a smooth, hard surface.

_____ 10. Formaldehyde and ethylene oxide are not effective against spores.
_____ 11. Pasteurization kills all the bacteria present in milk.
_____ 12. All bacteria must be destroyed because they all cause disease.
_____ 13. An infectious disease is any disease caused by the growth of microorganisms.
_____ 14. An antiseptic is a mild disinfectant used on the skin.
_____ 15. The antiseptic technique was developed by Lister in the late 1800s.

Multiple Choice

1. A bactericide would be effective against
   a. viruses
   b. endospores
   c. bacteria
   d. all of the above
2. Pasteurization is a good example of
   a. sterilization
   b. disinfection
   c. tyndallization
   d. antiseption
3. A combination of freezing and drying of microbes is called
   a. desiccation
   b. disinfection
   c. lyophilization
   d. hemolysis
4. The organisms found in the Great Salt Lake are
   a. thermophilic
   b. barophilic
   c. mesoduric
   d. halophilic
5. In a hypertonic solution the osmotic pressure
   a. increases
   b. stays the same
   c. diffuses
   d. decreases
6. An effective disinfectant must be effective against
   a. fungal spores

   b. _Mycobacterium tuberculosis_
   c. _Pseudomonas_ species
   d. hepatitis viruses
   e. all of the above
7. _Clostridium perfringens_ is the causative agent of
   a. tetanus
   b. leprosy
   c. gas gangrene
   d. ringworm
8. The most effective method of sterilization is
   a. moist heat combined with pressure
   b. chemical
   c. boiling
   d. dry heat combined with pressure
9. Sulfonamide drugs are considered
   a. bacterial
   b. sporicidal
   c. bacteriostatic
   d. viristatic
10. Modern chemotherapy began with the development of
   a. penicillin
   b. Prontosil
   c. salvarsan
   d. sulfanilamide
11. Thermal death time is
   a. time required to kill all cells at a given temperature

b. temperature that kills all cells in a given time
c. time and temperature needed to kill all cells
d. all of a–c choices
e. none of a–c choices

12. Asepsis refers to
    a. no organisms are present
    b. procedures that reduce spread of microorganisms
    c. barrier to infection is maintained

d. sterility of materials is maintained
e. all of a–d choices

13. The usual autoclaving temperature is
    a. 100°C
    b. 62.8°C
    c. 50°C
    e. 15°C
    e. 121°C

Chapter 6

Human and Microbial Interactions

Objectives

After studying this chapter, you should be able to

1. Discuss the importance of indigenous microflora and where it is found
2. List four types of symbiotic relationships
3. Differentiate between mutualism and commensalism and give examples of each
4. Describe one parasitic relationship
5. Discuss the factors related to the pathogenicity of microbes
6. Describe the ecological interrelationships of plants, animals, and microorganisms.

New Words

Antibiosis (an-tee-buy-oh'-sis). An antagonistic relationship

Bacillus (bah-sil'-lus). A rod-shaped bacterium

Commensalism (co-men'-sal-izm). A relationship in which one member benefits and the other is unaffected in any way

Indigenous (in-di'-gen-us). Native, natural, normal, inate, as in "indigenous microflora."

Infection (in-feck'-shun). The growth of parasitic microorganisms in a host

Mutualism (mew'-chew-al-izm). A relationship in which both organisms benefit

Parasitism (par'-uh-sit-izm). A relationship in which an organism benefits at the expense of the host organism

Pathogen (path'-o-jen). A microorganism that produces disease in the host

Spirochete (spy'-row-keet). A spiral-shaped bacterium

Symbionts (sim′-bee-yonts). Organisms living together

Symbiosis (sim′-bee-oh′-sis). A constant relationship between two or more unlike species of organisms

Synergism (sin′-er-jizm). A mutualistic relationship in which organisms accomplish together what neither could do alone

Indigenous Microflora

The indigenous microflora, or normal flora, of a person includes all the microbes that normally are found on or within the human body. These microorganisms include bacteria, fungi, protozoa, and viruses. A fetus has no indigenous microflora. During and after delivery a newborn is exposed to many microorganisms from the mother, the food, the air, and everything that touches the infant. Both harmless and helpful microbes take up residence on the skin, at all the body openings, and in the mucous membranes that line the digestive tract (mouth to anus) and the urogenital tract. In these areas the moist, warm environment provides excellent conditions for growth. The conditions for proper growth (moisture *p*H, temperature, oxygen supply, nutrients) vary throughout the body; thus, the types of resident normal flora differ from one part to another. Blood, lymph, and most internal organs should be free of microorganisms. See Table 6–1 for a list of the indigenous microflora frequently found within and on the human body.

Only a few types of microbes establish themselves as indigenous microflora because most of the organisms in our external environment do not find the body to be a suitable host. In addition to the *resident* microflora, *transient* microflora take up temporary residence in humans. The body is constantly exposed to the flow of microorganisms from the outside, and these transient microbes frequently are attracted to the moist body areas. These microbes are temporary "guests" for many reasons: they may be washed from the external areas by bathing; they may not be able to compete with the resident microflora; they may fail to survive in the acid or alkaline environment of the area; or they may be flushed out in excretions, such as urine, feces, tears, and perspiration.

Destruction of the resident microflora disturbs the balance established between the host and its microorganisms. Prolonged therapy with certain antibiotics often destroys the normal intestinal microflora; diarrhea is usually the result of such an imbalance, which, in turn, leaves the body more susceptible to secondary invaders. When the number of normal resident microbes is greatly reduced, opportunistic invaders may establish themselves within those areas. One important opportunist usually found in small numbers near the body openings is the yeast, *Candida albicans*, which, in the absence of sufficient numbers of other resident microflora, may grow unchecked in the mouth, vagina, or lower intestine, causing the disease candidiasis (also known as thrush or moniliasis; see Fig. 2–23).

Table 6–1. Locations of Microorganisms Normally Found in Humans

Normal Flora	Skin	Eye	Ear	Mouth	Nose	Respiratory Tract	Intestine	Urogenital Tract
Bacteria								
Bacillus spp.	+	−	−	+	−	−	+	−
Bacteriodes	+	−	−	+	+	+	+	+
Borrelia spp.	−	−	−	+	−	−	−	+
Clostridium spp.	+	−	−	−	−	−	+	+
Coliforms	+	−	−	−	−	+	+	+
Escherichia coli	−	−	−	−	−	−	+	+
Corynebacterium spp.	+	+	+	+	+	+	+	+
Fusobacteriuim spp.	−	−	−	+	−	−	+	−
Haemophilus influenzae	−	+	+	−	+	+	−	−
Klebsiella pneumoniae	−	−	−	−	+	−	+	−
Lactobacillus spp.	+	−	+	+	−	−	+	+
Leptotrichia	−	−	−	+	−	−	−	+
Micrococcus spp.	+	−	−	+	−	−	+	−
Mycobacterium spp.	−	−	+	−	−	−	−	+
Mycoplasmas (PPLO)	−	−	−	+	+	+	+	+
Neisseria spp.	−	+	−	+	+	+	−	+
Proteus spp.	−	−	−	−	−	−	+	+
Pseudomonas aeruginosa	−	−	+	−	−	−	+	−
Staphylococci	+	+	+	+	+	+	+	+
S. aureus	+	−	+	+	+	−	−	−
S. epidermidis	+	+	+	+	+	−	−	−
Streptococci	+	+	+	+	+	+	+	+
S. mitis	+	+	−	+	+	−	−	−
S. pneumoniae	−	+	+	+	+	−	−	−
S. pyogenes	+	+	+	−	−	−	−	−
Veillonella spp.	−	−	−	+	−	−	+	−
Fungi								
Actinomyces spp.	−	−	−	+	−	−	−	−
Candida albicans	+	+	−	+	−	−	+	+
Cryptococcus spp.	+	−	−	−	−	−	−	−
Protozoa	−	−	−	+	−	−	+	+
Viruses	+	−	−	+	+	+	+	−

+, present; −, absent

Microflora of the Skin

The resident microflora of the skin consists primarily of bacteria and fungi. The number and species of microorganisms present depends on many factors. Moist, warm conditions in hairy areas where there are many sweat and oil glands, such as under the arms and in the groin, stimulate the growth of staphylococci, streptococci, diphtheroids, aerobic spore-forming bacilli, nonpathogenic mycobacteria, gram-negative enteric bacilli (*Echerichia coli*), as well as the fungi *Candida albicans* and *Cryptococcus*. Dry, calloused areas of skin have few bacteria, whereas the moist folds between the toes and fingers support many bacteria and fungi. The surface of the skin near the mucosal openings of the body (the mouth, eyes, nose, anus, and genitalia) is inhabited by bacteria present in their secretions.

Frequent washing with soap and water removes most of the potentially harmful transient microorganisms harbored in sweat, oil, and other secretions from moist body parts. All persons involved in patient care must be particularly careful to keep their skin and clothing as free of transient microbes as possible, to help prevent personal infections and to avoid transferring the pathogens to patients. Such persons should always remember that most infections following burns, wounds, and surgery result from the growth of resident or transient skin microflora in these susceptible areas.

Microflora of the Mouth

The mouth and throat have an abundant and varied population of microorganisms. These areas provide the moist, warm mucous membranes that furnish excellent conditions for microbial growth. Bacteria thrive especially well in particles of food and in the debris of dead epithelial cells around the teeth. The peculiar anatomy of the oral cavity and the throat affords shelter for numerous anaerobic and aerobic bacteria. Anaerobic microorganisms flourish in the gum margins, in cervices between the teeth, and in the deep folds (crypts) on the surface of the tonsils.

The list of microbes that have been isolated from normal human mouths reads like a manual of the main groups of microorganisms. It includes cocci, bacilli, and spirilla, as well as yeasts, moldlike organisms, protozoa, and viruses. The first such list was made by Leeuwenhoek in 1690.

Most miroorganisms normally found in the mouth and throat are beneficial (or at least harmless); these include the diphtheroids, bacteroids, lactobacilli, and micrococci. Others, such as certain streptococci and staphylococci, are potentially pathogenic opportunists and are frequently associated with disease. Some people carry virulent pathogens in their throats but do not have the diseases associated with the pathogens, such as diphtheria, meningitis, pneumonia, and tuberculosis. Thse people are "healthy carriers" who are resistant to these pathogens, but can transmit the pathogens to susceptible persons.

Food remaining on and between the teeth provides a rich nutrient medium for the growth of the many oral bacteria. Carelessness in dental hygiene allows growth of these bacteria, with development of dental caries (tooth decay) and gingivitis (gum disease). These bacteria include species of *Actinomyces, Lactobacillus, Streptococci, Neisseria,* and *Veillonella.*

Many α-hemolytic streptococci are indigenous normal inhabitants of the mouth and oropharynx. When β-hemolytic streptococci are present, however, the person should be treated with an antibiotic to destroy these pathogens that may cause "strep" throat and its complications.

Microflora of the Ear and Eye

The middle ear and inner ear are normally sterile, whereas the outer ear and the auditory canal contain the same types of microorganisms as are found on moist skin areas, such as the mouth and the nose. When a person coughs, sneezes, or blows his nose, these microbes are carried along the eustachian tube and into the middle ear where they can cause infection. Infection can also develop in the middle ear when the eustachian tube does not open and close properly to maintain correct air pressure within the ear.

Many microorganisms are found in the external opening of the eye, in the conjunctiva that lines the eyelid, and in the tears. But these microbes are not a frequent cause of disease because the intact membranes serve as a barrier. These mucous membranes are constantly flushed by the tears, which contain an enzyme called lysozyme that destroys bacteria. The indigenous microflora in the eye area includes species of *Staphylococcus, Streptococcus,* and *Corynebacterium,* as well as *Branhamella (Neisseria) catarrhalis.*

Microflora of the Respiratory Tract

The respiratory tract consists of the nose, pharynx (throat), larynx (voice box), trachea, bronchi, bronchioles, and alveoli. The lower respiratory tract, below the larynx, is normally free of microbes because the mucous membranes and lungs have defense mechanisms that efficiently remove the invaders. Thus, staphylococci, streptococci, *Pseudomonas* species, or yeasts found in sputum specimens would indicate either an infectious disease of the lungs or specimen contamination by the indigenous microflora of the upper respiratory tract.

The membranes of the upper part of the tract, which includes the nasopharynx and the oropharynx, provide a suitable environment for the growth of many species of *Streptococcus, Staphylococcus, Neisseria, Corynebacterium,* and other microorganisms and yeasts. In susceptible persons, many of these opportunists can quickly cause disease.

Microflora of the Urogenital Area

The normal kidney, ureters, and bladder are sterile. However, the external opening of the urethra houses many normal microflora, such as nonpathogenic *Neisseria* species, staphylococci, enterococci, diphtheroids, mycobacteria, mycoplasms, enteric (intestinal) gram-negative rods, yeasts, and viruses. As a rule, these organisms do not invade the bladder, because it is constantly flushed by the acidic urine; however, persistent, recurring urinary infections can develop with obstruction or narrowing of the urethra and with infrequent urination, which allows the invasive organisms to multiply and cause urinary tract infections. Chlamydias and mycoplasms are frequent causes of nongonococcal urethritis (NGU). All of these organisms are easily introduced into the urethra by sexual intercourse.

The reproductive systems of both men and women are normally sterile, with the exception of the vagina; here the flora varies with the stage of sexual development. During puberty and following menopause, the vaginal secretions are alkaline, supporting the growth of various diphtheroids, streptococci, staphylococci, and coliforms (enteric gram-negative rods); through the childbearing years, the vagina secretions are acidic, encouraging the growth mainly of lactobacilli, along with a few α-hemolytic streptococci, staphylococci, diphtheroids, and yeasts.

The *Neisseria* species, particularly *Neisseria gonorrhoeae* (also called the gonococcus), can survive the acidic environment of the vagina and the penis; hence, they may be harbored by infected persons who show no symptoms of gonorrhea. This disease, which is readily transmitted through sexual contact, is asymptomatic (causes no symptoms) among 80% of infected women and among 20% of infected men.

Microflora of the Gastrointestinal Tract

The acidic environment of the stomach prevents the growth of normal indigenous microflora. However, a few microbes, protected by foods, manage to pass through the stomach during periods of low acid concentration. Also, when the amount of acid is reduced in the course of diseases such as stomach cancer, certain bacteria may be found in this site.

Normally, in the upper portion of the small intestine, the duodenum, few microflora exist because bile inhibits the growth of most microbes, but many are found in the lower part of the small intestine. The most abundant organisms include many species of *Staphylococcus*, *Lactobacillus*, *Streptobacillus*, *Veillonella*, and *Clostridium perfringens*.

The colon, or large intestine, contains large numbers of microorganisms growing on the food wastes collected there. Obligate anaerobic bacteria make up most of the colon population, including gram-positive *Clostridium* species and gram-negative *Bacteroides* and *Fusobacterium* species. Normally, less than 10% of the large intestine microflora are facultative anaerobes that are easily grown in the laboratory, including *Eschierichia coli, Enterobacter aerogenes,* and species of *Proteus, Pseudomonas, Streptococcus, Lactobacillus,* and *Mycoplasma.* Also, many fungi, protozoa, and viruses are found in the intestine. Usually these normal microflora are opportunists, often causing disease only when they lodge in the other areas or when the balance among the microorganisms is upset.

Beneficial Roles of Indigenous Microflora

Many benefits are derived by humans from the symbiotic relationship established with their normal microbial population. Some nutrients, particularly vitamins K, B_{12}, pantothenic acid, pyridoxine, and biotin are obtained from secretions of the coliform bacteria.

Evidence also indicates that these indigenous microbes provide a constant source of irritants and antigens to stimulate the immune system. Thus, the immune complex responds more readily by producing antibodies to other foreign invaders and substances, enhancing protection against disease-producing agents. It appears that by merely occupying a place and using the nutrients present, these normal microflora prevent other microorganisms that may be pathogenic from establishing a site of infection. This protection is maintained by competition for food, controlled pH and oxygen levels, and antibiotic production by certain of the resident microbes.

When the delicate balance of the various species in the population of indigenous microflora is upset by antibiotic or other chemotherapy, many complications may result. Certain microorganisms may flourish out of control, such as the yeast that is the cause of candidiasis. Also, diarrhea and intestinal upsets may occur. Frequently, cultures of *Lactobacillus* in yogurt or present in medications are prescribed to reestablish and stabilize the microbial balance.

Symbiotic Relationships

The relationship between normal microflora and the human host is an excellent example of *symbiosis.* This term is the name given to a general relationship between organisms living in close proximity. The symbionts (the organisms that live together) are two or more organisms of unlike species. The relationship may be beneficial, harmless, or harmful to one, several, or all of the symbionts. The types of relationships outlined in the following sections demonstrate that the pathogenicity of a microbe can be represented as a balance between the virulence of the pathogen and the resistance of the host. These factors are further discussed in later chapters.

Mutualism   In the symbiotic relationship called mutualism, both organisms benefit and, in fact, depend on each other metabolically. An example is the intestinal bacterium *Escherichia coli,* which obtains nutrients from food materials ingested by the host and produces vitamin K to be used by the host. Vitamin K is a blood-clotting factor that is essential in humans. Also, some protozoa live symbiotically in the intestine of the termite and enable the termite to digest the wood it eats by breaking down the wood cellulose into nutrients to be absorbed and used. In turn, the termite provides food and a place for the protozoa to live. Without these protozoa, the termite would die of starvation. A stable marriage could also be thought of as a mutualistic relationship.

In some mutualistic relationships, two organisms work together to produce a result that neither could accomplish alone. This is called *synergism*, or a synergistic relationship. The fusiform bacillus and the spirochete, which together cause the disease trench mouth, represent such a relationship. Also, the nitrogen-fixing bacteria and the roots of legumes where they exist have a true synergistic relationship, because each depends on the other for nutrients.

Commensalism   A relationship in which one member is benefited but the host organism is neither benefited nor harmed is called commensalism. These organisms "eat at the same table" in close proximity, but are not dependent on each other. Most of the normal microflora of humans are considered to be commensals, in that the microbes are provided nutrients and housing with no effect on the welfare of the host.

Neutralism   Indiffernce, or neutralism, exists when organisms occupy the same niche but do not affect each other, as with many bacteria that live in the human mouth and intestines. However, sometimes waste products of one microorganism can destroy certain neighboring bacteria. This situation is called *antagonism* or *antibiosis*. Penicillium mold growing on a culture plate of certain strains of staphylococci inhibits the growth of the staphylococci by producing penicillin.

Parasitism   The relationship in which an organism benefits at the expense of the host organism is called parasitism. Depending on the parasite and the circumstances, the damage may be slight or it may be fatal. However, the "wise" parasite does not kill its host but rather takes only the nutrients it needs to exist. Intestinal

Insight: Lyme Disease in the United States

Although Lyme disease has been prevalent in Europe since the 1800's, it was first recognized and named in the U.S. in 1975 when 39 children and 12 adults developed arthritislike symptoms in Old Lyme, Connecticut. The etiologic agent was found at the site of a deer tick bite. This pathogen, a spirochete, was named, *Borrelia burgdorferi*, after the scientist, Willy Burgdorpher, who first isolated and described this corkscrew-shaped bacteria.

The most frequent vector carrying the spirochete from large animals and rodents to humans is a reddish brown deer tick (*Ixodes dammini*), which is about the size of the eye of a needle. The western black-legged tick, *I. pacificus*, which serves as the vector in the northwestern U.S., is dark brown and the size of a poppy seed.

This disease has been identified in 43 states but has been reported most commonly in the northeast and northwest sections of the United States. Over 8,000 cases were reported in 1990. The disease is called the "great imitator", because it is so easy to misdiagnose, since the symptoms imitate those of many other diseases. Lyme disease symptoms usually occur in three stages. The early localized stage symptoms may occur within hours after the individual is bitten by an infected tick. At the site of the tick bite, a localized redness (erythema migrans) occurs. This ring-shaped rash is usually more than 5 cm in diameter. Simultaneously other flulike symptoms (headache, fever, chills, fatigue, aches and pains) develop, lasting about a week. In some people, this stage may be asymptomatic.

Months after the first stage, symptoms disappear, and the more severe second stage, or early disseminated stage, begins, including skin blotches, malaise, fatigue, enlarged lymph nodes, abnormal heart rhythms, joint and muscle pain, and encephalomyelitis with numbness and psychological problems. This secondary stage may last for weeks or months and then disappears.

Several months or years later, the third stage, or late persistent infection, symptoms may appear. The symptoms of this tertiary stage may include arthritis with swelling, pain and stiffness of the large joints, debilitating fatigue, chronic encephalomyelitis, and neuropathy with subtle mental disorders. During pregnancy, the spirochetes may cross the placental barrier and cause cardiac and neurological damage in the developing fetus.

Early diagnosis via antibody assays and treatment with amoxicillin, doxycycline, or cephalosporin can help relieve the pain and suffering for many patients with Lyme disease.

The best approach to the prevention of infection is the avoidance of tick infested areas. Always wear a hat, long-sleeved shirt, and long pants cinched at the ankle. Use a tick repellant containing DEET (diethyltoluamide) on skin and clothing, and always check yourself for ticks when returning from a walk in the woods. Remove any attached ticks with tweezers, apply a disinfectant, and observe the area for development of a rash. If a rash or other flulike symptoms develops following a tick bite, consult your physician.

worms, such as pinworms and tapeworms, and external parasites, such as mites, lice, and ticks, usually cause only minor damage in humans. The presence of these multicellular parasites in or on a host is referred to as an *infestation*, whereas invasion and multiplication of the unicellular parasites (microorganisms) that cause cellular damage is called an *infection* by pathogens.

Pathogenic Relationships   When parasitic microorganisms cause damage to the host during the infection process, a pathogenic relationship exists. The pathogen may be only a displaced commensal; for example, the staphylococci that normally inhabit the skin can cause an infection when the skin is wounded or burned. It may be a highly virulent airbone pathogen, such as the common cold virus, or it may be carried in food and water such as the dysentery pathogen. An *opportunist* is a pathogen that causes disease only in a host who is physically impaired or debilitated, because his normal defenses against disease are weakened. Pneumonia developing in a bedridden patient is another example of a pathogenic relationship. Thus, in the normal course of events, the opportunist microbe is harmless; it moves in to cause damage when an abnormal situation develops, such as a wound or a burn or the destruction of the normal microflora by antibiotic therapy (see Fig. 6–1).

Nonpathogenic Microbes   Microbes that never cause disease or do so only in rare circumstances in an extremely susceptible host are referred to as nonpathogenic microorganisms.

Microbial Ecology

Ecology is the systematic study of the interrelationships of various organisms to other organisms and to their shared environment. The interactions of microorganisms with animals, plants, and other microbes have far-reaching effects on our lives. We are all aware of diseases caused by microbial infections; this is just one example of the effects of one type of organism on another. Most of these relationships in nature are beneficial rather than harmful.

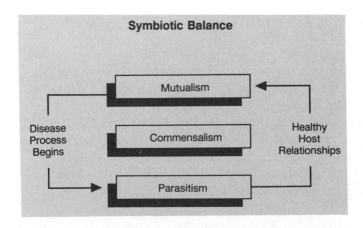

Figure 6–1. The dynamic symbiotic balance may shift toward the parasitic/ pathogenic disease state if the host defenses are reduced with an accompanying rise in host susceptibility. Recovery from disease occurs with a shift toward mutualism and commensalism.

Bacteria are exceptionally adaptable and versatile and are found on the land, in all waters, in every animal and plant, and even in other microorganisms. Some bacteria and fungi serve a valuable function by recycling back into the soil the nutrients from dead, decaying animals and plants, as discussed in Chapters 1 and 4 (see Fig. 1–3). The free-living fungi and bacteria that decompose dead organic matter into inorganic materials are called saprophytes. The inorganic nutrients that are returned to the soil are used by autotrophic bacteria and plants for synthesis of cellular biochemicals necessary to their growth; the plants are eaten by animals, which eventually die and are recycled again with the aid of the saprophytes.

Good examples of the cycling of nutrients in nature are the nitrogen, carbon, oxygen, sulfur, and phosphorus cycles, in which the microorganisms play very important roles in the following manner. In the nitrogen cycle, the free atmospheric nitrogen (N_2) is converted by nitrogen-fixing bacteria and cyanobacteria into ammonia (NH_3), nitrite (NO_2^-), and nitrate (NO_3^-) compounds in the soil (Fig. 6–2). The plants then use the nitrate to build plant proteins; these proteins are eaten by animals, which then use them to build animal proteins. The excreted

Figure 6–2. The nitrogen cycle. Nitrogen of the air is converted by nitrogen-fixing bacteria and algae into ammonia, nitrites, and nitrates. These inorganic nitrogen compounds are also derived from the breakdown of fecal material, and from decaying plant and animal material. The nitrates are used as food nutrients by plants, which are eaten by animals. The cycle is completed by the denitrifying bacteria, which produce free nitrogen from the inorganic nitrogen compounds.

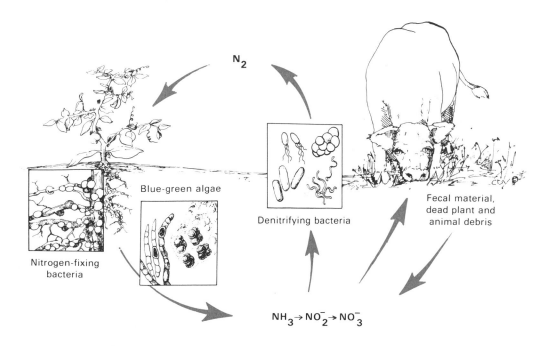

N_2

Blue-green algae

Denitrifying bacteria

Fecal material, dead plant and animal debris

Nitrogen-fixing bacteria

$NH_3 \rightarrow NO_2^- \rightarrow NO_3^-$

waste products (such as urea in urine) are converted by certain bacteria to ammonia. Also, the dead plant and animal debris and fecal material are transformed by the saprophytic fungi and bacteria into ammonia, nitrites, and nitrates for recycling by plants. To replenish the free nitrogen in the air, a group of bacteria called denitrifying bacteria convert nitrites and ammonia to atmospheric nitrogen (N_2). Thus, the cycle continues.

The nitrogen-fixing bacteria are of two types, free-living and symbiotic ("living together"). The symbiotic bacteria live in and near the root nodules of plants called legumes — alfalfa, clover, peas, soy beans, and peanuts (Fig. 6–3). These plants are often used in crop-rotation techniques by farmers to return nitrogen compounds to the soil and thus avoid the loss of nutrients.

The types and amounts of microorganisms living in the soil depend on many factors: amount of decaying organic material, available nutrients, moisture present, oxygen available, acidity, temperature, and the waste products of other microbes present. Likewise, the types and number of harmless microbes that live on and within the human body depend on the pH (acidity), moisture, nutrients, antibacterial factors, and the presence of other microorganisms.

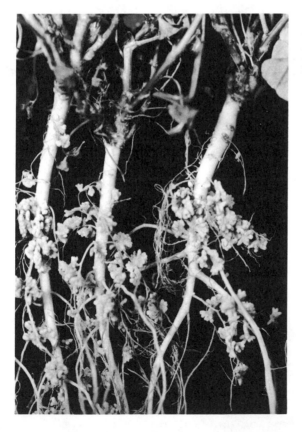

Figure 6–3. Bacterial nodules on the roots of a legume. (Lechavalier HA, Pramer D: The Microbes. Philadelphia, JB Lippincott, 1970)

Summary

The interrelationships of the organisms, plants, animals, and microbes, are discussed in this chapter. You will become aware of how necessary the microorganisms are for the survival of humankind in this environment. Apparently by mutation, some of the harmless microorganisms have developed the ability to invade other organisms and cause disease. These are the opportunists and the true pathogens.

Study Outline

I. Indigenous microflora of humans.
  A. Skin
  B. Mouth
  C. Ear and eye
  D. Respiratory tract
  E. Urogenital area
  F. Gastrointestinal tract
II. Symbiotic relationships
  A. Definition of symbiosis
  B. Mutualism
    1. Synergism
  C. Commensalism
  D. Neutralism
    1. Antagonism
  E. Parasitism
    1. Infestation
    2. Infection
    3. Pathogens
    4. Opportunists
    5. Nonpathogens
III. Microbial ecology
  A. Cycling of nutrients
    1. Nitrogen cycle
  B. Factors affecting types and amounts of microbes

Problems and Questions

1. What relationship exists between humans and their indigenous microflora?
2. Where would you find symbiotic relationships in your environment?
3. What are the differences between mutualism, commensalism, neutralism, antagonism, and parasitism?
4. Why are the microbial decomposers so necessary for life on earth?
5. What factors control the number of microorganisms in the soil and on the human body?

Self Test

After you have read Chapter 6, examined the objectives, studied the new words, reviewed the study outline and answered the questions at the end of the chapter, complete the following self tests.

Matching Exercises

Complete each statement from the list of words provided with each section.

Symbiotic Relationships

symbiotic   mutualism   synergism
antibiosis   pathogen   opportunist
symbionts   commensalism   neutralism
parasite   infestation   infection

1. A parasitic microorganism that causes damage to its host is called a _pathogen_ .

2. An organism that lives on or within a host organism is called a ~~symbiont~~ _parasite_ .

3. If a parasite is multicellular, like pinworms, the host has an _infestation_ .

4. If the parasite is a single-celled microbe, the host has an _infection_ .

5. When two organisms live together they live in a _symbiotic_ relationship.

6. The two organisms that live together are termed _symbionts_ .

7. If both organisms benefit from the relationship, they live in a state of _mutualism_ .

8. If the two organisms work together to produce an effect, they live in a state of _synergism_ .

9. If one organism secretes a material that damages or repels another organism, the two organisms live in a state of _antibiosis_ .

10. The secretion of penicillin by a *Penicillium* mold in an area where bacteria are established would be an example of _antibiosis_ .

11. When two organisms live together without harming or benefiting each other, the relationship is termed _neutralism_ .

12. If the growth of one organism benefits another one, the relationship is one of _commensalism_ .

True or False (T or F)

_F_ 1. All normal microflora are nonpathogens.

_T_ 2. Newborn infants acquire their first resident microflora organisms as they pass through the birth canal.

_T_ 3. The saprophytes aid in the cycling of nutrients, which provides plants with proper carbon, oxygen, sulfur, phosphorus, and nitrogen sources.

___ 4. Nitrogen-fixing protozoa change free nitrogen from the air into ammonia, nitrites, and nitrates.

___ 5. Legumes, like alfalfa and clover, help fertilize the soil because of the bacteria that live on and in their roots.

___ 6. The yeast *Candida albicans* is a normal microflora organism that may become an opportunist.

___ 7. The cool, dry areas of the skin support the growth of most indigenous microflora of the skin.

___ 8. Wound and burn infections are frequently caused by resident microflora.

___ 9. Careless dental hygiene encourages dental caries and gingivitis.

___ 10. Beta-hemolytic streptococci are responsible for "strep" throat, scarlet fever, and rheumatic fever.

___ 11. The lysozyme found in saliva and tears helps to destroy bacteria.

Multiple Choice

1. Symbionts could also be identified as
   a. opportunists
   b. parasites
   c. mutualists
   d. all of the above

2. Normal microflora that are facultative anaerobes are most apt to be found
   a. in the stomach
   b. in the mouth
   c. on the skin
   d. in the large intestine

3. The presence of the intestinal bacterium *Escherichia coli* as resident microflora is an example of
   a. mutualism
   b. neutralism
   c. parasitism
   d. commensalism

4. The normal microflora of the blood might be
   a. *Streptococcus*
   b. *Proteus*
   c. *Staphylococcus*
   d. none of the above

5. Nitrate compounds in the soil are utilized by plants to
   a. synthesize carbohydrates
   b. give off nitrogen
   c. build plant proteins
   d. neutralize toxins

6. *Escherichia coli* is a normal inhabitant of the
   a. intestinal tract
   b. vagina
   c. urinary tract
   d. mouth

7. The synthesis of vitamins B and K by enteric bacteria is an example of
   a. commensalism
   b. mutualism
   c. opportunism
   d. infection

8. Indigenous microflora that are harmless are called
   a. aerobes
   b. commensals
   c. opportunists
   d. parasites
   e. cytopathogenic

9. The greatest microbial population on the skin is
   a. *Staphylococcus*
   b. *Streptococcus*
   c. *Diplococcus*
   d. *Klebsiella*
   e. *Neisseria*

10. A gram-negative faculative bacterium you would expect to see in fecal material is
    a. bacteriophage
    b. plasmid
    c. *Klebsiella*
    d. β-hemolytic streptococcus
    e. *Escherichia coli*

11. A microbe that lives on its host and gives no evidence of benefit or harm is known as a (an)
    a. symbiont
    b. commensal
    c. leech
    d. opportunist

Chapter 7

Microbes versus Humans

Objectives

After studying this chapter, you should be able to

1. Differentiate between infectious, communicable, and contagious disease
2. List six reasons why an infection may not occur when a pathogen is present
3. Discuss the disease process
4. Define acute and chronic disease
5. State the difference between primary and secondary diseases
6. State the difference between local and generalized infections
7. List three factors associated with the virulence of a pathogen
8. List and discuss eight factors that affect the pathogenicity of bacteria
9. Write the meaning of the following terms: *epidemiology, epidemic, endemic,* and *pandemic*
10. Describe the difference between sporadic and nonendemic diseases
11. List three factors that contribute to an epidemic
12. List six reservoirs of infection
13. List five modes of disease transmission
14. Discuss the procedure for stopping an epidemic

New Words

Amebiasis (ah-me-buy'-uh-sis). A disease caused by a protozoan, *Entamoeba histolytica*

Arthropod (ar'-throw-pod). A phylum classification of animals including insects, mites, lice, ticks, and fleas

Coagulase (co-ag'-you-laze). An enzyme that clots plasma around bacteria

Collagenase (col-lodge'-in-aze). An enzyme that breaks down collagen in connective tissue

Endemic (en-dem'-ick). A disease present in normal numbers in a community

Epidemic (ep-i-dem'-ick). More than the normal number of cases of a disease in a community at a particular time

Fibrinolysin (fy-brin-oh'-li-sin). An enzyme that breaks down fibrin clots

Fomite (fō'-mite), pl. *fomites* (fo'-mi-teez). An object such as a book or an item of clothing that is not in itself harmful but that is able to harbor pathogenic organisms and thus serve as an agent for transmission of an infection

Hemolysin (he-moll'-uh-sin). An enzyme that breaks down red blood cells

Hyaluronidase (high-al-your-on-uh-days). An enzyme that breaks down connective tissue

Leukocidin (lew-co-side'-in). An enzyme that destroys white blood cells

Pandemic (pan-dem'-ick). A worldwide epidemic

Parenteral injection (pear-ren'-ter-al). Intramuscular or intravenous

Pathogenicity (path-oh-gin-iss'-city). The ability of an organism to cause disease

Streptokinase (strep-tow-kine'-aze). An enzyme that aids streptococci to invade the body by dissolving blood clots

Toxigenicity (tox-uh-gin-iss'-city). The ability of a pathogen to produce a toxin, causing damage to the host

Toxin (tox'-in). A toxic or damaging substance

Vector (veck'-tore). A carrier (especially an arthropod) of pathogenic organisms from one host to another

Virulence (veer'-you-lence). The properties of an organism that make it pathogenic

Disease and Infections

There are many diseases that are not caused by pathogens. Included among them are those caused by malfunction of an organ, such as diabetes and hyperthyroidism; those caused by a vitamin deficiency, such as scurvy and rickets; those caused by an allergic response, such as asthma and hay fever; and those caused by uncontrolled cell growth, such as tumors and cancer. However, this chapter focuses on the many infectious diseases caused by the growth of pathogens on and in living tissues.

The ability of a pathogen to invade and infect the host, cause damage, and produce disease is termed its *virulence*. Those microbes that can cause disease with relative ease are referred to as *virulent* pathogens; microorganisms incapable of causing disease, except in rare circumstances, are described as *avirulent*. Within a single genus and species, some strains may be virulent and others avirulent, as determined by the genetic characteristics of the microorganism. Thus, when a person is exposed to a pathogen, whether a disease results depends on many factors, including the host's resistance and the virulence of the microorganism.

The potential for infections always exists when organisms live in a parasitic relationship. When a pathogen finds the appropriate places and conditions in which it can grow and cause damage, it produces an infectious disease.

An *infection* occurs when a pathogenic microbe is able to multiply in the tissues where it lodges. Thus, an *infectious* disease results from the growth of a pathogenic microorganism. A *communicable* disease can be transmitted from one person to another, as with measles, gonorrhea, and diphtheria. A *contagious* disease is a communicable disease that is easily transmitted from person to person via droplets in the air, such as occurs with the common cold and influenza.

The severity of an infectious disease and the amount of damage it causes are determined by the host's ability to resist invasion and to neutralize the damaging enzymes and toxins from the pathogen.

$$\text{Severity of infection} = \frac{\text{microbial virulence}}{\text{host defenses}}$$

Why Infection Does Not Always Occur

Many people exposed to pathogenic microbes do not get sick for numerous reasons:

1. The microbe may alight in the wrong place and be unable to multiply. For example, when a respiratory pathogen falls on the skin, it may be unable to grow because the skin lacks the necessary warmth, moisture, and nutrients required for the growth of the particular microbe.
2. Many pathogens must be able to attach to specific host receptor sites before they can multiply and cause damage.
3. Antibacterial factors that destroy or inhibit the growth of microbes may be present, for example, as lysozyme in tears, saliva, and perspiration.
4. The normal flora may inhibit the growth of the foreign microorganism in regions such as the mouth, vagina, and intestine by occupying the space and using the available nutrients.
5. The microbes already growing in the region may produce antibacterial factors (called bacteriocidins) that have a local antibiotic effect, as when streptococci inhibit the diphtheria pathogen.
6. Antibodies may be present because the person had previously had the infection or had been immunized against it. These antibodies attack and destroy the pathogen before it can multiply.
7. Phagocytes present in the mucous membranes may engulf and destroy the invader.

The Development of Infection

Infection occurs when pathogens are able to enter the host, attach, adhere, multiply, and cause damage to the tissues of the host.

The body responds to the infection via the inflammatory process (Fig. 7–1). The symptoms of inflammation are swelling (edema), redness, heat (fever), and pain. The swelling is due to the escape of large quantities of fluid from the highly permeable capillaries. The area becomes reddened because more blood is brought to it to fight the infection. The heat is caused by increased metabolic activity in the cells. Pain usually results from pressure on the nerve endings. Phagocytes rush in to help destroy the invaders and to rid the area of dead tissue. Pus is often found at the site of inflammation; it consists of lymph, serum, tissue cells, dead leukocytes, and sometimes bacteria.

The production of antibodies begins slowly; the body attempts to isolate the infection by forming a connective tissue wall that inhibits deeper penetration by the pathogens around the site of infection. If the pathogen is pyogenic (pus-forming), such as a staphylococcus or a streptococcus, the inflamed area contains much more pus than is normally present during the inflammatory process. Inflammation and antibody production are further discussed in Chapters 8 and 9, which are devoted to mechanisms of defense against disease.

The Disease Process

If the body wins the battle against the invading pathogens at the site of inflammation, the local infection is stopped. The person then has some antibodies to protect the body against a later similar infection, but the individual may become a

Figure 7–1. The development of infection and the inflammatory process. The symptoms of inflammation include swelling, redness, heat, and pain. Pus may also be present whether or not pyogenic bacteria are present.

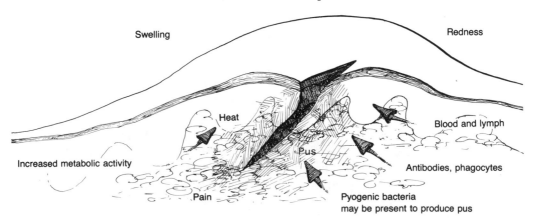

"carrier" if all of the pathogens have not been destroyed. A person may recover from a sore throat without complications, but may harbor a few resistant pathogens (become a carrier) and transmit them to others.

Clinical disease occurs when the body's primary defenses lose the battle with the pathogen. The disease may be a *local* infection in which the pathogen is confined to a single area; this is the situation in diphtheria, "staph" boils or carbuncles, "strep" throat, tuberculosis, primary syphilis, and gonorrhea. But if the pathogen is not stopped at the local level, it may emerge from this *focal* site to invade the tissues or be carried by the phagocytes to other organs or by the bloodstream as a *generalized* or *systemic* infection; this occurs in systemic streptococcal infection, staphylococcal septicemia, and meningitis.

A disease may be acute or chronic, or it may be both, beginning as an acute response that becomes a chronic illness. An *acute* disease has a rapid onset followed by a rapid recovery, as with measles, mumps, and influenza. A *chronic* disease is one of long duration and slow onset, such as tuberculosis, leprosy (Hansen's disease), and syphilis. Some diseases, such as gonorrhea, often have an acute inflammatory phase and then become chronic, causing slow deterioration of the infected tissues.

A disease may also reach a stage in which there are no symptoms (asymptomatic disease); it is then known as a *latent infection* or considered to be in a *latent stage*; tuberculosis, syphilis, gonorrhea, and herpes cold sores are examples. In tuberculosis, when the tubercles of *Mycobacterium tuberculosis* are successfully walled off in the lungs, the symptoms disappear temporarily; the infection then is said to be latent. Syphilis progresses through primary, secondary, latent, and tertiary stages (Fig. 7 – 2). The lesion, or chancre, of the primary stage appears at the site of entry of the spirochete *Treponema pallidum*. A few weeks after the spirochete has invaded the bloodstream, the chancre disappears, and the symptoms of the secondary stage arise, including rash, fever, and lesions of the mucous membranes. This is the most contagious stage of syphilis. These symptoms also disap-

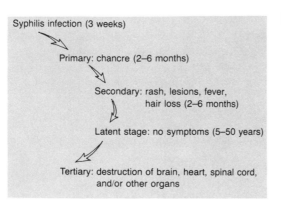

Figure 7 – 2. Stages of syphilis.

pear after a few weeks when the disease enters the latent stage, which may last from 1 to 50 years and may cause a few or no symptoms. In tertiary syphilis, the organism causes destruction of the organ where it had been hiding: the brain, the heart, or bone tissue.

Gonorrhea, caused by *Neisseria gonorrhoeae*, is often an *asymptomatic disease* in the early phase when the organism lives in the mucous membranes of the urogenital tract, rectum, or mouth. After many months, during which the organism causes damage, scarring, and construction of the fallopian tubes or vas deferens, localized pain is experienced. Gonorrhea is very contagious by direct mucous membrane-to-mucous membrane transfer, usually sexual. It is particularly difficult to detect and control because it has been shown to be asymptomatic in most infected women and in many infected men.

Cold sores, or fever blisters, and venereal herpes are caused by the herpes virus. After the initial local infection, the viruses remain dormant (latent) inside the ganglion cells of the nervous system and may not cause another local lesion until some type of stress acts as a trigger. These stresses may be fever caused by illness; heat and ultraviolet rays from the sun (sunburn); a bruise; extreme cold; or an emotional upset.

An infection that is the first or original illness is called the *primary* disease, such as a cold or influenza. A *secondary* disease or infection is caused by a pathogen that can invade only a weakened person with lowered resistance. Examples of secondary diseases or infections are pneumonia and ear or sinus infections following a primary case of influenza.

Once exposure to the pathogen has occurred, the course of infectious disease has three periods: (1) the incubation period when there are no symptoms, (2) the period of illness with progression of symptoms, and (3) the convalescent period, disability, or death (fortunately the final stage is usually the convalescent period; Fig. 7–3). The communicable diseases are most contagious during the second period. For instance, in measles the incubation period lasts 10 to 12 days after the initial exposure to the virus. The early symptoms are much like those of a cold, with an eye infection and low-grade fever, and Koplik's spots (red with white

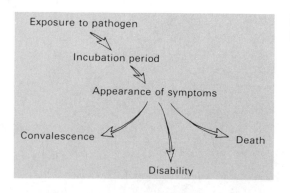

Figure 7–3. The course of infectious disease.

centers) inside the cheeks. During this early stage, the virus is easily transmitted in secretions from the eyes, nose, and mouth. As the illness progresses, a skin rash appears; it disappears during the convalescent stage. Usually, measles is considered contagious only from the time the fever begins until the second day of the rash. Complications are frequent because body defenses are lowered by the initial virus infection; thus, the virus and possibly opportunistic bacteria can invade deeper to cause pneumonia, ear and sinus infections, or encephalitis.

Although the patient may recover from the illness itself, permanent damage may be caused by the disease: brain damage may follow encephalitis or meningitis; paralysis may follow poliomyelitis; deafness may follow ear infections. This type of damage is caused by destruction of tissues in the affected area.

Mechanisms of Disease Causation

Virulence

The capacity of pathogens to cause disease (virulence) is related to their abilities (1) to infect the host or protect themselves against the body's defenses, (2) to invade and multiply in tissues, and (3) to cause damage or destruction to tissue. In other words,

$$virulence = infectivity + invasiveness + toxigenicity$$

Each species of pathogenic microbes has specific characteristics, including its unique metabolism, that determine its pathogenicity and virulence. It would be impossible to list every individual pathogen and its disease-causing mechanism in this text; in fact, the mechanism frequently is not completely understood. With these limitations in mind, we discuss some of the factors associated with virulence and pathogenicity.

The ability of a pathogen to settle on a susceptible tissue and to survive the shock of landing is largely a matter of chance. However, once it finds itself in a moist, warm environment, if it is to multiply successfully, it must be able to attach to the site (so that it is not flushed away) and it must be able to resist the body's bacteriolytic enzymes, antibodies, and phagocytes.

Bacterial Morphologic Characteristics Associated with Infection

Some structural aspects of pathogens actually enable them to attach to tissues in certain areas of the host and to survive so that they may multiply, thus causing an infection. These structures include capsules, flagella, and pili.

Capsules Capsules are often regarded as a portion of the cell envelope (including cell membrane, cell wall, and outer slime layer). Capsular constituents vary

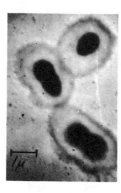

Figure 7–4. Electron micrograph of *Streptococcus pneumoniae*, type 1. The capsule has been reacted with a specific antibody (Qwellung reaction) to enhance its visibility. (Mudd S, et al: J Exp Med 78:327, 1943. By copyright permission, Rockefeller University Press)

among the different species of procaryotes. Many bacteria have slimy capsule layers, consisting of polysaccharides only; others have proteins within the polysaccharide capsule. Both serve to enable the bacteria to attach to tissues and to resist phagocytic digestion (Fig. 7–4). Most bacteria infecting the body have some type of capsule, but it is frequently not observable when they are grown on an artificial medium.

Some colonies of bacteria secrete polysaccharide fibers (glycocalyx) to increase adherence to teeth and mucous membranes. This additional polysaccharide layer also protects the colony from antibodies, phagocytes, and other antimicrobial agents.

The cell envelope of group A *Streptococcus pyogenes* contains a certain antigenic protein (protein M), that appears to be antiphagocytic, and other substances that aid the organism in adhering to pharyngeal cells.

Flagella   Although flagella serve useful functions by making certain bacteria motile, they also can aid bacteria in invading the aqueous areas of the body. In spite of the flushing action and continuous peristaltic movement of the ureters, some flagellated pathogens are able to reach the kidney where they cause serious infections and complications.

Pili and Fimbriae   Frequently, the piliated pathogens are able to adhere to cells within mucous membranes to establish an infection when other pathogens cannot; for example, *Neisseria gonorrhoeae* with pili attaches to urethral cells and multiplies, whereas other pathogens are flushed away by urination. Enterotoxigenic *Escherichia coli*, with its many fimbriae (pili), is able to attach to cells in the intestine where it multiplies and secretes the exotoxins that cause gastroenteritis. (See Figure 2–9 for an example of a piliated *E. coli*).

Enzymes Associated with Invasiveness

Some pathogens excrete enzymes that increase their ability to invade body tissues. These substances include (1) coagulase, (2) streptokinase, (3) hyaluronidase, and (4) collagenase. Note that the *-ase* ending always indicates that the material is an enzyme, that is, it catalyzes (speeds up) a particular reaction.

Coagulase   Pathogenic staphylococci are noted for the production of the extracellular (outside the cell) enzyme coagulase. This enzyme enables the staph organisms to clot plasma and thereby to form a sticky coat of fibrin around themselves for protection. In the laboratory, the coagulase-positive staphylococci cause citrated blood plasma to clot.

Streptokinase   Sometimes referred to as fibrinolysin, streptokinase has the opposite effect of coagulase. Streptokinase lyses, or dissolves, a fibrin clot that covers a wound, thus enabling the streptococci to invade and spread throughout the body. A similar enzyme produced by staphylococci is called *staphylokinase*.

Hyaluronidase   The spreading factor, as hyaluronidase is sometimes called, enables pathogens to spread through connective tissue by breaking down the tissue's hyaluronic acid. It is secreted by several pathogenic species of staphylococcus, streptococci, clostridia, and pneumococci.

Collagenase   The enzyme collagenase breaks down collagen, the supportive protein found in tendons, cartilage, and bones. *Clostridium perfringens*, which causes gas gangrene, spreads deeply within the body by secreting collagenase and hyaluronidase.

Toxins and Enzymes Associated with Toxigenicity

The ability to damage host tissues may depend on the excretion of hemolysin, leukocidin, and exotoxins. Endotoxins (*endo* = within), which are an integral part of the pathogen's cell wall, may also be toxic to the host.

Hemolysin   Hemolysin (*hemo* = blood; *lysis* = breakdown or dissolution) causes damage to the host's red blood cells, the erythrocytes. This hemolysis of red blood cells in blood agar is useful as a diagnostic tool for identifying α-hemolytic and β-hemolytic streptococci. The pathogenicity and invasiveness of the streptococci may not depend on the amount of hemolysin produced, although it is certainly related to the amount of damage the organisms can cause to the host.

Leukocidin   Leukocidin, the enzymelike exotoxin (*exo* = outside) that is secreted by some staphylococci and streptococci, causes destruction of the white blood cells, the *leukocytes*. The lytic effect of leukocidin has been observed on a laboratory slide of leukocytes in the presence of streptococci.

Lecithinase   The alpha (α) toxin of *Clostridium perfringens* is called lecithinase. It is destructive to the cell membranes of red blood cells and other tissues.

Exotoxins   Bacterial exotoxins are usually proteins secreted by living (vegetative) pathogens. Exotoxins are often described by the target organs they affect. The most toxic exotoxins are *neurotoxins*; they cause nerve destruction in botulism and diphtheria and spasmodic muscle contractions (tetany) in tetanus. *Enterotoxins*, those toxins that affect the vomiting centers of the brain and cause gastroenteritis, are secreted by *Staphylococcus aureus*, *Vibrio cholerae*, *Shingella dysenteriae*, and a few other enteric pathogens. Some new strains of *E. coli* are known to produce an enterotoxin causing a form of dysentery. Symptoms of toxic shock syndrome are caused by exotoxins (C and F) secreted by staphylococci. The *exfoliations* of these organisms cause the epidermal layers of the skin to slough away, and *erythrotoxins* cause rash and redness in the skin. Pathogens of diphtheria secrete toxins that affect the heart muscles (cardiotoxins), nerves (neurotoxins), and kidneys (nephrotoxins).

Endotoxins   The cell walls of certain gram-negative bacteria contain endotoxins that cause disease when the bacteria are present in large numbers. With the destruction and death of the bacteria in the digestive tract, the lipopolysaccharide and protein molecules in the cell wall cause fever, vomiting, and diarrhea. Diseases associated with endotoxins include dysentery, meningitis, typhoid fever, gonorrhea, and cholera.

Endotoxins may destroy phagocytes, upset the water and salt balance in the intestine, and weaken the infected host by dehydration (because of water loss in diarrhea); as a result, the person is a prime target for secondary infections.

Pathogenicity and Virulence

In summary, all of the terms presented thus far in this chapter concerning the pathogenicity and virulence of pathogens are useful in discussing general concepts of disease causation. Pathogenicity and virulence are sometimes used synonymously, but this is not entirely accurate; virulence refers to the degree of pathogenicity.

Pathogenicity refers to the ability of a species or genus of microorganisms to produce disease. This implies that some avirulent strains or species may exist within those groups. For instance, some avirulent strains of *N. gonorrhoeae*, *Corynebacterium diphtheriae*, and *Myobacterium tuberculosis* have been identified.

Virulence depends on infectivity, invasiveness, and toxigenicity; therefore, one might observe that pathogens that occur in large numbers or that are highly infective but low in invasiveness might produce a large carrier rate. This large group of pathogens would include the opportunists found among the indigenous microflora. Likewise, if the infectivity of a pathogen were low but its invasiveness and toxigenicity were high, sporadic outbreaks of the disease would occur.

The production of toxic products by pathogens is the most influential factor in their pathogenicity. Toxin-producing bacteria differ greatly in the amount of exotoxin they produce, depending on growth conditions. For example, virulent strains of some pathogens become avirulent when grown in the laboratory under artificial conditions; some virulent encapsulated pathogens lose their ability to produce capsules when grown on artificial media in the laboratory, as has been shown to occur in gonococci. Also, some toxin producers cease producing exotoxins on artificial media.

These changes can be regarded as the pathogen's response to different environments. On a completely artificial medium in the incubator where a constant temperature is maintained, optimal conditions exist for the microorganisms. Plenty of nutrients are present; the temperature is ideal; no overcrowding occurs from other microbes; and no phagocytes or antibodies exist; thus, pathogens have no need to arm themselves with capsules and toxins, as they do when attempting to grow in human tissues.

It should also be noted that virulence usually increases in pathogens that are transmitted from animal to animal and human to human, which explains why virulence may increase during an epidemic. This factor may also account for the relatively high virulence of pathogens in a hospital environment, where there is a continuously changing population of susceptible persons. Rampaging hospital staphylococcal infections are caused by virulent staphylococci that continue to mutate and to become resistant to the antibiotics used in ever greater varieties and numbers to fight infections.

Epidemiology and Disease Transmission

Epidemiology is the science that deals with the frequency and distribution of diseases and the factors that contribute to the spread of disease. These contributing factors include the virulence of the pathogen; susceptibility of the population because of overcrowding, lack of immunization, or inadequate sanitation procedures; and the mode of transmission of the pathogen.

Several terms are used to describe the prevalence of disease in an area at a particular time: endemic, epidemic, pandemic, sporadic, and nonendemic. Each term is discussed in this section.

Endemic Diseases

Endemic diseases are those that are constantly present in a community, usually involving only a few people. The number of cases increases and decreases at various times, but the disease never dies out completely. The endemic infections that occur regularly in the United States include tuberculosis, staphylococcal and streptococcal infections, and viral diseases, such as the common cold, influenza, chickenpox, and mumps. Tuberculosis remains endemic in the world as well as in the United States, particularly among the poor, who live in crowded conditions; however, the number of deaths has been greatly reduced by drug therapy. In some parts of this country, plague (caused by *Yersinia pestis*) is endemic among rats, prairie dogs, and other rodents; as a result, endemic plague in humans is occasionally observed. The actual incidence of an endemic disease at any particular time depends on a balance among several factors: environment, the genetic susceptibility of the population, behavioral factors, the number of people who are immune, the virulence of the pathogen, and the reservoir or source of infection (Fig. 7–5).

Epidemic Diseases

Infections that are usually endemic may become epidemic. An *epidemic* is defined as more than the normal number of cases of a disease in an area within a particular period (see Fig. 7–6).

A current example of a historically important epidemic of a new disease is the acquired immunodeficiency syndrome (AIDS) epidemic of the 1980s and 1990s (Fig. 7–7). Evidently, a mutant virus was picked up from monkeys by African natives. It was transmitted among Africans via mucous membranes, semen, and blood, usually by sexual contact or by blood transfer. From Africa, the disease spread to Haiti, from where the virus was carried to New York, Miami and many other parts of the United States. The virus then spread among the homosexual males and intravenous drug-using communities and through blood banks to hemophiliacs. Finally, the occurrence of AIDS cases among the heterosexual population and children has increased throughout the world. The virus was quickly isolated and indentified as (human T-cell lymphotrophic virus, type 3 (HTLV–III)

Figure 7–5. Factors influencing endemic disease.

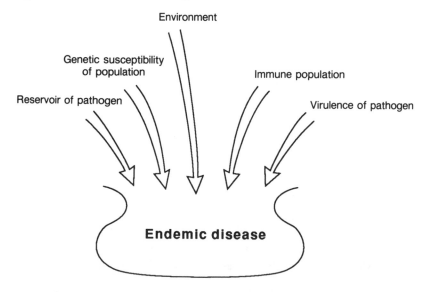

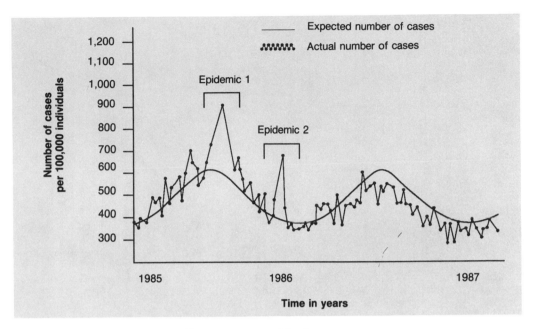

Figure 7–6. A graph illustrating two epidemics.

lymphadenopathy-associated virus (LAV), and later named human immunodeficiency virus (HIV) by international agreement. In 1990, over 3 million people in the United States were believed to be infected, and at least 20%, were expected to develop the symptoms of AIDS in the next few years. All will probably die, unless new treatments are developed. This sexually transmitted or blood-borne virus has a long incubation period during which it destroys the T4 helper lymphocytes, crippling the immune system so that most victims succumb to secondary infections (see Chapters 9 and 10). One significant outcome of this epidemic is the increased awareness of other sexually transmitted diseases (gonorrhea, syphilis, herpes).

Another example of a disease becoming epidemic is the 1976 occurrence of a respiratory illness following an American Legion convention in Philadelphia, Pennsylvania (Legionnaires' disease, or legionellosis). The organism was finally isolated, identified, and named *Legionella pneumophilia* (Fig. 7–8). Other such epidemics have been identified through constant surveillance and accumulation of data by the U.S. Centers for Disease Control (CDC). Epidemics usually follow a specific pattern in which the number of cases of a disease increases to a maximum and then decreases rapidly, because the number of susceptible and exposed individuals is limited.

Epidemics may occur in communities that have not been previously exposed to a particular pathogen. People from populated areas who travel into isolated com-

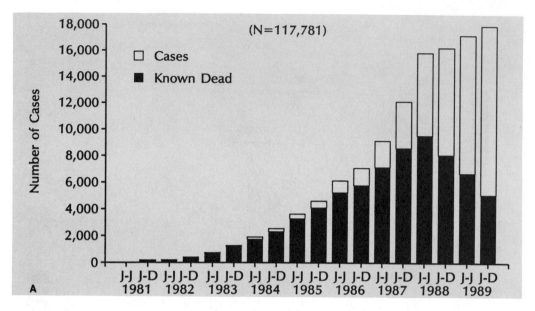

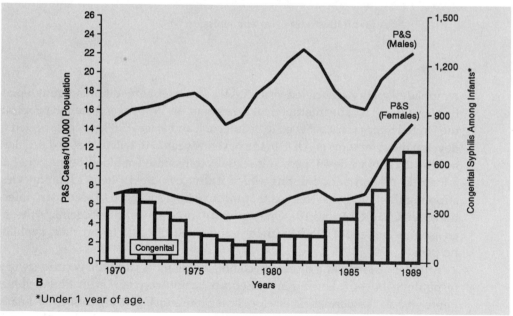

Figure 7–7. (*A*) Acquired immunodeficiency syndrome (AIDS)—Cases and known deaths, by 6-month periods of report to CDC, United States, 1981–1989. (*B*) Syphilis, congenital (under 1 year) and primary and secondary (P&S)—By sex, United States, 1970–1989. (Centers for Disease Control. Summary of notifiable diseases, United States, 1989. Morbidity and Mortality Weekly Report, 1989;38[54].)

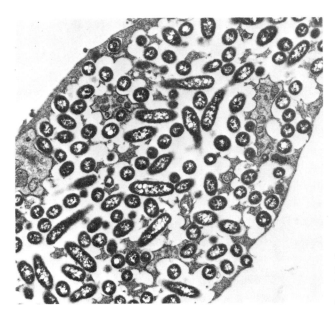

Figure 7–8. *Legionella pneumophila* cultured in human embryonic lung fibroblasts. (Courtesy of Mae C. Wong, Centers for Disease Control, Atlanta, Georgia)

munities frequently introduce a new virulent pathogen to susceptible natives of that community; then the disease spreads like wildfire. There have been many such examples described in history. The syphilis epidemic in Europe in the early 1500s was caused by a highly virulent spirochete carried back from the West Indies by Columbus's men in 1492. Also, measles and tuberculosis introduced to native Americans by early explorers and settlers almost destroyed many tribes. Recently, we have observed devastating outbreaks of measles and other contagious diseases in Australia, Africa, Greenland, and other relatively isolated areas.

In communities in which normal sanitation practices are relaxed, allowing fecal contamination of water supplies and food, epidemics of typhoid, cholera, giardiasis, and dysentery frequently occur. Visitors to these communities should be aware that they are more susceptible to these diseases, because they never developed a natural immunity by being exposed to them during childhood.

In the 1970s, gonorrhea reached epidemic proportions in the United States and most of the world because no immunity remains after the disease is cured (Fig. 7–9). This disease runs rampant in a promiscuous, mobile society. The use of birth control pills makes women more susceptible by changing the environment of the vagina. Also, the careless use of penicillin allowed the gonococcus to mutate into penicillin-resistant strains, (penicillinase-producing-Neisseria gonorrheae, PPNG) making control by penicillin more difficult. An effective vaccine might produce antibodies to prevent the pathogen from adhering to mucous membranes. An additional complicating factor is that this disease is asymptomatic in 80% of infected women and 20% of infected men; that is, the gonococcus lives and multiplies in the urogenital areas yet produces no symptoms. As noted in Fig-

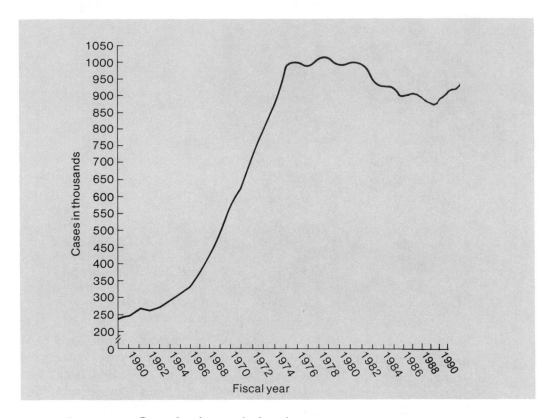

Figure 7–9. Gonorrhea has reached epidemic proportions in the United States; the graph shows the number of reported cases. (Prepared from data provided by U.S. Public Health Service, Centers for Disease Control, Atlanta, Georgia)

ure 7–9, a significant reduction in the number of cases has occurred during the herpes and AIDS epidemics since 1980.

Diseases such as the various types of influenza occur in many areas during certain times of the year and involve most of the population because the immunity developed is usually temporary. Thus, the disease recurs each year among those who are not revaccinated or naturally resistant to the infection. The recent epidemics have been caused by influenza type A (H1 N1), type A (H3 N2), and type B.

Pandemic Diseases

A *pandemic* is a worldwide epidemic of a specific disease. Pandemics of influenza ("flu") have been recorded in 1898, 1917–1918, 1955, 1968, 1972, 1975, and 1978. Recent influenza pandemics are often named for the point of origin or first recognition, such as the Taiwan flu, Hong Kong flu, London flu, Port Chalmers flu, and the Russian flu.

Sporadic and Nonendemic Diseases

Certain diseases follow neither the endemic nor the epidemic pattern but occur only sporadically; these are *sporadic* diseases, such as tetanus, gas gangrene, and botulism. Diseases that are controlled as a result of immunization and sanitation procedures are termed *nonendemic*; these include smallpox, poliomyelitis, and diphtheria (in most parts of the world). Occasionally, outbreaks of these controlled diseases occur where vaccination programs have been neglected for one reason or another.

The communicability of pathogens relies entirely on the survival of infectious agents during their transfer from one host to another. Thus, health professionals should be thoroughly familiar with pathways of transfer and sources of potential pathogens. For instance, a hospital staphylococcal epidemic begins when aseptic conditions are relaxed and a carrier of a staphylococcal infection introduces the organism to the many susceptible patients (babies, surgical patients, and debilitated persons). Such an epidemic may quickly spread from one person throughout the entire hospital population.

Reservoirs of Infectious Agents

The sources of microorganisms that cause infectious diseases are many and varied. They are known as *reservoirs of infection*. A reservoir of infection is any site where the pathogen can multiply or merely survive until it is transferred to its host. Reservoirs of infection may be living hosts or inanimate objects or materials.

Living animal reservoirs include humans, horses, cattle, pigs, cats, dogs, wildlife, insects, ticks, mites, and many others. Humans may acquire pathogens from other humans and animals, which may or may not be diseased; through direct contact and bites; by eating meat or other products from diseased animals; or through the bites of mosquitoes, flies, fleas, mites, ticks, and other arthropod vectors. The most important reservoir of human infections is man himself, because many human pathogens are species specific, which means they can cause disease in only one species of animal; thus, human pathogens usually cause disease only in humans.

Some people who do not have the disease may harbor the pathogen and transmit it to susceptible people who then develop the disease symptoms. Those who "carry" the pathogen without manifesting symptoms are called *carriers*. Human carriers are infected with the pathogen, but they are asymptomatic. *Active carriers* have recovered from the disease but continue to harbor the pathogen indefinitely. *Passive carriers* carry the pathogen without having the disease. *Convalescent carriers* harbor the pathogen during their recovery from the disease. Usually, the respiratory secretions and the intestinal or urinary excretions are the vehicles by which the disease agent is transferred to food and water and directly to many other persons. Human carriers are very important in the spread of staphylococcal and streptococcal infections as well as in the spread of hepatitis, diphtheria, dysentery, meningitis, and the sexually transmitted diseases.

The inanimate reservoirs of infection include air, soil, food, milk, water, as well as fomites, including articles of clothing, bedding, eating and drinking utensils, and hospital equipment, such as bedpans, and urinals, that are easily contaminated by pathogens from the respiratory tract, intestinal tract, and the skin of patients. Air is contaminated by dust, smoke, and respiratory secretions of humans expelled into the air by breathing, blowing, sneezing, and coughing. The most highly contagious diseases are those such as colds and influenza, in which the respiratory viruses can be transmitted through the air on droplets of water or by the hands to another person. Dust particles also can carry spores of certain bacteria and dried bits of human and animal excretions that contain pathogens. Bacteria cannot multiply in the air but can be easily transported to a warm, nutrient site for growth via airborne particles. All personnel in hospitals and other facilities where housekeeping is done for large numbers of people must be especially aware of air currents that carry dust and pathogens throughout the facility. Great care must be taken by the nursing and hospital staff to prevent transmission of pathogens to patients, causing a nosocomial (hospital-acquired) infection.

Modes of Disease Transmission

There are five principal modes of transfer of pathogens from an infected person to a susceptible person (Fig. 7–10 and Table 7–1).

- Direct person-to-person contact with the skin of a diseased person or carrier
- Direct mucus-to-mucus contact by kissing or sexual intercourse
- Indirectly through droplets or dust in the air
- Indirect contamination of food and water by fecal material, dead or live animals, soil, and other sources
- Blood contamination indirectly by arthropod and other animal vectors and directly by parenteral injection by nonsterile syringes and needles, as well as by intravenous transfusions and kidney dialysis.

Most diseases transferred by direct contact are those in which the causative organism can be carried on the skin; usually the pathogen is transferred by the hands and face. Many viruses and opportunistic bacteria are thus transferred and cause colds, influenza, staphylococcal and streptococcal infections, pneumonia, tuberculosis, polio, and diphtheria. In hospitals, this mode of transfer is particularly prevalent. Even the dysentery organisms, *Salmonella* and *Shigella*, can be transferred by the fecal material on the hands of one person to the hands, mouth, and food of another.

The mucus-to-mucus mode of transfer by kissing or sexual intercourse has been called the venereal route because sexually transmitted diseases (STD), such

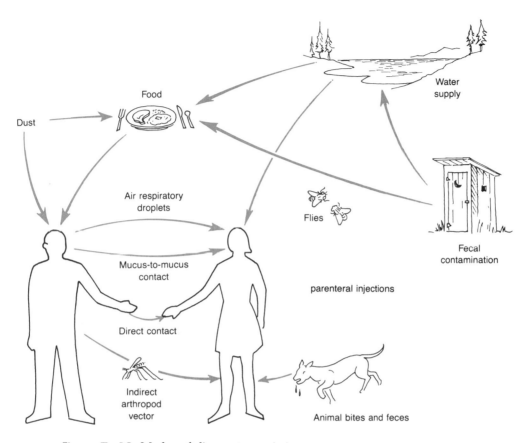

Figure 7–10. Modes of disease transmission.

as syphilis and gonorrhea, can be transmitted only in this manner. However, many other pathogens, including the herpes and AIDS viruses, may also be transmitted to others in this manner.

Most of the contagious airborne diseases are due to respiratory pathogens carried in droplets of moisture to susceptible people. Some respiratory pathogens may dry as they settle in dust particles and be carried long distances through the air and into a building's ventilation system (as observed in the Legionnaires' disease epidemic). Improperly cleaned inhalation therapy equipment can easily transfer these pathogens from one patient to another. Diseases that may be transmitted in this manner include colds, influenza, measles, mumps, chickenpox, smallpox, and pneumonia. Psittacosis or parrot fever is a respiratory infection that may be acquired from infected birds. Also, some fungal respiratory diseases (*e.g.*, histoplasmosis) are frequently transferred via dried bird feces.

Indirect transfer of organisms to a susceptible person frequently occurs through contamination of foods and water. Human and animal fecal materials

Table 7 – 1.   Common Routes of Transmission

Route of Exit	Route of Transmission or Entry	Disease
Skin	Skin discharge → air → respiratory tract	Chicken pox, colds, influenza, measles, staph and strep infections
	Skin to skin	Impetigo, eczema, boils, warts, syphilis
Respiratory	Aerosol droplet inhalation Nose or mouth → hand or object → nose	Colds, influenza, pneumonia, mumps, measles, chicken pox, tuberculosis
Gastrointestinal	Feces → hand → mouth Stool → soil → food → mouth	Gastroenteritis, hepatitis, salmonellosis, shigellosis, typhoid fever, cholera, giardiasis, amebiasis
Salivary	Direct salivary transfer	Herpes cold sores, infectious mononucleosis, AIDS, tuberculosis, strep throat
Genital secretions	Urethral or cervical secretions	Gonorrhea, herpes, *Chlamydia* infection
	Semen	Cytomegalovirus infection, AIDS, syphilis, warts
Blood	Transfusion or needle prick	Hepatitis B; cytomegalovirus infection; malaria, AIDS
Zoonotic	Insect bite	Malaria, relapsing fever
	Animal bite	Rabies, plague
	Contact with carcasses	Tularemia, anthrax,
	Arthropod	Rocky Mountain Spotted fever; Lyme disease, typhus, encephalitis, yellow fever, malaria

from outhouses, cesspools, and feed lots often are carried into water supplies. Improper disposal of sewage and inadequate treatment of drinking water contribute to the spread of fecal and soil pathogens. Food and milk may be contaminated by careless handling, which allows pathogens to enter from dust particles, dirty hands, hair, and respiratory secretions. If these pathogens and bacterial spores are not destroyed by proper processing and cooking, food poisoning can develop.

Diseases frequently transmitted through foods and water are tuberculosis, botulism, staphylococcal and streptococcal infections, diarrhea caused by *Salmonella* and *Shigella* species, typhoid fever, amebiasis (caused by an ameba), giardiasis (diarrhea caused by *Giardia*), and trichinosis (caused by *Trichinella* worms in pork).

Normally the blood is sterile; thus, the discovery of organisms in the blood indicates the presence of a pathogen. A *vector* is necessary to carry pathogens from the blood of one person to another. Living vectors are animals, usually arthropods (ticks, fleas, lice). Included among the arthropod vectors are insects such as mosquitoes and flies, which bite an infected person or animal, then carry the pathogens to a healthy individual.

To better understand this mode of transmission, let us consider the tick. (If you own a dog, you probably have a well-placed fear of ticks.) The pathogen involved is *Rickettsia rickettsii*, which causes Rocky Mountain spotted fever (see Chapter 2). The organisms are widespread among the animal population and among ticks themselves. If an infected tick bites a person, the pathogen may be injected, causing an infection. Ticks may also carry the pathogens of Q fever, typhus, Lyme disease and tularemia. In similar fashion, body lice and head lice are the vectors of epidemic typhus, trench fever, relapsing fever, trachoma, impetigo, and even cholera. The blood-sucking fleas carry the pathogens of plague and endemic typhus. Deer flies transmit tularemia, and tsetse flies carry African sleeping sickness. Certain strains of mosquitoes transmit malaria, encephalitis, and yellow fever.

Many pets and other animals are important reservoirs of *zoonoses* (infections of animals transmissible to humans). Dogs, cats, bats, skunks, and other animals are known vectors of rabies, transmitting the rabies virus to man via the saliva injected when they bite. Salmonellosis and shigellosis are frequently acquired from the feces of turtles, dogs, and poultry. Cat and dog bites easily transfer *Pasteurella*, *Staphylococcus*, and *Streptococcus* species into the tissues where severe infections may result. Toxoplasmosis, a protozoan disease carried by cats and other animals, may cause severe brain damage to the fetus when contracted by a woman during the first 3 months of pregnancy. This infective agent can be contracted from cat feces in cat litter boxes as well as from infected raw meats.

Common inanimate vectors of blood and internal infections are the instruments and apparatus handled by medical personnel, most often nonsterile syringes, needles, and solutions, and blood-processing equipment such as kidney dialyzers and blood-transfusing apparatus (Fig. 7–11). One reason disposable sterile tubes, syringes, and various other types of single-use hospital equipment have become very popular is that they are effective in preventing blood infections. Any blood disease can be transferred by improperly sterilized instruments and equipment. Hepatitis, syphilis, malaria, AIDS, and systemic staphylococcal infections are the diseases most often seen. Individuals using illegal intravenous drugs easily transmit these diseases to each other by sharing needles and syringes.

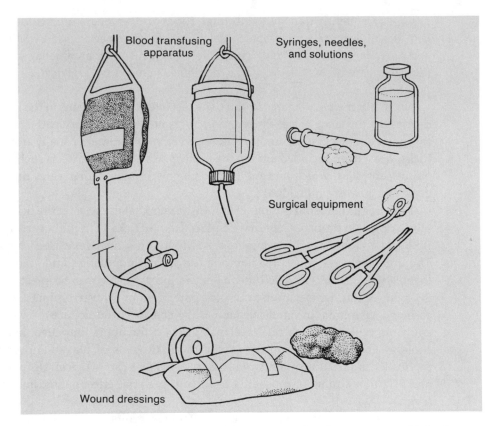

Figure 7–11. Medical instruments and apparatus are inanimate vectors of infection.

Control of Epidemic Diseases

The World Health Organization and the U.S. Public Health Service constantly strive to prevent epidemics and to identify and eliminate those that do occur. One way in which health personnel and community workers participate in this massive program is by reporting cases of communicable diseases to the proper agencies. They also can help to educate the public by describing the transmission of diseases, by explaining proper sanitation procedures, by identifying and attempting to eliminate reservoirs of infection, by carrying out measures to isolate diseased persons, by participating in immunization programs, and by helping to treat sick persons. Through measures like these, diphtheria, poliomyelitis, and smallpox have been practically eliminated in most parts of the world. Everyone in our society should contribute in whatever way possible to eliminate infectious diseases from the human environment.

Insight: Eradication of Poliomyelitis

The Pan-American Health Organization (PAHO) established a plan for eradicating the transmission of wild poliovirus from the Western Hemisphere in 1985. PAHO's program strategy included (1) achievement and maintenance of high levels of poliomyelitis immunization, (2) detection of all new cases of acute flaccid paralysis, (3) a rapid response to all new cases of paralysis.

The rates of reported paralytic poliomyelitis declined markedly, with a doubling in oral poliovirus vaccine (OPV) administration to young children, through 1989. The aggressive approach to case detection combined with immediate action to control outbreaks has contributed to the containment of wild poliovirus within the two remaining areas of risk: northwestern Mexico and the northern Andean subregion.

Each of the countries in the Region of the Americas needs to continue to investigate properly all cases of acute flaccid paralysis, and stool specimens obtained from persons with suspected polio must be submitted to the laboratory in good condition, because the ultimate diagnosis rests with the laboratories. The current level of effort must be sustained if polio is to be eradicated from the Americas by 1991 and from the world by the year 2000.

Insight Figure 7–1. Oral polio vaccine coverage in children 1 year of age and rate* of reported paralytic poliomyelitis by year—the Americas, 1969–1989. (Data from Morbidity and Mortality Weekly Report, 1990; 39 [33]. U.S. Department of Health and Human Services, Public Health Service, Centers for Disease Control, Atlanta, Georgia).

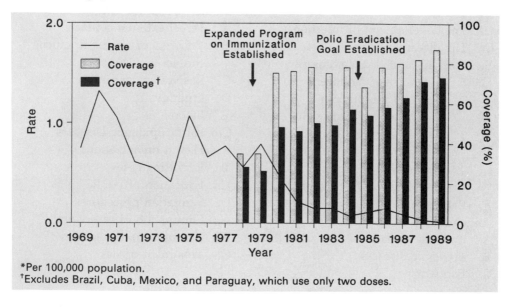

*Per 100,000 population.
†Excludes Brazil, Cuba, Mexico, and Paraguay, which use only two doses.

Summary

It is important to understand the factors that enable pathogens to invade tissues and cause disease. When individuals are exposed to pathogens, these microorganisms may or may not be able to cause disease. Disease causation depends on the natural resistance of the individual and virulence, infectivity, invasiveness, and toxicity of the pathogens. The natural defenses of the human body include the skin, mucous membranes, bacteriolytic secretions, normal flora, phagocytes, antibodies, and the process of inflammation. Pathogenic microorganisms are more able to resist phagocytosis and the inflammatory response than nonpathogens. Also, many secrete enzymes to invade and cause damage to tissues. Thus, they may overwhelm and win the battle against the normal body defenses to cause disease in localized areas or throughout the body.

The frequency and distribution of cases of infectious diseases and the factors that contribute to the spread of these diseases constitute the field of epidemiology. The factors that contribute to the occurrence of epidemics include the virulence of the pathogen, the susceptibility of the population, the sanitation practices, and the ways by which the pathogens are transmitted. To irradicate certain diseases and to prevent epidemics, all of these factors must be considered.

Study Outline

I. Disease and Infections
    A. Types of infections
    B. Why infection does not always occur
    C. The development of infection
    D. The disease process
    E. Mechanics of disease causation
        1. Virulence of pathogen
        2. Bacterial morphology associated with infectivity
        3. Enzymes associated with invasiveness
        4. Toxins and enzymes associated with toxigenicity
    F. Pathogenicity and virulence

II. Epidemiology
    A. Endemic diseases
    B. Epidemic diseases
    C. Pandemics
    D. Sporadic diseases
    E. Nonendemic diseases
    F. Reservoirs of infectious agents

III. Modes of Disease Transmission
    A. Direct external contact
    B. Venereal or mucus-to-mucus contact
    C. Respiratory or air
    D. Enteric
    E. Blood

IV. Control of Epidemic Diseases
    A. Health organizations
    B. Reporting cases
    C. Education of public
    D. Sanitation procedures
    E. Elimination of reservoirs
    F. Immunization programs
    G. Treatment of sick

Problems and Questions

1. Define *infectious*, *communicable*, and *contagious disease*. Why are some diseases more contagious than others?
2. List several ways that the human body resists infection by foreign invaders.
3. Define and illustrate the following terms used to describe infectious diseases: (a) acute, (b) chronic, (c) latent, (d) primary, (e) secondary, (f) local, (g) systemic.
4. Name three phases in the course of infectious diseases.
5. On what general properties does virulence and pathogenicity depend?
6. Compare exotoxins with endotoxins. List some diseases produced by each.
7. Name some general types of exotoxins.
8. Define and give examples of epidemic, endemic, pandemic, sporadic, and nonendemic diseases.
9. In what way do infected persons who carry pathogens but have no symptoms influence epidemics?
10. Discuss how the reservoirs of infection could be reduced or destroyed.
11. How could each of the five modes of transmission be interrupted to prevent diseases transmitted in that way?
12. If you were called to a distant island to stop an epidemic, what measures would you take?

Self Test

After you have read Chapter 7, examined the objectives, studied the new words, reviewed the study outline, and answered the questions at the end of the chapter, complete the following self test.

Matching Exercises

Complete each statement from the list of words provided with each section.

Infectious Diseases

communicable   contagious   infectious
inflammation   virulence

1. The ability of a pathogen to produce disease may depend on the pathogen's _virulence_.
2. The body tissues respond to damage or infections by a process called _inflammation_.

3. A disease that results from dietary deficiencies, such as rickets, is not a/an _contagious_ disease. *infectious*

4. A disease caused by the growth of microorganisms is a/an _infectious_.

5. Diseases that are very easily transmitted, such as colds, are called _communicable_ *contagious*

6. Diseases that result from close contact with the infected person are termed _communicable_ diseases.

7. The symptoms fever, redness, swelling, and pain are indications of a/an _inflammation_.

Types of Disease States

local	generalized	latent
acute	chronic	primary
secondary	asymptomatic	carrier
systemic		

1. When the infection is confined to a single area it is _local_.

2. During the course of a disease the pathogen may be walled off or hidden in certain organs; then the infection is _latent_.

3. If the pathogen is present and detectable but there are no symptoms of the disease, it is _asymptomatic_.

4. A disease that has a rapid onset and a rapid recovery period is _acute_.

5. If the disease is characterized by slow onset and long duration, it is _chronic_.

6. A person who has recovered from a disease but who still harbors the pathogens that may be transmitted to others is known as a _carrier_.

7. An infection that has invaded the bloodstream has become _generalized_ and thus is a _systemic_ infection.

8. A _primary_ infection, such as influenza, may leave the individual in a weakened condition so that a _secondary_ infection may occur because the body defenses are at a low level.

Disease Causation

capsule	coagulase	streptokinase
fibrinolysin	staphylokinase	hyaluronidase
collagenase	exotoxins	leukocidin
endotoxins	hemolysin	

1. Very toxic proteins that are secreted by living pathogens that cause diseases such as botulism, tetanus, and diphtheria are _exotoxins_.

2. The protective coating outside the cell wall of an organism, which may protect it from a phagocytosis, is a _capsule_.

3. An enzyme secreted by a pathogen that enables it to spread through connective tissue by breaking down the hyaluronic acid is _hyaluronidase_.

4. Some bacteria cause disease because their cell walls are very toxic to humans. This toxic material, which is part of the bacterial cell, is an _endotoxin_.

5. An enzyme secreted by some bacteria that clots plasma around the bacterial cell is _coagulase_.

6. Streptococci and some staphylococci can break down a fibrin blood clot by secreting _streptokinase_, which could also be called _fibrinolysin / staphylokinase_.

7. Red blood cells are lysed by _hemolysin_ when α- and β-hemolytic streptococci are grown on blood agar.

8. Some streptococci and staphylococci are able to destroy white blood cells by secreting _leukocidin_.

9. An enzyme that destroys collagen in tendons and cartilage is _collagenase_.

Epidemiology

epidemic	endemic	pandemic
sporadic	nonendemic	

1. An epidemic that spreads throughout the world is _pandemic_.

2. When more than a normal number of cases of a disease occur in a specific area during a certain time, the disease has reached _epidemic_ proportions.

3. Those diseases, such as smallpox, that do not occur in most countries are _nonendemic_.

4. Certain diseases, such as botulism, that occur only occasionally are _sporadic_.

5. Some diseases are usually present in an area, but the numbers of cases vary with the season and month of the year. These diseases are _endemic_.

6. In most areas colds and influenza are _endemic_.

7. In the United States diphtheria has been controlled as a result of immunization programs; it is a/an _nonendemic_ disease.

8. In recent years gonorrhea has become _epidemic_ in the United States and _pandemic_ in the world.

Reservoirs of Infection

carriers   venereal   vectors
arthropods   fomites   respiratory
fecal material   pathogens

1. Small animals such as insects, ticks, fleas, mites, and lice that transfer pathogens by their bites are _arthropods_. _vectors_
2. Pathogens may be transferred to a susceptible patient via the bed clothes, urinals, towels, or sheets of another sick patient. These items are _fomites_
3. Food, milk, and water supplies are easily contaminated with human _fecal material_ containing enteric pathogens.
4. Contaminated syringes, needles, and other hospital equipment frequently serve as inanimate _vectors_ of disease agents.
5. The most contagious diseases are usually transferred by droplets of moisture in the air and by dust; these particles often carry _respiratory pathogens_.
6. Persons who transmit pathogens to other susceptible people but who have no symptoms of the disease themselves are _carriers_.
7. Pathogens that must be transmitted by mucus-to-mucus contact are the ones that cause _venereal_ diseases, such as syphilis and gonorrhea.
8. Rocky Mountain spotted fever and tularemia are transmitted from wildlife to man by the bite of infected ticks, which are _arthropods_.
9. Hepatitis and syphilis are often transmitted by blood transfers in which the blood as well as the needles are _vectors_.

True or False (T or F)

_T_ 1. Infectious diseases are those caused by the growth of pathogenic microorganisms.

_T_ 2. The virulence of a pathogen depends on its ability to infect, invade, and damage the host.

_T_ 3. A communicable disease is one that can be transmitted from one person to another by direct contact.

_F_ 4. When a pathogen lands on the skin, it immediately starts to grow and cause a sore.

_T_ 5. A carrier is a person who carries a pathogen and may give it to others but does not have symptoms of the disease caused by that pathogen.

_T_ 6. An acute disease, such as gonorrhea, may become a chronic one.

_T_ 7. In the latent stage, herpes cold sores are not apparent.

8. Gonorrhea is never asymptomatic.
9. Pneumonia and ear infections are usually primary diseases.
10. Streptokinase helps staphylococci break down blood clots.
11. The actual number of cases of an endemic disease depends on many factors, including the environment.
12. Hospital staphylococcal epidemics are usually caused by the hospital personnel.
13. Gonorrhea has never been epidemic in the United States.
14. Living hosts or inanimate objects may be reservoirs of infection.
15. Man is the most important reservoir of infection for human diseases.
16. Arthropod vectors are all insects that carry pathogens.
17. All species of mosquitoes carry malaria parasites.
18. Body lice may be vectors of epidemic typhus, trachoma, and impetigo.
19. Improperly sterilized syringes, needles, and blood transfusion and dialysis equipment are frequently the sources of blood infections such as systemic staphylococcus and hepatitis.
20. The best way to prevent an epidemic is to isolate all sick people.
21. An endemic disease can become an epidemic.
22. *Legionella pneumophila* is the causative agent in an endemic disease.
23. Toxoplasmosis is an example of zoonoses.

Multiple Choice

1. Measles is a disease considered to be
   a. avirulent
   b. communicable
   c. contagious
   d. secondary
2. Syphilis is caused by
   a. *Staphylococcus aureus*
   b. *Yersinia pestis*
   c. *Treponema pallidum*
   d. *Streptococcus syphilitis*
3. Leprosy would be an example of a disease that is
   a. acute
   b. local
   c. chronic
   d. viral
4. *Clostridium botulinum* is pathogenic because of its
   a. exotoxin
   b. endospore

   c. endotoxin
   d. capsule
5. An example of a systemic disease would be
   a. herpes cold sores
   b. "staph" septicemia
   c. ear infections
   d. sinusitis
6. Diseases are usually most contagious during the
   a. convalescent period
   b. latent period
   c. period of illness
   d. incubation period
7. Enterotoxins that cause gastroenteritis are secreted by
   a. *Haemophilus ducreyi*
   b. *Vibrio cholerae*
   c. *Pseudomonas aeruginosa*
   d. *Bordetella pertussis*

8. Virulence indicates
   a. the ability to resist disease
   b. the production of toxins
   c. the ability to produce disease
   d. high rate of reproduction
9. Endotoxins tend to affect the cells of the
   a. skin
   b. heart
   c. vascular system
   d. intestinal tract
10. An example of a sporadic disease is
    a. tuberculosis
    b. tetanus
    c. influenza
    d. poliomyelitis
11. A passive carrier
    a. is recovering from the disease
    b. is an inanimate vector
    c. has never had the disease but carries the pathogen
    d. has recovered from the disease but still carries the pathogen

12. Tulaemia, typhus, and Rocky Mountain spotted fever are transmitted by
    a. inanimate vectors
    b. direct skin contact
    c. poor hygiene
    d. arthropod vectors
13. Smallpox is nonendemic primarily because of
    a. the avirulence of the organism
    b. the mutagenic properties of the organism
    c. immunization programs
    d. the increased number of passive carriers
14. Reservoirs of infection are
    a. only inanimate objects
    b. any site where pathogens survive
    c. only living hosts
    d. only fomites

Chapter 8

Preventing the Spread of Communicable Diseases

Objectives

After studying this chapter, you should be able to

1. List the six factors that have contributed to an increase in hospital-acquired (nosocomial) infections
2. List areas in the hospital where nosocomial infections are most probable
3. List several types of patients who are extremely vulnerable to infectious diseases
4. Write a brief description of reverse isolation and source isolation
5. Briefly describe the important procedures to follow in universal precautions
6. Discuss the role of the health worker in the collection of specimens
7. List the types of specimens that usually must be collected from patients
8. Discuss the general precautions that must be observed during the collection and handling of specimens
9. Describe the proper procedure for obtaining specimens
10. Discuss the importance of quality control in a microbiology laboratory
11. List the sources of water contamination
12. Describe how water and sewage are treated
13. Discuss how epidemics are controlled and prevented

New Words

Clostridium botulinum (clos-strid'-ēe-um bot-you-lin'-um). The species of anaerobic bacteria that causes botulism, a toxic food poisoning

Clostridium perfringens (clos-trid'-ee-um per-frin'-genz). A species of
   anaerobic bacteria that causes gas gangrene and food poisoning
Nosocomial (nos-o-ko'-me-al). Of hospital origin
Proteus (pro'-tea-us). A genus of intestinal pathogens
Staphylococcus aureus (staff-fill-oh-cock'-us or'-ee-us). A species of bacteria
   that causes boils, wound infections, and hospital "staph" infections
Streptococcus pneumoniae (strep-toe-cock'-us new-moan'-ee-aye). A species
   of bacteria that causes pneumonia and meningitis

Prevention of Hospital Infections

How Hospital Infections Develop

The importance of microbiology to those who work in the health-related occupations can never be overemphasized. Whether working in a hospital, an institution, a medical or dental clinic or as caring for sick persons in their homes, all
health workers must follow the same procedures to prevent the spread of communicable diseases.

Thoughtless or careless actions when giving patient care can cause preventable
infections. Infections associated with hospitalization are of two types: community-acquired infections or hospital-acquired (nosocomial) infections. According
to the Centers for Disease Control (CDC), community-acquired infections are
those present or incubating at the time of hospital admission. All other hospital
infections are considered nosocomial, including those that erupt within 14 days of
hospital discharge. Iatrogenic infections are those caused as a result of treatment
by a physician or surgeon.

Preventable nosocomial infection often adds several weeks to the patient's stay
in the hospital and may give rise to serious complications or even result in the patient's death. Cross-infections transmitted by hospital personnel, including physicians, are not infrequent; this is particularly true when hospitals and clinics are
overcrowded and the staff is overworked. However, these infections *can* be
avoided through proper care and the disciplined use of aseptic techniques and
precautions.

Nurses and physicians play major roles in preventing nosocomial infections;
nevertheless, respiratory therapists, physical therapists, laboratory technicians,
occupational therapists, radiologic technologists, dental hygienists, dentists, and
all others who deal with patients must be equally knowledgeable about methods
of preventing the spread of pathogens. Members of the hospital housekeeping
staff or the central supply department and those who prepare, dispense, and dispose of food as well as administrative personnel and those who dispose of medical wastes can help to prevent cross-contamination among patients or, through
their carelessness, can contribute to the spread of diseases. Of course, sick and debilitated hospitalized patients are much more susceptible to even minor oppor-

tunistic pathogens than are the healthy people caring for them. In all situations, health workers must protect themselves from infectious agents as well.

The number of nosocomial infections has increased during the past 25 years to over 1 million cases per year despite the availability of new disinfectants and antibiotics. There are many reasons for this situation: (1) the indiscriminate use of broad-spectrum antibiotics, which may allow opportunistic pathogens to mutate and become antibiotic-resistant; (2) a false sense of security about the effectiveness of antibiotics, with a corresponding neglect of aseptic techniques and precautions; (3) lengthy, more complicated types of surgery; (4) overcrowding of hospitals and shortage of staff; (5) increase in both numbers and types of hospital workers who often are not aware of the importance of routine infection control and aseptic and sterile techniques; (6) increased use of anti-inflammatory and immunosuppressant agents, such as radiation, steroids, anticancer chemotherapy, and antilymphocytic serum and (7) the use of medical devices. The presence of even one of these factors is sufficient to enable opportunistic pathogens to rush in and cause problems; taken together, they are the cause of approximately 60% of hospital-acquired infections. The most prevalent opportunistic bacteria are *Staphylococcus aureus*, *Escherichia coli*, *Streptococcus pneumoniae*, and *Pseudomonas* and *Klebsiella* species, which cause most wound, burn, respiratory, and surgical infections.

Medical devices that support or monitor basic body functions contribute greatly to the success of modern medical treatment. By passing normal defensive barriers, these devices provide microorganisms access to normally sterile body fluids and tissues. The risk of bacterial or fungal infection is related to the degree of debilitation of the patient and the design and management of the device. The most common nosocomial infections are urinary infections associated with the use of urinary catheters. Thus, it is advisable to discontinue the use of urinary catheters, vascular catheters, respirators, and hemodialysis as soon as medically feasible.

The emergency room, operating room, delivery room, nursery, and the central supply area are the most critical areas from the standpoint of disease transmission. In the emergency room, many patients, carrying unknown pathogens, are rushed in and treated quickly to halt a life-threatening situation; in haste, the emergency room attendants may neglect to protect themselves and others by failing to use the recommended precautions. In the operating theater and delivery areas, particular care must be taken because portals of entry into the body are readily accessible to pathogens. The nursery is critical because newborns have very little resistance to disease. The central supply department must take great care not to distribute contaminated materials or supplies, since these might expose patients to a myriad of pathogens.

In a hospital, the most vulnerable patients are (1) newborn and premature babies; (2) women in labor and delivery; (3) surgical and burn patients; (4) diabetic and cancer patients; (5) those receiving treatment with steroids, anticancer drugs, antilymphocyte serum, and radiation; (6) those with a deficient immune response, as in AIDS and (7) patients who are paralyzed or who are undergoing renal dialysis or catheterization. These patients' normal defense mechanisms are not working properly.

The greatest risk to health workers who handle blood and body fluids is the transmission of Hepatitis B (HBV) and/or the human immunodeficiency virus (HIV). Control of these viruses requires meticulous attention to procedures that prevent direct contact with blood, such as the use of gloves and gowns.

Nosocomial viral infections are frequently ignored because most hospitals lack adequate viral diagnostic laboratories. Influenza virus, respiratory syncytial virus, and other respiratory viruses have been shown to spread in hospitals via direct contact or droplet inhalation. Other highly infectious viruses that cause measles and chickenpox may cause outbreaks among susceptible patients and hospital staff.

General Control Measures

Using general principles of sanitation, disinfection, and sterilization, a general state of cleanliness must be maintained throughout the hospital or institution. Each area, from the trash disposal area to the operating rooms, must be thoroughly cleaned and disinfected to prevent the growth and spread of micro-organisms.

Hospitals vary greatly in their specific requirements for the maintenance of medical asepsis, but there is general agreement about sanitary methods for handling food and dishes, proper cooking and storage of food, proper disposal of waste products and contaminated materials, proper hand-washing and personal hygiene of hospital personnel, proper use of gown and mask in isolation rooms, proper washing and sterilization of hospital equipment, proper use of disposable equipment, and proper disinfection of a room after the patient has been discharged.

Prevention of Airborne Contamination   Respiratory infections are most often transmitted through the air. Observe the following measures to decrease the number of pathogens transmitted by this means:

- Cover the mouth and nose when coughing or sneezing.
- Limit the number of persons in a room.
- Remove the dirt and dust from floor and furniture by damp dusting.
- Open the room to fresh air and sunlight whenever possible.
- Roll linens together carefully to prevent dispersal of microbes in the air.
- Remove bacteria from the air by a filtered air-conditioning system.

Handling Food and Dishes Contaminated food provides an excellent environment for the growth of pathogens. Most often, human carelessness is responsible for this contamination: failure to take precautions with fecal material, handwashing, flies and insects, dust, dirt, and domestic animals and pets. The microbes most frequently carried in food are *Staphylococcus* species (from skin and dust), *Clostridium botulinum* (from dust and dirt), *Clostridium perfringens* (from dust, dirt, and hands), *Salmonella* species (from feces, hands, flies, and pets), *Shigella* species (from feces, hands, flies, and pets), *Proteus* species (from feces, hands, flies, and pets), and *Pseudomonas* species (from dirt, hands, and contaminated equipment).

Regulations for safe handling of food and dishes are not difficult to follow. They include

- Using high quality fresh food
- Properly refrigerating and storing food
- Properly washing, preparing, and cooking food
- Properly disposing of uneaten food
- Thoroughly washing hands and fingernails before handling food and after visiting a restroom
- Properly disposing of nasal and oral secretions in tissues
- Covering hair and wearing clean clothes and aprons
- Providing periodic health examinations for kitchen workers
- Prohibiting anyone with an infection or intestinal upset from handling food or dishes
- Keeping all kitchen equipment and all other equipment scrupulously clean
- Rinsing and then washing dishes in a dishwasher in which the water temperature is above 80°C (176°F)

Handling of Fomites As previously described, fomites are any articles or substances other than food that may harbor and transmit microbes. Examples of fomites are dishes, bedpans, urinals, thermometers, washbasins, bed linen, and clothing and other personal patient items. Transmission of pathogens by these items may be prevented by observing the following rules:

- Use disposable equipment and supplies wherever possible.
- Disinfect or sterilize equipment as soon as possible after use.
- Use individual equipment for each patient.
- Use an individual thermometer for each patient and store each thermometer in a disinfectant solution.
- Empty bedpans and urinals, wash them in hot water, and store them in a clean cabinet between uses.
- Place bed linen and soiled clothing in bags to be sent to the laundry.

Hand-Washing   Hand-washing is the single most important aseptic precaution. Hands should be kept clean at all times and should be washed before and after each patient contact to preclude carrying pathogens from one patient to another. A disinfectant soap containing hexachlorophene is often used to control staphylococci. Common-sense rules that one should always follow include

- Use of gloves or tongs to handle contaminated materials
- Wash hands with disinfectant soap before and after contact with a patient
- Rinse hands under running water
- Dry hands and apply antiseptic lotion to prevent chapping

Infection Control Procedures

Medical and Surgical Asepsis

Following the lessons learned by Semmelweis and Lister in the 19th century, we know that contamination of wounds is not inevitable and that we must prevent microorganisms from reaching susceptible areas, a concept referred to as asepsis, which may be medical or surgical in nature. The techniques used to achieve asepsis depend on the site, the circumstances, and the environment.

Once basic cleanliness is achieved, it is not difficult to maintain asepsis. The goal of medical asepsis is to exclude all pathogenic microorganisms from the immediate environment. Medical asepsis includes all the precautionary measures necessary to prevent direct transfer of pathogens from person to person and indirect transfer of pathogens through the air or on instruments, bedding, equipment, and other inanimate objects (fomites).

In the hospital, medical asepsis is practiced using sterile equipment, dressings, medications, and any items that could transfer microorganisms to susceptible sites. Invasive procedures, such as drawing blood, giving injections, catheter insertion, cardiac catheterization, and lumbar punctures, must be performed under strict aseptic precautions. The most controlled and strict aseptic procedures must be applied in the operating room and surgical area. The goal of surgical asepsis is to exclude *all* microorganisms from the immediate environment. Surgical aseptic techniques include those practices that make and keep all objects and the area itself sterile. These practices are necessary during all surgical procedures, as well as any other procedure that involves exposure of the deep body tissues, to prevent the entry of any microorganisms into those tissues.

The surgical area of the patient's skin must be shaved and thoroughly cleansed and scrubbed with soap and antiseptic. If the surgery is to be extensive, the surrounding area is covered with a plastic film or sterile cloth drapes so that a sterile surgical field is established. The surgeon and all surgical assistants must scrub for 10 minutes with a disinfectant soap and cover their clothes, mouth, and hair, because these might shed microorganisms onto the operative site. These coverings include sterile gloves, gowns, caps, and masks. All instruments, sutures, and dressings must be sterilized; as soon as they are contaminated, they must be discarded and replaced with sterile ones. Any instruments or equipment that cannot be autoclaved must be properly disposed of. All needles, syringes, and sharps must be placed in appropriate containers.

The floors, walls, and all equipment in the operating room must be cleaned and disinfected before each use. Proper ventilation must be maintained to ensure that fresh, filtered air is circulated throughout the room at all times.

Universal Precautions   HBV and HIV are occasionally transmitted from patients to medical staff. Blood and blood products are the primary mode of transmission of these viruses in the medical field, although the usual means of transmission is by sexual contact; by contaminated needles, transplants, or transfusions; and by infected mothers' transmission of the virus to their infants.

In the medical setting, all patients are considered potentially infectious for HIV, HBV, and other bloodborne pathogens. For this reason "universal precautions" have been recommended by the CDC to prevent transmission of these bloodborne pathogens in health care units. Transmission of hepatitis B is more likely than transmission of HIV. Of primary concern is contact with the patient's blood or mucosal surfaces or penetration of the skin, i.e., needle sticks. The universal precautions demand the use of gloves, gowns, masks, and sometimes goggles during high risk procedures, such as suctioning, bronchoscopy, surgery, and many emergency or dental procedures.

Universal precautions include but are not limited to the following procedures:

- Hands should always be washed before and after contact with patients. Hands should be washed even when gloves are used. If hands come into contact with blood, body fluids, or human tissue, they should be washed with soap and water.
- Gloves should be worn when contact with blood, body fluid, tissues, or contaminated surfaces is anticipated.
- Gowns are indicated if blood splattering is likely.
- Masks and protective goggles should be worn if aerosolization or splattering is likely to occur such as in certain surgical procedures, wound irrigations, and bronchoscopy
- The need for emergency mouth-to-mouth resuscitation and mouth pieces should be minimized by strategically locating resuscitation bags or other ventilation devices where they are available for use in areas where they may be needed.
- Sharp objects should be handled cautiously to prevent accidental cuts or punctures. Used needles should not be bent, broken, reinserted into their original sheath, or unnecessarily handled. They should be discarded intact immediately after use into an easily accessible, impervious needle disposal

container. All needle stick accidents, mucosal splashes, or contamination of open wounds with blood or body fluids should be reported immediately.

- Blood spills should be cleaned up promptly with a disinfectant solution, such as a 1:10 dilution of chlorine bleach.
- All patients' blood specimens should be considered biohazardous.

Although universal precautions apply to blood and other body fluids containing visible blood, they should also be applied to other tissues and fluids, such as semen and vaginal secretions, cerebrospinal fluid, synovial fluid, pleural fluid, peritoneal fluid, pericardial fluid, and amniotic fluid. The risk of transmission from these fluids is unknown, and epidemiologic studies are currently inadequate to assess the potential risk to health care workers from occupational exposure to them.

Universal precautions do not apply to feces, nasal secretions, sputum, sweat, tears, urine, vomitus, and saliva, unless they contain visible blood. The risk of transmission of HIV and HBV from these fluids and materials is extremely low; however, some of the excretions are a potential source for nosocomial and community infections.

Although universal precautions do not apply to saliva, general infection control practices should be observed, including wearing gloves for examination of mucous membranes and for endotracheal suctioning and hand-washing after exposure to saliva to further reduce the minute risk of salivary transmission of HIV and HBV. However, special precautions, including the use of gloves and masks, must be observed for dental procedures.

The implementation of universal precautions does not eliminate the need for other category- or disease-specific isolation precautions, such as enteric precautions for infectious diarrhea or isolation for pulmonary tuberculosis. Universal precautions are intended to supplement rather than to replace other recommendations for routine infection control, such as hand-washing and using gloves to prevent gross microbial contamination of hands. These guidelines are published by the Centers for Disease Control, Atlanta, Georgia in the *Morbidity and Mortality Weekly Report* (MMWR).[1]

Isolation of Patients

Patients are placed in isolation for one of two reasons: (1) to prevent the spread of pathogens to other susceptible people, or (2) to protect a very susceptible patient from exposure to pathogens.

---

[1] Published in August 1987 and June 24, 1988 in MMWR and available through National AIDS Information Clearinghouse, P.O. Box 6003, Rockville, MD 20850.

Reverse Isolation   Certain patients are especially vulnerable to infection; among them are patients with severe burns, those who have leukemia, patients who have received a transplant, immunodeficient persons, and those receiving radiation treatments. Premature babies are also highly susceptible. All such patients are protected through isolation procedures. This type of isolation is referred to as reverse isolation. The room must be thoroughly cleaned and disinfected before the patient is admitted. Those entering the room must wear sterile gowns and masks to prevent depositing microorganisms into the room from their clothes or their respiratory tract. Proper handwashing procedures must also be followed before entering the room.

Source Isolation   Whenever possible, patients with contagious diseases should be isolated in private air-conditioned rooms with a private bath (Fig. 8–1, Table 8–1). In this manner infectious agents are isolated within a definite area, and thereby spread of the pathogens to other patients is prevented. Isolation procedures should be determined by

- The mode of transmission of the disease from one person to another
- The location of the pathogen causing the infection, its portal of exit (intestinal, respiratory, or wound drainage), and its portal of entry
- The virulence of the pathogen and its susceptibility to antibiotics

Isolation Techniques   Isolation techniques are designed to immediately destroy the pathogenic organisms in the infectious discharges of the patient. Nondisposable items are disinfected, with a minimum of handling, then cleaned thoroughly and resterilized. If the patient's infection involves spore-forming bacteria such as those found in gas gangrene and tetanus, then contaminated equipment must be autoclaved to destroy the spores before the item can be reused. Disposable equipment must be incinerated or thoroughly autoclaved before disposal.

Hand-washing   Doctors, nurses, and other hospital personnel entering the room must be particularly careful to wash their hands before and after caring for a patient. Hand contact with door knobs, telephones, elevator buttons, and furniture easily transmits pathogens to and from the patient. Fingernails should be kept short and clean, and jewelry should not be worn in an isolation room.

Gowns   In every isolation room, gowns should be used. A clean fresh gown should be available for each person who enters the isolation room on each occasion and discarded after each use. To be protective, gowns should be large enough to be fastened securely. They must be kept dry—remember that a moist environment is required for growth of pathogens, so if an area is moist, the pathogens may gain access to clothing worn under the gown.

Strict Isolation

Visitors—Report to Nurses' Station
Before Entering Room

1. Private Room—*necessary*; door must be kept closed.

2. Gowns—must be worn by all persons entering room.

3. Masks—must be worn by all persons entering room.

4. Hands—must be washed on entering and leaving room.

5. Gloves—must be worn by all persons entering room.

6. Articles—must be discarded, or wrapped before being sent to Central Supply for disinfection or sterilization.

Enteric Precautions

Visitors—Report to Nurses' Station
Before Entering Room

1. Private Room—necessary for children only.
2. Gowns—must be worn by all persons having direct contact with patient.
3. Masks—not necessary.
4. Hands—must be washed on entering and leaving room.
5. Gloves—must be worn by all persons having direct contact with patient or with articles contaminated with fecal material.
6. Articles—special precautions necessary for articles contaminated with urine and feces. Articles must be disinfected or discarded.

Protective Isolation

Visitors—Report to Nurses' Station
Before Entering Room

1. Private Room—*necessary;* door must be kept closed.
2. Gowns—must be worn by all persons entering room.
3. Masks—must be worn by all persons entering room.
4. Hands—must be washed on entering and leaving room.
5. Gloves—must be worn by all persons having direct contact with patient.

Wound & Skin Precautions

Visitors—Report to Nurses' Station
Before Entering Room

1. Private Room—desirable.
2. Gowns—must be worn by all persons having direct contact with patient.
3. Masks—not necessary except during dressing changes.
4. Hands—must be washed on entering and leaving room.
5. Gloves—must be worn by all persons having direct contact with infected area.
6. Articles—special precautions necessary for instruments, dressings, and linen.

Respiratory Isolation

Visitors—Report to Nurses' Station
Before Entering Room

1. Private Room—*necessary;* door must be kept closed.
2. Gowns—not necessary.
3. Masks—must be worn by all persons entering room if susceptible to disease.
4. Hands—must be washed on entering and leaving room.
5. Gloves—not necessary.
6. Articles—those contaminated with secretions must be disinfected.
7. Caution—all persons susceptible to the specific disease should be excluded from patient area; if contact is necessary, susceptibles must wear masks.

Figure 8–1. Hospital precaution signs used for the protection of patients, staff, and visitors. (Volk WA, Wheeler MF: Basic Microbiology, 5th ed. Philadelphia, Harper & Row, 1984)

Table 8–1. Isolation Techniques Used in Hospitals to Prevent Spread of Infection in Hospitals

Isolation	Route of Transmission	Isolation Techniques	Diseases
Strict	All	Private rooms, gowns, gloves, masks, sterilize all contaminated articles	Congenital rubella, chicken pox, plague (pneumonic), generalized staphylococcal infections
Respiratory	Respiratory	Private rooms, masks, contaminated articles	Measles, pertussis, tuberculosis
Enteric	Enteric, from feces	Private rooms, gowns, gloves, contaminated articles	*Salmonella*, *Shigella*, hepatitis
Contact	Contact with lesions, infected wounds	Private rooms, gowns, gloves, masks	Infected burns, draining wounds
Blood and body fluid	Contact with blood or body fluids	Private room	Hepatitis or human immuno-deficiency virus infections
Protective	Staff to patient	Universal precautions, private rooms, masks	Extensive burns; immuno-suppressed

Masks Masks generally are not worn outside the operating room. However, if a patient is isolated because of a respiratory infection, the patient should be masked whenever it is necessary to go for treatment in other parts of the hospital. Personnel working closely with an isolated respiratory patient may wish to wear masks for self-protection. Remember that wet masks are not effective. Used masks should be promptly discarded or laundered and autoclaved. Hands should be washed again after touching a used mask.

Gloves The type of latex or vinyl gloves selected should be appropriate for the task being performed.

1. Use sterile gloves for procedures involving contact with normally sterile areas of the body.
2. Use examination gloves for procedures involving contact with mucous membranes and for other patient care or diagnostic procedures not requiring sterile gloves, unless otherwise indicated.
3. Change gloves between patient contacts.
4. Do not wash or disinfect surgical or examination gloves for reuse. Disinfectants may cause deterioration and washing with surfactants may allow liquids to penetrate the barrier through undetected holes in the glove.
5. Use general-purpose utility gloves for housekeeping chores involving potential blood contact and for instrument cleaning and decontamination procedures. Utility gloves may be decontaminated and reused but should be discarded if there is evidence of deterioration.

Hospital Infection Control

All hospitals are required by the regulatory agencies to have a formal infection control program. This program may vary slightly from hospital to hospital, but all must have an infection control committee and an epidemiology service. The infection control committee consists of representatives from the medical and surgical services, as well as the laboratory, pathology, nursing, hospital administration, housekeeping, food services, central supply, and other hospital departments. The chairman is usually an infectious disease specialist, pathologist, microbiologist, or one knowledgeable about infection control. The committee periodically reviews the hospital's infection control procedures and incidence of nosocomial infections. It is a policy-making and review body that may take drastic action when epidemiologic circumstances warrant.

The epidemiology service is the part of the infection control committee that is charged with patient surveillance, environmental surveillance, investigation of outbreaks and epidemics, and education of the hospital staff regarding infection control. In many hospitals, these activities are actually performed by the infection control nurse or epidemiologist.

Even though every department of the hospital or institution endeavors to maintain aseptic conditions, the total environment is constantly bombarded with microbes from the outside. These must be controlled for the protection of patients.

Hospital personnel (members of the infection control committee or nurse) entrusted with this aspect of health care diligently and constantly work to maintain the proper environment. The microbiology laboratory cooperates to keep constant watch over asepsis within the hospital and consults, as necessary, with various personnel to ensure the maintenance of aseptic conditions throughout the hospital. Laboratory tests can demonstrate the presence and location of contaminating microbes as well as the effectiveness of the disinfection processes. The laboratory should also be able to trace the sources of infections and make recommendations to prevent recurrence. In case of an epidemic, the infection control committee notifies city, county, and state health authorities so they can concentrate their efforts toward bringing the epidemic to an end.

Medical Waste Disposal

General Regulations   According to the Occupational Health and Safety Administration Standards, medical wastes must be disposed of properly. These standards include the following:

1. Any receptacle used for putrescible (decomposable) solid or liquid waste or refuse must be constructed so that it does not leak and must be maintained in a sanitary condition. This receptacle must be equipped with a solid, tight-fitting cover, unless it can be maintained in a sanitary condition without a cover.
2. All sweepings, solid or liquid wastes, refuse, and garbage shall be removed to avoid creating a menace to health and shall be removed as often as necessary to maintain the place of employment in a sanitary condition.
3. The infection control program must address the handling and disposal of potentially contaminated items.

Sharp Instruments; Reusables and Disposables   These items must be disposed of in the following manner:

1. Needles shall not be recapped, purposely bent or broken by hand, removed from disposable syringes, or otherwise manipulated by hand.
2. After use, disposable syringes, scalpel blades, and other sharp items must be placed in puncture-resistant containers for disposal.
3. These containers must be easily accessible to all personnel needing them and must be located in all areas where needles are commonly used, as in areas where blood is drawn, including patient rooms, emergency rooms, intensive care units, and surgical suites.
4. The containers must be constructed so that the contents will not spill if knocked over and will not cause injuries.

Laboratory Specimens   All specimens of body fluids must be put in a well-constructed container with a secure lid to prevent leaking during transport and must be disposed of in an approved manner. Contaminated materials used in laboratory tests should be decontaminated before processing or be placed in bags and disposed of in accordance with institutional policies for disposal of infectious waste.

Specimen Collection, Processing, and Testing

It would not be feasible in a book of this size to give a complete discussion of collection, handling, and processing of specimens. Only a few important concepts are discussed here.[2]

Role of Health Care Personnel

Extreme care must be taken by those involved in the collection, handling, and processing of specimens to be examined for the presence of microorganisms. The microbiological analysis can be only as reliable as the quality of the specimen allows. When specimens are properly collected and handled, (1) the causative microorganisms may not be found or may be destroyed, (2) overgrowth by indigenous microflora may mask the pathogen, and (3) contaminants may interfere with the identification of the pathogens.

A close working relationship among the members of the health care team is essential for the proper identification of pathogens. When the attending physician recognizes the clinical symptoms of a possible infectious disease, certain specimens and clinical tests may be requested. The clinical microbiologist who performs the laboratory microbial analysis must provide adequate collection materials and instructions for their proper use. The doctor, nurse, medical technologist, or other qualified health care worker must perform the collection procedure properly, and then the specimen must be transported quickly to the laboratory where it is cultured, stained, analyzed, and identified. Laboratory findings must then be conveyed to the attending physician as quickly as possible to facilitate the prompt diagnosis and treatment of the disease.

Proper Collection of Specimens

When collecting specimens, these general procedures should be followed:

1. All specimens should be collected in a sterile manner. This requires that they be put into a sterile container to prevent contamination by indigenous microflora and airborne microorganisms.
2. The material should be collected from the site where the suspected organism is most likely to be found and where the least contamination is likely to occur.
3. Specimens should be obtained before antibiotic therapy has begun. If this is not possible, the laboratory should be informed of which antibiotic is being used.

[2]For more detailed information, refer to *Manual of Clinical Microbiology*, 3rd ed, Chap 6, American Society for Microbiology, Washington, D.C. 1991; or to *Collection, Handling, and Shipment of Microbiological Specimens*, U.S. Department of Public Health, Publication #976, Washington, D.C., 1973.

4. The acute stage of the disease is the appropriate time for the collection of most specimens. Some viruses, however, are more easily isolated during the onset stage of the disease.

5. Specimen collection should be performed with care and tact to avoid harming the patient, causing discomfort, or causing undue embarrassment. If the specimen, such as sputum or urine, is to be collected by the patient, clear and detailed instructions should be given.

6. A sufficient quantity of the specimen should be obtained to allow enough material for all diagnostic tests that need to be performed. The amount should be indicated by the physician or laboratory microbiologist.

7. Specimens should be protected from heat and cold, and promptly delivered to the laboratory so the results of the analysis will be a valid representation of the organisms present at the time of collection. If delivery is delayed, some delicate pathogens will die. Obligate anaerobes die when exposed to the air. Also, the indigenous microflora may overgrow the pathogens, which may inhibit or kill them. Delay of delivery considerably decreases the chances of isolating the pathogen.

8. Dangerous specimens must be handled with even greater care to avoid contamination of the ward messenger, patients, nurses, and other hospital personnel. Such dangerous specimens are usually placed in a sealed plastic bag for immediate transport to the laboratory.

9. All specimen containers must be cleaned, sterilized, and properly stored to avoid contamination of the specimen by microbes and harmful chemicals from the container.

10. After the specimen is collected, the container must be properly labeled and accompanied by the appropriate laboratory instructions written on the requisition. The label must identify the patient and the source of the specimen (*e.g.*, throat, wound). The requisition must give the date, time of collection, doctor's name and address, and laboratory tests requested. The laboratory also should be given any additional clinical information that will aid in performing the appropriate analyses.

11. Specimens should be collected and delivered to the laboratory as early in the day as possible to allow the technicians time to process the material, especially if the hospital or clinic does not have 24-hour laboratory service. Many hospitals require the laboratory technicians to collect specimens for immediate evaluation.

Types of Specimens Usually Required

Special techniques in collection and handling are required to obtain specific types of specimens.

Blood   Normally, the blood is sterile. Organisms found in the blood usually indicate a disease condition although temporary, transient bacteremias may occur following oral surgery, etc. Therefore, extreme care must be taken to use sterile technique for drawing the blood into a sterile blood-collecting bottle containing an anticoagulant.[3] After locating a suitable vein, disinfect the skin with 70% ethyl alcohol, then 2% tincture of iodine, or similar antiseptic, allowing it to dry. Apply a tourniquet and withdraw 10 ml to 20 ml of blood with a 21-gauge needle into a sterile container, such as the Vacutainer®, containing an anticoagulant. The blood sample should be transported promptly to the laboratory and cultured in a specially prepared growth medium. If necessary, the blood sample may be refrigerated up to 2 hours before it is cultured.

In many infectious diseases, bacteremia (bacterial blood infection) may be found during certain stages. In this circumstance at least three blood samples should be taken an hour apart. These diseases include bacterial meningitis, typhoid fever and other salmonella infections, pneumococcal pneumonia, urinary infections, endocarditis, brucellosis, tularemia, plague, anthrax, syphilis, and wound infections by β-hemolytic streptococci, staphylococci, and other invasive bacteria. A severe septicemia caused by gram-negative rods is frequently found in patients following gastrointestinal and urological surgery.

Urine   Urine, like blood, is normally sterile; however, it is usually contaminated by the indigenous microflora of the urethra during urination. The contamination can be reduced by collecting a midstream "clean-catch" urine specimen. The area around the urethra is cleansed by washing with soap and rinsing with water. With the glans penis or labial folds separated, the urethra is flushed with the first portion of urine; then the middle portion of the urine is caught in a sterile container. In some circumstances the physician may prefer to collect a catheterized specimen or to use the suprapubic needle aspiration technique to obtain a sterile sample of urine.

A urinary tract infection is indicated if the number of bacteria in a midstream clean-catch urine specimen exceeds 100,000 organisms per milliliter (org/ml), as normal urine may contain less than 10,000 org/ml.

Urine specimens must be processed within an hour or refrigerated at 4°C (39.2°F) to prevent continued bacterial growth until they can be analyzed (within 5 hours). The presence of two or more bacteria per $1,000\times$ microscopic field of a Gram-stained smear indicates bacteriuria with 100,000 organisms per ml, or more.

Cerebrospinal Fluid   Spinal fluid specimens must be collected into a sterile tube by a "spinal tap" under surgically aseptic conditions. This difficult procedure is performed by a physician. Meningitis and meningoencephalitis can be caused by

---

[3] Many satisfactory blood collecting systems are available from suppliers such as Becton, Dickinson and Company, Rutherford, NJ; Hyland Laboratories, Costa Mesa, CA; Difco Laboratories, Detroit, MI; BBL-Bioquest, Cockeysville, MD; and others.

a variety of microbes, including bacteria, fungi, protozoa, and viruses. Because the meningococci are susceptible to cold temperatures, the specimen must be cultured immediately and not refrigerated. Specimens to be further examined for viruses may be kept frozen at $-20°C$ $(-4°F)$.

Sputum Sputum may be collected by allowing the patient to spit coughed-up mucus into a sterile wide-mouthed bottle with a lid, warning the patient not to contaminate the sputum with saliva from the oral cavity. If proper mouth hygiene is maintained, the sputum may not be severely contaminated with oral microorganisms. If tuberculosis is suspected, extreme care in handling the specimen should be exercised because one could easily be infected with the agent. Sputum specimens usually may be refrigerated for several hours without loss of the pathogens.

However, the physician may wish to obtain a better specimen by bronchial aspiration through a bronchoscope or by inserting a needle into the trachea below the glottis (transtracheal aspiration). Needle biopsy of the lungs may be necessary for diagnosis of *Pneumocystis carinii* (in AIDS) and for mycobacterial, fungal, and viral pathogens.

Mucous Membrane Swabs Sterile polyester swabs are used to take specimens of exudates and secretions of the throat, nose, ear, eye, urogenital openings, rectum, wounds, operative sites, and ulcerations. Cotton swabs are no longer used because the fatty acids in the cotton inhibit the growth of some microorganisms. Handy, sterile, disposable collection units can be obtained from many supply houses. Each unit contains a sterile polyester swab in transport medium in a sterile tube. With this setup the organisms are kept alive and protected during transportation to the laboratory.

Genital swabs should be inoculated immediately onto Thayer-Martin chocolate agar plates and incubated in a CO_2 (carbon dioxide) environment; or they should be inoculated into a tube or bottle (e.g., Transgrow®) that contains CO_2 while the bottle is held in an upright position to prevent the loss of CO_2. These cultures should be incubated at $35°C$ $(95°F)$ overnight, then shipped to the public health diagnostic facility for positive identification of gonococci.

Feces Ideally, fecal specimens should be collected at the laboratory and processed immediately to prevent a decrease in temperature, which allows the pH to drop, causing the death of many *Shigella* and *Salmonella* species; or the specimen may be placed in a container with a preservative that maintains a pH of 7. In some cases the specimens are collected anaerobically if *Clostridium* species are suspected to be present.

Since the majority of fecal bacteria are anaerobic gram-negative rods, the specimen should be cultured anaerobically and aerobically. In intestinal infections, the pathogens frequently overwhelm the normal microflora so that they are the major organism seen in smears and cultures. Direct microscopic examination and serologic tests may be performed to identify gram-negative and gram-positive bacteria (enterotoxigenic and invasive *E. coli, Salmonella* spp., *Shigella* spp., *Clostridium perfringens, Clostridium difficile, Vibrio cholerae, Campylobacter* spp., and *Staphylococcus* spp.) fungi (*Candida*), protozoa (*Giardia, Entamoeba*), and other parasites.

Shipping Specimens

Occasionally, a specimen must be sent to a laboratory in another city for identification. Such specimens should be shipped by the fastest means available. If they are sent by mail, viral cultures must be quick-frozen and shipped in dry ice. Pathogenic bacteria must be so labeled on the outside of the package. They should be cultured on solid agar in a tube, which is capped, with tape around the cap. The glass tube should be wrapped in cotton or bubble wrap and placed in a metal can and then in a cardboard mailing box. These specimens should be sent by first-class mail.

Identification and Drug Sensitivity of Pathogens

After the pathogen from a specimen has been isolated, the main remaining tasks are to identify the organism and determine its sensitivity to antibiotic treatment.

Types of Tests

By performing a few simple tests on a pure culture of a pathogen, at least the genus to which the organism belongs can be determined. The Gram stain enables the laboratory worker to describe the Gram reaction (positive or negative); morphology (cocci, bacilli, or spirilla); grouping (pairs, chains, tetrad, or cluster); and whether or not it produces spores. By observing a culture on solid agar, one can describe the shape, consistency, size, and color of the colony as well as whether it is an anaerobe or an aerobe. The use of certain selective and differential media, such as EMB (eosin methylene blue), and a few simple biochemical tests, such as those for catalase or oxidase, substantially helps determine the genus and species of the organisms. The final determination may be made by serotyping, if necessary.

Many laboratories make use of the new multiple-test systems available from Analytab Products, Inc.; Roche Diagnostics; BBL-Bioquest; and many others. Each system has certain advantages and disadvantages, but in general, they are faster, more comprehensive, and easier to use than the conventional methods. Care should be taken to evaluate each before one is adopted as the accepted analysis. Many of these identification systems are read and evaluated by computers, greatly increasing the speed and accuracy of the tests.

Antibiotic Sensitivity

One of the most helpful tests for the physician is the disk antibiotic-sensitivity method described by Kirby and Bauer. In this test, the pure culture of the organism in tryptose phosphate broth is streaked evenly for complete coverage on a Mueller-Hinton agar plate. The disks that have permeated with various antibiotics are then placed on the agar plate and the plate is incubated at 37°C (98.6°F) under the proper conditions (Figs. 8–2, 8–3).

For gram-positive bacteria, disks of tetracycline, penicillin, ampicillin, vancomycin, streptomycin, erythromycin, lincomycin, kanamycin, neomycin, or oxacillin might be used. For gram-negative bacteria, disks of tetracycline, ampicillin, streptomycin, kanamycin, neomycin, nitrofurantoin, or colistin, as well as many other new antibiotics, might be used. Within 24 hours the diameter of the zones of inhibition around each disk should be measured in millimeters. These measurements must then be compared with the size of zone on a Kirby-Bauer chart, which indicates sensitivity or resistance of the organism.

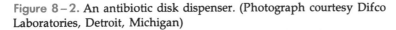

Figure 8–2. An antibiotic disk dispenser. (Photograph courtesy Difco Laboratories, Detroit, Michigan)

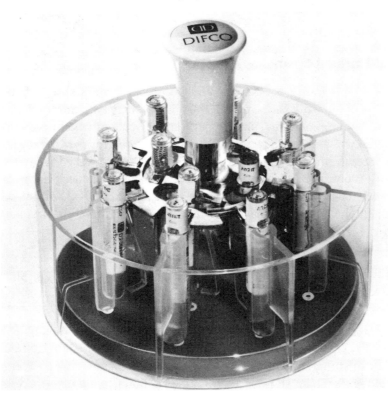

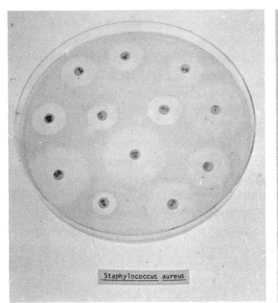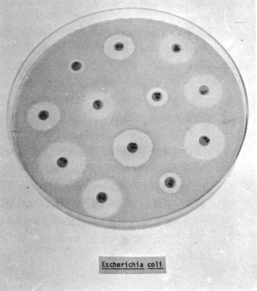

Figure 8 – 3. Paper disks impregnated with various antibiotics are dropped onto the surface of inoculated plates. The antibiotic diffuses into the medium, inhibiting the growth of organisms sensitive to the antibiotic. (Volk WA, Wheeler MF: Basic Microbiology, 4th ed. Philadelphia, JB Lippincott, 1984)

Quality Control in the Laboratory

A quality control program is necessary in any laboratory to monitor the reliability and the quality of the work performed. In the microbiology laboratory, all media, reagents, and staining solutions should be evaluated frequently for effectiveness. Also, all equipment should be maintained and monitored for performance. Refrigerators, freezers, incubators, and water baths should be checked for accuracy of temperature control. By constant surveillance and frequent checking, the efficiency and reliability of the laboratory work can be maintained so that other members of the hospital team have confidence in the information supplied to them from the laboratory.

Environmental Disease Control Measures

Public Health

Massive networks involving the World Health Organization (WHO), public health agencies at all levels, and community groups work together to coordinate preventive health programs and to maintain constant surveillance for sources and causes of epidemics. The WHO also develops international regulations for disease

Insight: Cholera Epidemic of 1991

Cholera has long been present in Africa, Asia, and Europe but had not been reported in South America during this century until January 1991, when cholera appeared simultaneously in several coastal cities of Peru. Sporadic cases have been reported in the United States since 1973; these cases were associated with the consumption of undercooked crabs and raw oysters harvested domestically in the Gulf of Mexico. In 1988, raw oysters shipped from the Gulf Coast caused single cases of cholera in six states, but in the United States, secondary transmission from imported or domestic cases is unlikely because of the availability of safe drinking water and proper treatment of sewage. Only one outbreak has been traced to fecal contamination and that was on a floating oil rig in the Gulf of Mexico.

During the first 4 months of 1991, there were 169,255 cholera cases and 1,244 deaths in Peru that were reported to the Pan-American Health Organization; cholera also spread to Ecuador, Chile, Columbia, Brazil, and Mexico, as a result of poor sanitation and crowded living conditions. Several confirmed cases appeared in Florida, New Jersey, and other parts of the U.S., via travelers who ate raw oysters and crabmeat in Ecuador, Columbia, and Mexico. However, no secondary cases had been reported in the U.S. as of July, 1991.

The risk of tourist's acquiring cholera is considered extremely low, but the number of cases in travelers returning from Ecuador and Mexico emphasizes the need for travelers to epidemic areas to follow the precautions described for prevention of travelers' diarrhea. The general rule "boil it, cook it, peel it, or forget it" is important to remember. Tourists to infected areas should not consume (1) unboiled or untreated water and ice made from such water; (2) raw or partially cooked fish and shellfish; (3) food and beverages from street vendors; and (4) uncooked vegetables. Travelers should eat only hot, cooked foods or fruits they peel themselves. Carbonated bottled water and carbonated soft drinks are usually safe if no ice is added.

Cholera vaccination, which protects approximately 50% of vaccinated persons for 3–6 months, is not recommended for travelers and is not a substitute for scrupulously choosing food and drink in countries with poor sanitation. (From *Morbidity and Mortality Weekly Report*, vol. 40 (287–289), 1991. U.S. Department of Health and Human Services, Public Health Service. Centers for Disease Control, Atlanta, Georgia.)

control and standardization of drugs and plays an active part in the distribution of technical information. When an epidemic strikes, teams of epidemiologists are sent to the scene to investigate the situation and assist in bringing the outbreak under control. Because of this assistance, many countries have been successful in their fight to control smallpox, diphtheria, malaria, tracheoma, and numerous other diseases. In fact, it appears that smallpox may be completely eradicated from the face of the earth; hence, smallpox vaccination of a population or of international travelers may no longer be required.

In the United States, the Department of Health and Human Services administers the U.S. Public Health Service and the Centers for Disease Control, which assist state and local health departments in the application of all aspects of epidemiology. Through the valiant efforts of these agencies working with local physicians, nurses and other health workers, educators, and community leaders, many diseases are no longer endemic in the United States. A list of the diseases that no longer pose a serious threat to the community would include diphtheria, smallpox, typhoid fever, and cholera.

The prevention and control of epidemics is a never-ending community goal. To be effective, it must include measures to

- Increase host resistance through development and administration of vaccines that induce active immunity and maintain it in susceptible persons.
- Ensure that persons who have been exposed to a pathogen are protected against the disease; for instance, injections of gamma globulin or antisera are effective against outbreaks of diphtheria.
- Segregate, isolate, and treat those who have contracted a contagious infection to prevent the spread of pathogens to others.
- Identify and control the potential reservoirs and vectors of infectious diseases. This control may be accomplished by prohibiting "healthy carriers" from working in restaurants, hospitals, and other institutions where they may transfer pathogens to susceptible people, and by instituting effective sanitation measures to control diseases transmitted through water supplies, sewage, and food, including milk.

Water Supplies and Sewage Disposal

Water is the single most essential resource necessary for the survival of humanity. The main sources of community water supplies are surface water from rivers, natural lakes, and reservoirs, and groundwater from wells. However, two types of water pollution are present in our society that are making it increasingly difficult to provide safe water supplies; these come from chemical and biological sources. *Chemical pollution* of waters occurs when industrial installations dump waste products into local waters without proper pretreatment, when pesticides are used indiscriminately and when chemicals are expelled in the air and carried to earth by rain. The main source of *biological pollution* is waste products of humans—

fecal material and garbage — which swarm with pathogens. The pathogens of cholera, typhoid fever, bacterial and amebic dysentery, giardiasis, infectious hepatitis, and poliomyelitis can all be spread through contaminated water. Waterborne epidemics today are the result of failure to make use of the available existing knowledge and technology. In those countries that have established safe sanitary procedures for water purification and sewage disposal, outbreaks of typhoid fever, cholera, and dysentery only rarely occur.

Source of Water Contamination   Rainwater falling over a large area collects in lakes and rivers and thus is subject to contamination by soil microbes and raw fecal material. For example, an animal feed lot located near a community water supply source harbors innumerable pathogens, which are washed into lakes and rivers. A city that draws its water from a local river, processes it, and uses it, but then dumps inadequately treated sewage into the river at the other side of town may be responsible for a serious health problem in another city downstream on the same river. The city downstream must then find some way to rid its water supply of the pathogens. In many communities, untreated raw sewage and industrial wastes are dumped directly into local waters; then, a storm or a flood may result in contamination of the local drinking water with sewage (Fig. 8–4).

Groundwater from wells also can become contaminated. To prevent such con-

Figure 8–4. Sources of water contamination.

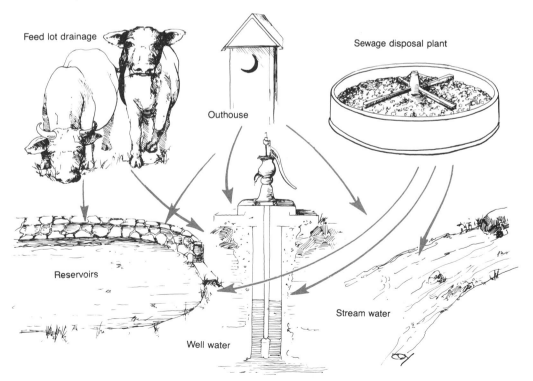

Feed lot drainage

Outhouse

Sewage disposal plant

Reservoirs

Well water

Stream water

tamination, the well must be dug deep enough to ensure that the surface water is filtered before it reaches the level of the well. Outhouses, septic tanks, and cesspools must be situated in such a way that the surface water passing through these areas does not carry fecal microbes directly into the well water. With the growing popularity of trailer homes in recent years, a new problem has arisen because of trailer sewage disposal tanks that are located too near the water supply.

In some very old cities where the water pipes are cracked and the sewage pipes leak, the sewage has easy access to the water pipes wherever there is a break in the pipe at a point just before it enters the dwelling. This is often the case in the older cities of the world.

Water and Sewage Treatment   Water must be properly treated to make it safe for human consumption. It is interesting to trace the many steps involved in such treatment (Fig. 8–5). The water first is filtered to remove large pieces of debris such as twigs and leaves. Next, it is held in sedimentation ponds where the addition of alum coagulates bacteria and organic materials, which then settle more rapidly. The water is then filtered through sand filters to remove the remaining bacteria and other small particles. Finally, chlorine gas or sodium hypochlorite is added to a final concentration of 0.2 to 1.0 part per million (ppm); this kills most remaining bacteria.

In the laboratory, water can be tested for fecal contamination by checking for the presence of coliform bacteria (*E. coli*). These bacteria normally live in the human intestine, thus, their presence in drinking water is a sure sign that the water was subjected to fecal contamination.

Figure 8–5. Steps in water treatment.

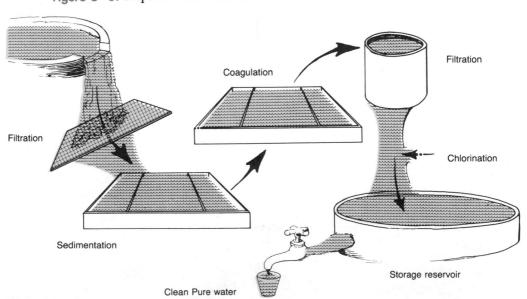

If one is unsure about the purity of drinking water, boiling for 20 minutes destroys any pathogens present. It can then be cooled and used.

When sewage is adequately treated in a disposal plant, the water it contains can be returned to lakes and rivers to be recycled. Raw sewage consists mainly of water, fecal material including intestinal pathogens, and garbage and bacteria from the drains of human habitations. In the sewage disposal plant, large debris first is filtered out; then the bacteria break down some of the organic material. Next, the "activated sludge," which includes the solid matter and bacteria, is settled out in a settling tank. In some communities, the sludge is heated to kill the bacteria, then dried and used as fertilizer. The remaining liquid is filtered and chlorinated so that the effluent water can be returned to the rivers or oceans. In some desert cities where water is at a premium, the effluent water from the sewage disposal plant is distilled so that it can be returned directly to the drinking water system. In some other cities, the effluent water is used to irrigate lawns; however, it is expensive to install a separate water system for this purpose.

Summary

People such as health personnel who are in contact with many infectious diseases must be aware of the necessary preventive measures to inhibit the spread of communicable diseases. They must prevent cross-infections from themselves and the hospitalized, contagious patients to susceptible patients such as newborns and women in delivery, as well as surgical, diabetic, cancer, and paralyzed patients. Health workers must also use precautions to protect themselves against blood-borne pathogens from patients.

Collecting laboratory specimens properly is of utmost importance for identifying the causative agent. Special techniques are necessary for the handling of blood, urine, spinal fluid, sputum, and mucous swabs to prevent contamination and assure survival of the pathogens. The microbiology laboratory plays an important role in the identification of diseases, selection of antibiotics, and maintenance of quality control in the hospital. The national, state, and local health authorities are important agencies that help to prevent and control epidemic diseases. The spread of enteric and waterborne pathogens may be prevented by appropriate water and sewage treatments.

Study Outline

I. Prevention of hospital infections
    A. How hospital infections develop
        1. Hospital-acquired community-acquired infections
        2. Protection of patients

II. Specimen collection, processing, and testing
    A. Role of health care personnel
    B. Proper collection of specimens
    C. Shipping procedures

D. Identification and drug
    sensitivity of pathogens
E. Quality control
III. Environmental disease control
      measures
A. Public health authorities
B. Water supplies and sewage
    disposal
    1. Water pollution
    2. Water and sewage treatment

3. Protection of health care
    workers
B. General control measures
C. Infection control procedures
    1. Medical and surgical asepsis
    2. Universal precautions
    3. Patient isolation
D. Hospital infection control
E. Medical waste disposal

Problems and Questions

1. What groups of people are responsible for the development of
    nosocomial infections?
2. How can hospital infections be eliminated or reduced in number?
3. Which patients are most susceptible to nosocomial infections?
4. Which pathogens are most frequently found in nosocomial infections?
5. Why are universal precautions necessary and how have they changed
    nursing procedures.
6. What are the differences between surgical and medical asepsis?
7. Who must be notified to help control an epidemic?
8. How can you be hurt by collecting and handling laboratory specimens?
9. In what ways can the specimen be contaminated?
10. Why should the nurse not locate the vein after the skin has been
    disinfected when she is taking a blood specimen?
11. Which pathogens might be found in a blood sample?
12. How would you prepare a pathogenic specimen for shipping to a
    distant laboratory?
13. How would you determine which antibiotic would be most effective
    against a certain pathogen?
14. How could you determine which pathogen you had isolated from a
    throat culture?
15. How is water treated to make it safe for human consumption?
16. If a laboratory test showed that *Escherichia coli* were present in a
    sample of drinking water, what would this indicate?

Self Test

After you have read Chapter 8, examined the objectives, studied the new words,
reviewed the study outline, and answered the questions at the end of the chapter,
complete the following self test.

Matching Exercises

Complete each statement from the list of words provided

aseptic	surgical	sterilization
sterile	sanitation	reverse isolation
medical	disinfection	

1. The technique used to avoid all microorganisms is the
   _____ technique and is accomplished by
   _____ .

2. The _____ technique is used to exclude all
   microorganisms from surgical areas to maintain _____
   asepsis.

3. To maintain _____ asepsis, _____
   technique is employed to exclude all pathogens from the area.

4. _____ of dressings and _____ of the skin
   is used to maintain _____ asepsis while dressing a wound.

5. The practical application of sanitary measures and cleanliness is termed
   _____ .

6. Patients with severe burns and organ transplants are protected from
   hospital infections by _____ _____ .

True or False (T or F)

____ 1. Hospital infections can be avoided by the proper awareness and
   use of aseptic techniques.

____ 2. Sick and debilitated patients are much more susceptible to
   opportunistic pathogens than are healthy individuals.

____ 3. Because of the new disinfectants and antibiotics, the incidence of
   hospital-acquired infections has decreased.

____ 4. Many health care workers are not adequately aware of the
   importance of aseptic and sterile techniques and universal
   precautions.

____ 5. The operating and delivery rooms are always clean, so no special
   precautions are necessary to protect the patient.

____ 6. Patients receiving steroids, anticancer drugs, antilymphocyte sera,
   and radiation treatments are usually resistant to hospital-acquired
   infections.

____ 7. Medical asepsis includes all the precautionary measures necessary
   to prevent the transfer of pathogens from person to person,
   including the indirect transfer of pathogens through the air or on
   inanimate objects.

_____ 8. Contaminated foods provide an excellent growth medium for pathogens.

_____ 9. *Staphylococcus aureus* is one of the main pathogens spread by the hands and mouths of hospital workers.

_____ 10. Isolation techniques are used to protect everyone in the hospital from contagious diseases.

_____ 11. Damp or wet masks are just as effective as dry ones.

_____ 12. The microbiology laboratory should constantly monitor aseptic conditions in the hospital.

_____ 13. Smallpox may be totally eradicated owing to the efforts of the public health authorities.

_____ 14. All the pathogens can be identified in the clinical laboratory, even in the presence of many contaminants.

_____ 15. If the specimen is improperly collected, unnecessary contamination may mask the disease-causing agent.

_____ 16. Laboratory findings must be conveyed to the attending physician as soon as possible to aid in the diagnosis and treatment of the diseases.

_____ 17. The specimens most likely to yield the pathogens are collected before antibiotic therapy begins.

_____ 18. Aerobic microbes die when exposed to the air.

_____ 19. Dangerous specimens should be placed in a sealed container for immediate transport to the laboratory.

_____ 20. The label on the specimen should identify only the patient.

_____ 21. Staphylococci are a part of the normal flora of the blood and spinal fluid.

_____ 22. A septicemic condition indicates that there are pathogens in the blood.

_____ 23. Sputum specimens may be refrigerated for several hours without loss of pathogens.

_____ 24. Genital swabs for gonorrhea must be inoculated immediately onto Thayer-Martin media and incubated in the presence of carbon dioxide.

_____ 25. Only the people who work in hospitals are responsible for the prevention and control of epidemics.

Multiple Choice

1. "Nosocomial" refers to
   a. the patients' condition on hospital admission
   b. the physician's health status
   c. infection that develops in a patient during hospitalization
   d. infection that develops in staff
   e. none of a–d choices

2. "Fomite" refers to
   a. inanimate materials
   b. sputum contamination of a fork

c. bandages from infected
    surgical site
d. contaminated bedpan
e. all of a–d choices

3. Reverse isolation would be
   appropriate for
   a. a patient with tuberculosis
   b. a patient who has had minor
       surgery
   c. a patient with glaucoma
   d. a patient with leukemia

4. The microorganism most apt to
   cause nosocomial infections is
   a. *Yersinia pestis*
   b. *Bacillus anthracis*
   c. *Staphylococcus aureus*
   d. *E. coli*

5. Housekeeping and central supply
   personnel contribute to hospital
   asepsis by
   a. restricting contact with patients
   b. protecting themselves from
       infectious organisms
   c. using techniques to prevent
       cross-contamination
   d. all of the above

6. During strict isolation
   a. a double room is desirable
   b. gloves must be worn by
       everyone having contact with
       the infected area
   c. masks are necessary only
       during dressing changes
   d. masks must be worn by all
       persons entering the room

7. Using a clean-catch specimen, a
   urinary tract infection is indicated by
   a. less than 100 org/ml
   b. more than 1000 org/ml

c. any bacteria present
d. more than 10,000 org/ml

8. For an antibiotic sensitivity test,
   the test plate should be
   a. streaked for isolated colonies
   b. incubated 35°C
   c. read after 48 hours
   d. stored in an anaerobic chamber

9. Spinal fluid specimens
   a. are easily obtained
   b. must be inoculated onto
       Thayer-Martin agar plates
   c. are cultured aerobically and
       anaerobically
   d. must be cultured immediately
       for evidence of meningococci

10. All specimens should be
    a. refrigerated
    b. promptly delivered to the
        laboratory
    c. given time to grow
    d. obtained after onset of drug
        therapy

11. Polyester swabs are used
    a. to clean skin before blood
        collection
    b. to take specimens of throat,
        ear, and nose secretions
    c. for anaerobic organisms
    d. for none of the above

12. Raw sewage should be
    a. treated to be safe enough only
        for nonhuman uses
    b. treated sufficiently to be used
        as drinking water
    c. cleaned of most debris and
        some bacteria
    d. none of the above

Chapter 9

Human Defenses Against Disease

Objectives

After studying this chapter, you should be able to

1. List and describe the nonspecific defenses of the human body, or the first line of defense
2. Define phagocytosis, the body's second line of defense
3. List the various types of phagocytic cells
4. Describe the process of inflammation
5. Describe the immune response, or third line of defense
6. Define *antigen, antibody,* and *immunoglobulin*
7. Differentiate between active and passive immunity
8. Compare natural and artificial immunity
9. List three ways in which vaccines are prepared
10. Draw a graph representing the primary and secondary antibody responses to antigens
11. Differentiate between immediate and delayed hypersensitivity
12. Define autoimmunity and give examples
13. List five serological tests used to determine the presence of a specific antibody in human serum

New Words

Agglutination (uh-glue-ten-ay'-shun). The clumping of cells following reaction with antibodies

Allergen (al'-ur-jen). An antigen that causes an allergic reaction

Allergy (al'-ur-gee). A disease resulting from exposure to an antigen

Anamnestic response (an-am-nest'-tick). Memory response following antigen exposure in sensitized individuals

Anaphylactic shock (an-na-fill-lack'-tick). A severe allergic reaction that may result in death

Antibody (an-tea-body). A glycoprotein produced by lymphocytes in response to antigens

Antigen (an'-ti-gin). A foreign substance that stimulates the production of antibodies

Antitoxin (an-tea-tock'-sin). An antibody that neutralizes a toxin

Arthus reaction (ar'-thus). An immune complex skin reaction at the site of repeated injections

Attenuated (uh-ten'-you-ay-ted). An adjective meaning weakened, less pathogenic, used to describe certain microorganisms

Autoimmune disease (au-to-i-mūn'). A disease in which the body produces antibodies to its own tissues

Chemotaxis (keem-oh-tacks'-sis). Movement of cells in response to a chemical substance (the attraction of phagocytes to an area of injury)

Complement (com'-ple-ment). A blood serum protein group involved in inflammation, chemotaxis, and lysis of bacteria

Hapten (hap-ten'). A small, nonantigenic molecule that becomes antigenic when combined with a large molecule

Histamine (hiss'-tuh-mean). Potent chemical released from cells during some immune reactions, causing swelling and inflammation

Hypersensitivity (hi-purr-sens-uh-tiv'-it-tea). A cell-mediated immunological reaction that causes tissue destruction or inflammation

Immunoglobulin (im'-mew-no-glob'-you-lin). An antibody

Interferon (in-ter-fear'-on). Antiviral, soluble protein substances produced by cells infected with an animal virus; also regulates immune function (Interferon is cell-specific and species-specific, but not virus-specific.)

Lymphokines (lim'-fo-kines). T-cell secretions following antigenic stimulation

Precipitin (pre-sip'-i-tin). The precipitation of soluble antigenic material by the specific antibody

Serological tests (sero-o-lodge'-eh-cal). Serum antigen-antibody tests used for diagnostic purposes

Nonspecific Mechanisms of Defense

Humans and lower animals have survived on earth for millions of years because they have many built-in mechanisms of defense against harmful microorganisms and the infectious diseases caused by them. The ability of any animal to resist these invaders and recover from disease is due to many complex interacting functions within the body.

Humans have three lines of defense against bacteria, viruses, fungi, and other parasitic organisms. The first two lines of defense are nonspecific, that is, the body attempts to destroy all types of substances that are foreign to it. However, the third line of defense, the immune response, is very specific. Antibodies are formed in response to the presence of particular foreign substances. These foreign substances are called antigens because they cause the production of specific antibodies (*anti*-"against"; *gen*-"to produce, born"). The immune response is discussed in more detail later in this chapter.

Nonspecific defense mechanisms are general in nature and serve to protect the body against most harmful substances. One of the nonspecific defenses is innate, or inborn, resistance observed among some species of animals, among some races of humans, and among some persons who have a natural resistance to some diseases. Innate or inherited characteristics make these people and animals more resistant to some diseases than to others. Resistance to cholera is an example of species resistance. Human beings can contract human cholera but not chicken cholera. The exact factors that produce this innate resistance are not well understood but are probably due to chemical, physiological, and temperature differences between the species, as well as the general state of physical and emotional health of the person and the environmental factors that affect certain races and not others.

Although we are usually unaware of it, our bodies are, more or less, constantly in the process of defending against microbial invaders. Nonspecific defense mechanisms include such things as mechanical and physical barriers to invasion, chemical factors, microbial antagonism by our indigenous microflora, phagocytic host cells, fever, and the inflammatory response (Fig. 9–1).

Figure 9–1. Non-specific defenses against microbial invasion.

Non-specific
defenses against microbial invasion

Exposure to
microbes

Break in
skin

Intact
skin
barriers
secretions

Body openings
mucous
membrane
barriers

inflammation

capillaries

Chemical
defenses
pH
lysozyme
complement
interferon

phagocytes

Trapping
flushing

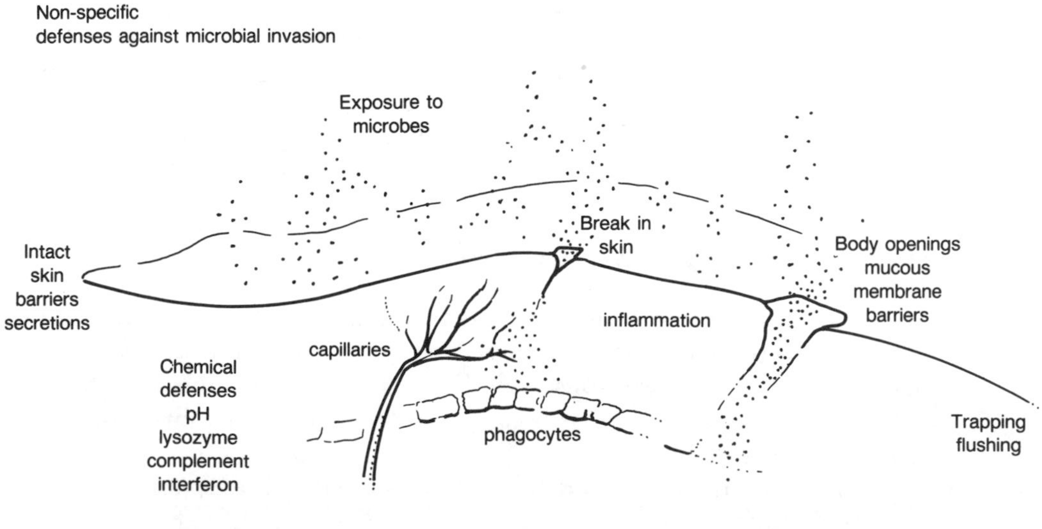

First Line of Defense

The body protects itself against invasion by foreign microorganisms and other substances by defending the body openings to the respiratory, digestive, urinary, and reproductive systems with mucous membranes that entrap the invaders. Also, the skin provides an unbroken and complete external covering for all other parts of the body.

The unbroken skin acts as a physical or mechanical barrier to pathogenic microorganisms; only when it is cut, abraded (scratched), or burned can they gain entrance. There are several factors that account for the skin's ability to resist pathogens. One is the skin's normal secretions, which destroy bacteria or inhibit their growth on its surface. These bactericidal secretions include acidic perspiration of the sweat glands and fatty acids of the oil glands. In addition, the pathogens may not be able to establish themselves and multiply because there are many microorganisms already living in the pores and in moist parts of the head, underarms, hands, feet, and perianal and urethral regions.

The respiratory system would be particularly accessible to invaders that could ride on dust or other particles inhaled with each breath, were it not for the hair, mucous membranes, and the irregular chambers of the nose that serve to trap much of the inhaled debris. The cilia (mucociliary covering) of the epithelial (surface) cells of the posterior nasal membranes, nasal sinuses, bronchi, and trachea sweep the trapped dust and microbes toward the throat, where they are swallowed or expelled by sneezing and coughing. Phagocytes (a type of white blood cells) in the mucous membranes may also be involved in this mucociliary clearance mechanism. Lysozymes and other enzymes that lyse or destroy bacteria are present in nasal secretions, saliva, and tears. The microflora usually residing in the nose and mouth may also serve a protective function.

The digestive system is protected, to a large degree, by the process of digestion, digestive enzymes, acidity of the stomach, and alkalinity of the intestine. Bile, which is secreted from the liver into the intestine, lowers the surface tension and causes chemical changes in the bacterial cell wall and membrane that make bacteria more digestible. Many invading microorganisms are trapped in the mucous lining of the digestive tract where they may be destroyed by bactericidal enzymes and phagocytes. The indigenous microflora that use available nutrients and occupy space in the intestines include *Escherichia coli, Enterobacter aerogenes, Enterococcus faecalis,* and many other enteric (intestinal) bacteria. Peristalsis and the expulsion of feces serve to flush the bacteria from the intestine, as well.

The urinary tract is usually sterile in healthy persons; therefore, urine drawn in an aseptic manner (via needle and syringe) should have no microorganisms present. Also, the reproductive system of the male and most of the reproductive organs in the female lack microflora. However, the indigenous microflora and pathogens from the anus and surrounding skin may grow in the vagina and vaginal opening and invade the urethral opening to the bladder. Microorganisms, (which act as opportunists in this circumstance) are continually flushed from these areas by frequent urination and expulsion of mucous secretions. Many bladder infections occur simply as a result of infrequent urination, especially failure to urinate after intercourse. Normally, the acidic urine and vaginal secretions also inhibit microbial growth. Many women who are taking certain oral contraceptives are particularly susceptible to some infections because those chemicals reduce the acidity of the vagina.

The prevention of colonization of potential microbial pathogens by the indigenous microflora of a given anatomical site is called *microbial antagonism*; this is another example of a nonspecific defense mechanism. The inhibitory capability of these microflora has been attributed to a competition for nutrients and the production of certain inhibitory substances. Examples of such inhibitory substances are the *colicins* produced by certain strains of *Escherichia coli*. Similar substances are produced by some strains of *Pseudomonas* and *Bacillus* species, as well as by other bacteria. Collectively these antibacterial substances (proteins), produced by other bacteria, are known as *bacteriocins*. The effectiveness of microbial antagonism is frequently decreased following prolonged administration of broad-spectrum antibiotics. The antibiotics reduce or eliminate certain members of the microflora (*e.g.*, the vaginal and gastrointestinal flora) and permit overgrowth by bacteria and/or fungi that are resistant to the antibiotic being administered. This overgrowth of organisms, *e.g.*, by *Candida albicans* or *Clostridium difficile*, is called a *superinfection*.

Second Line of Defense

The nonspecific cellular and chemical responses to microbial invasion are considered the second line of defense. Virulent pathogens that penetrate the first line of defense usually are destroyed by a series of defense mechanisms, including the inflammatory response. A complex sequence of events develops involving fever production, iron balance, cellular secretions (interferon, fibronectin, β-lysin, interleukins, prostaglandins, histamine), activation of serum proteins (complement, properdin), chemotaxis, phagocytosis, neutralization of toxins, and clean-up and repair of damaged areas. Each of these responses is addressed in this section.

Fever Production

A fever may be triggered by the pyrogenic (fever-producing) secretions of many infecting pathogens. The increased body temperature augments the host's defenses by (1) stimulating leukocytes to deploy and destroy the invaders; (2) reducing available free plasma iron, which limits the growth of pathogens that require iron for replication and synthesis of toxins; and (3) inducing the production of interleukin-1 (IL-1), which causes the proliferation, maturation, and activation of lymphocytes in the immunological response.

Iron Balance

The virulence of many bacteria is enhanced in the presence of free iron, used for the synthesis of exotoxins. In response to pathogenic invasion, some of the host's leukocytes produce interleukin-1 (an endogenous pyrogen). This substance induces the release of lactoferrin, which stimulates iron storage in the liver and thus reduces the free iron available for the pathogen.

Cellular Secretions

Interferons The α-, β-, and γ-interferons are produced by certain body cells (leukocytes, fibroblasts, and T-lymphocytes) when the cells are infected or stimulated by certain viruses, chlamydias, rickettsias, or protozoa and by the presence of some tumors and cancers. The interferons are secreted into the surrounding cells where they inhibit the synthesis of certain essential proteins that are necessary for the production of viruses and other pathogens within those cells. Thus, the spread of the infection is inhibited, allowing the other body defenses to fight the disease more effectively. In this way many viral diseases (*e.g.*, colds, influenza, and measles) are self-limiting in duration. Similarly, the acute phase of herpes simplex cold sores is of limited duration, but then the virus enters a latent phase and hides in nerve ganglion cells where it is protected until the person's defenses are down; thus, the cycle of disease is repeated.

The interferons, a group of small proteins, are not pathogen-specific, but they are species-specific, that is, they are effective only in the animals that produce them. Thus only human interferon is effective for humans. Human interferons are industrially produced by bacteria with recombinant DNA (with interferon genes inserted) and are used clinically for some viral infections, cancers, tumors, and immunodeficiency diseases.

Fibronectin This epithelial tissue secretion normally enables the cells to bind with collagen and other components of the extracellular matrix. It can also interact with certain bacteria (staphylococci, streptococci) to block their attachment to epithelial cells; thus, it aids in clearing and flushing these pathogens from the body.

β-lysin This polypeptide is released from blood platelets during an infection. It destroys gram-positive bacteria by disrupting the plasma membranes, causing lysis. It is also found inside phagocytes where it aids in the digestion of microbes.

Interleukins These polypeptides (IL-1, IL-2, IL-3) are secreted by antigen-stimulated *macrophages* (certain phagocytic white blood cells). They enhance T-lymphocyte activation, proliferation, and activity during the immune response.

Serum Proteins

Complement   A series of 11 proteins (C1–C9) found in normal blood serum constitute the complement system, which is so called because it is "complementary" to the action of antibodies in immune and allergic reactions. Complement is a nonspecific defense mechanism because it binds to many antigen-antibody complexes. Once bound, it becomes activated (1) to enhance the inflammatory response, (2) to aid in the destruction (lysis) of cells and microorganisms, (3) to attract phagocytes into the region (chemotaxis), and (4) to aid in neutralizing the toxins of certain microorganisms.

Properdin   The serum protein, properdin, works in tandem with complement C3 and C5 proteins in the absence of an antigen-antibody complex. It also enhances phagocytosis, inflammation, and the destruction of bacteria and certain viruses.

Prostaglandins   The prostaglandins are membrane-associated lipids, acting much like local hormones. They are biologically reactive in controlling platelet aggregation, immune response, inflammation, increased capillary permeability, pain production, diarrhea, autoimmune responses, and many other conditions in health and disease.

Phagocytosis

The process by which phagocytes surround and engulf (swallow) foreign material is called phagocytosis. Those foreign materials not needed by the body include dead cells, unused secretions (such as milk), dust, debris, and microorganisms. Phagocytes serve as the "clean-up crew" to rid the body of these unwanted and often harmful substances.

The white blood cells (leukocytes) that act as phagocytes are microphages and macrophages. Microphages are phagocytic *granulocytes*, including neutrophils, eosinophils, and basophils. The most efficient and abundant phagocytes are the neutrophils. Eosinophils become more plentiful and play a phagocytic role in allergic responses, whereas basophils become the mast cells in tissues involved in inflammatory reactions. Macrophages develop from monocytes during the inflammatory response to infections. These cells leave the blood and migrate to the infected area as *wandering macrophages* and are very efficient phagocytes. *Fixed macrophages*, or histocytes, are those macrophages that remain in tissues and organs and serve to trap foreign debris. They may be found in tissues of the reticuloendothelial system (RES); this defensive system includes cells in the liver (Kupffer cells), spleen, lymph nodes, and bone marrow, as well as the lungs (dust cells), blood vessels, intestines, and brain (microglia). Thus, it appears that the macrophages are more efficient scavenger cells than the neutrophilic microphages, but both are able to destroy most of the microorganisms they ingest.

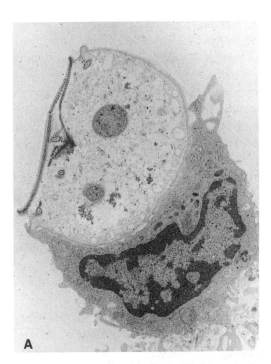

A

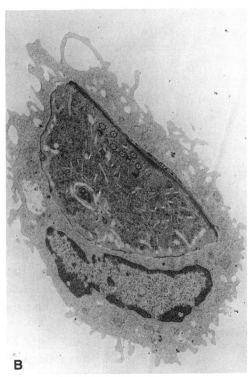

B

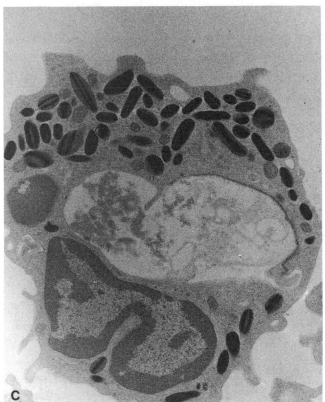

C

Figure 9–2. Phagocytosis of a Giardia trophozoite. (*A*) Attachment. (*B*) Ingestion. (*C*) Digestion. Note the cross sections of cilia in *A* and *B*, and the lysosomes in *C*. (From S. Koester and P. Engelkirk)

The principal function of the entire RES is the engulfment and removal of foreign and useless particles, living or dead, such as excess cellular secretions, dead and dying leukocytes, erythrocytes, and tissue cells, as well as foreign debris and microorganisms that gain entrance to the body.

Phagocytosis begins when a phagocyte moves to within 100 μm of a foreign object such as a bacterium. The phenomenon that causes the phagocyte to be attracted to the bacterium is called chemotaxis. This chemical attraction is not well understood but is the result of lymphokines produced by T lymphocytes and the activation of complement in many circumstances (as discussed later).

When the phagocyte touches a pathogen, the phagocyte's membrane indents (invaginates), and the phagocyte moves around the microbe until it surrounds the latter completely (Fig. 9–2). The membrane-bound vesicle that surrounds the pathogen, which is now inside the phagocyte, is called the phagosome, or phagocytic vacuole. The phagosome fuses with nearby lysosomes to form a digestive vacuole (phagolysosome), and killing and digestion of the microbe begins. Within 10 to 30 minutes after ingestion, the microorganism is killed by lactic acid and hydrogen peroxide from the lysosome. Then lysosomal digestive enzymes, including lysozyme and β-lysin, digest and degrade the carbohydrates, lipids, proteins, and nucleic acids. The products of this digestion, which may be used by cells as nutrients, are then absorbed into the cytoplasm. Undigested materials are retained within the membrane, thus the digestive vacuole becomes the residual body until the undigested wastes are expelled from the phagocyte.

It should be noted that not all bacteria engulfed by phagocytes are destroyed by the digestive enzymes. Usually encapsulated bacteria are resistant to digestion; thus, they may be carried to another part of the body before the phagocyte expels them. Also, some pathogens secrete an enzyme, leukocidin (discussed in Chapter 7), that destroys leukocytes, including the phagocytes that ingest them. Other pathogens, such as *Mycobacterium* species, are able to multiply within the phagosome and destroy the phagocyte. The causative agents of brucellosis and tularemia may remain dormant within the phagocyte for months or years before they escape to cause disease. These types of virulent pathogens usually win the battle with phagocytes. Unless antibodies are present to activate complement to aid in the destruction of these pathogens, the infection may progress unchecked (Fig. 9–3).

Inflammation

The body normally responds to any local injury, irritation, microbial invasion, or bacterial toxins by a complex series of events called inflammation. The purposes of the inflammatory response are to localize an infection, to prevent the spread of microbial invaders, to neutralize toxins, and to aid in the repair of damaged tissue (Fig. 9–4). In this process, all the nonspecific defenses come into play. These interrelated physiological reactions result in characteristic signs and symptoms of

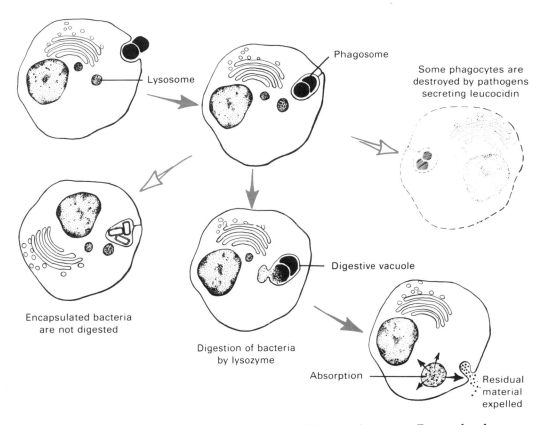

Figure 9–3. Not all pathogens are destroyed by the phagocytes. Encapsulated bacteria and bacteria that secrete leukocidin are two types that are not destroyed if antibodies are lacking.

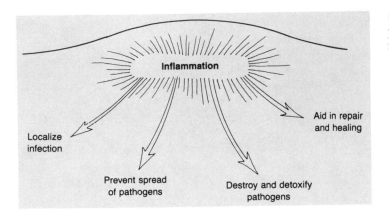

Figure 9–4. The purposes of inflammation.

inflammation: *edema* (swelling of the area), *redness, heat* (fever), *pain*, and often pus formation and occasional loss of function of the damaged area.

A complex series of physiological events occurs immediately after the initial damage to the tissue. Some of the injured cells (mast cells, basophils, and platelets) release certain chemicals (histamine, bradykinin, other kinins, and heparin) that increase the permeability of capillaries and venules, and prevent immediate clotting of the blood. Vasodilation and increased capillary permeability allow more blood (plasma, clotting agents, and cells) to enter the area, including more leukocytes for phagocytosis and antibody production. Macrophages are also attracted to the region by chemotaxis due to the secretions from damaged cells.

The surrounding tissue becomes engorged with fluids, and edema results. Red blood cells collecting in the irritated area cause redness. Metabolic heat is generated and fever is produced by increased cellular activity in the destruction and detoxification of foreign materials, microbes, dead cells (tissue and phagocytic), and toxic chemicals, including waste products released by invading microorganisms.

Pain or tenderness usually accompanies inflammation. It may result from actual damage of the nerve fibers because of the injury, from irritation by microbial toxins or other cellular secretions (such as prostaglandins), or from the edema causing increased pressure on the nerve endings (Fig. 9–5).

The accumulation of fluid and cells within the inflamed site is referred to as the *inflammatory exudate*. If the exudate is thick and yellow with many dead leukocytes, it is known as a purulent exudate or pus. However, it should be noted that in many inflammatory responses, such as arthritis or pancreatitis, there is no exudate and no invading microorganisms. When pyogenic (pus-producing) microor-

Figure 9–5. The inflammatory response.

1. Skin puncture
2. Histamine released
3. Capillaries dilate
4. Increased capillary permeability
5. Increased plasma in tissues
6. Increased phagocytosis of microorganisms and injured tissue
7. Fibrocytes wall off and heal area

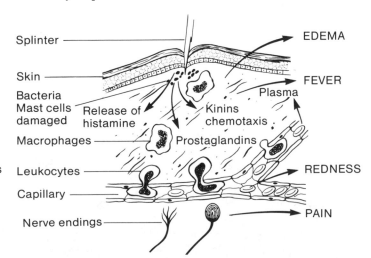

ganisms, such as some staphylococci and streptococci, are present, even more pus is produced as a result of the killing effect of the bacterial toxins on phagocytes and tissue cells. Most pus is greenish-yellow, but in infections caused by *Pseudomonas aeruginosa*, the exudate may be greenish-blue due to certain pigments (pyocyanin) produced by the bacteria.

When the inflammatory response is over and the body has won the battle, the phagocytes continue cleaning up the area and helping to restore order. The cells and tissues can then repair the damage and begin to function normally again in a homeostatic state, although some permanent damage and scarring may have occurred.

The lymphatic system, including the lymph fluid, lymphatic vessels, lymph nodes, and lymphatic organs (tonsils, spleen, and thymus gland), also plays an important role in defending the body against invaders. The primary functions of this system include draining and circulating intercellular fluids from the tissues and transporting digested fats from the digestive system to the blood. Also, macrophages and B- and T-cell lymphocytes in the lymph nodes serve to filter the lymph by removing foreign matter and microbes and by producing antibodies and other factors to aid in the destruction and detoxification of any invading microorganisms.

The body continually wages war against damage, injury, malfunction, and microbial invasion. The outcome of each battle depends on the person's age, hormonal balance, genetic resistance, and overall state of physical and mental health, as well as the virulence of the pathogens involved.

Immune Response to Disease: Third Line of Defense

The *immune response* is the third line of defense against pathogens. Usually, in this protective type of immunity, antibodies are produced by lymphocytes to bind with, inactivate, and destroy specific microorganisms. These humoral (circulating) antibodies are normally found in serum, lymph, and other body secretions where they readily protect against those specific pathogens that stimulated their formation. Thus, a person has an immunity to a particular disease because of the presence of specific protective antibodies that are effective against the causative agent of that disease. In addition, there are protective cell-mediated immune responses that do not involve the presence of antibodies.

Although the immune system protects against disease and aids in fighting cancer, it may also cause damage to its host, as you will learn from the following discussions on cell-mediated hypersensitivity and autoimmunity.

Immunity

Immunity is the resistance to disease due to the presence of antibodies to the causative pathogens (etiologic agents) of that disease. The innate, or native, resistance to disease found in certain individuals, races, and species of animals is not a type of immunity conferred by antibodies but, rather, is a resistance resulting from natural nonspecific factors. A person who is susceptible to a disease usually has inadequate levels of protective antibodies or insufficient nonspecific defenses, which may simply reflect a very poor state of health or the presence of an immunodeficiency disease.

Acquired Immunity

Immunity that results from the production or transfer of antibodies is termed acquired immunity. If the antibodies are formed by the lymphocytes of the protected person, the immunity is called *active acquired immunity*. In *passive acquired immunity*, antibodies are transferred from one person (or from an animal) to another person to temporarily protect the latter against infection (Table 9–1).

Active Acquired Immunity   People who have had a specific infection usually have some resistance to reinfection by the causative pathogen because of the presence of antibodies and stimulated lymphocytes. This is called *naturally acquired active immunity*. Symptoms of the disease may or may not be present when these antibodies are formed. Such resistance to reinfection may be permanent (as with mumps, measles, smallpox, diphtheria, whooping cough, poliomyelitis, plague, and typhoid fever), or it may be only temporary (as with pneumonia, influenza, gonorrhea, and streptococcal, and staphylococcal infections). There is no immunity to reinfection following recovery from syphilis and tuberculosis.

Artificially acquired active immunity is the second type of actively acquired immunity. It occurs when a person receives a vaccination, which is the administration of a vaccine that causes specific antibodies to be produced. Sufficient antigens of a pathogen are contained in the vaccine to enable the person to form antibodies against that pathogen before exposure to the disease. A good vaccine is one that (1) contains enough antigens to protect against infection by the pathogen; (2) contains antigens from all of the strains of the pathogen that cause that

Table 9–1.   Types of Acquired Immunity

Active		Passive	
Natural	*Artificial*	*Natural*	*Artificial*
Clinical or subclinical disease	Vaccines: Dead or extract Attenuated Toxoids	Congenital (across placenta) Colostrum	Antiserum Antitoxin Gamma globulin

disease (*e.g.*, three strains of virus cause "polio"); (3) is not too toxic; and (4) does not cause disease in the vaccinated person.

A successful vaccine for colds has not been developed, because so many different viruses cause colds. Maintaining a successful vaccine for influenza is also difficult; because the viruses continually change by mutation.

Vaccines are made from living or dead pathogens or from certain toxins they excrete (Fig. 9–6). In general, vaccines made from living organisms are most effective, but they must be prepared from harmless organisms that are antigenically closely related to the pathogens or from weakened pathogens that have been genetically changed so they are no longer pathogenic. The process of weakening pathogens is called attenuation. The smallpox (variola) vaccine is derived from the cowpox virus (vaccinia), which causes a mild pox infection in cattle and humans. Most other live vaccines are avirulent (nonpathogenic) mutant strains of pathogens that have been derived from the virulent organisms; this is done by growing them for many generations under various conditions or by exposing them to mutagenic chemicals or radiation. Pasteur developed the attenuated vaccine for rabies and Sabin developed the attenuated oral vaccine for poliomyelitis. Other attenuated living vaccines include those for measles (rubeola), mumps, German measles (rubella), yellow fever, and typhus.

Vaccines made from dead pathogens, which have been killed by heat or chemicals, can be produced faster and more easily, but they are less effective than live vaccines because the antigens on the dead cells are usually less effective and produce a shorter period of immunity. The dead vaccines are safer to use during the

Figure 9–6. Sources of vaccines.

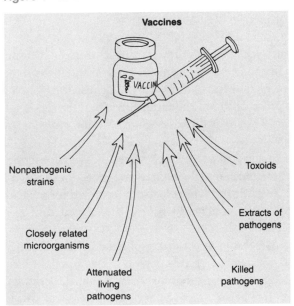

experimental phase of vaccine production because of the remote possibility that an avirulent strain of a living organism may revert to the virulent strain before the strain's stability has been proved. For example, the first poliomyelitis virus vaccine, which was developed by Jonas Salk, contained the killed organisms of three strains of polioviruses, which had to be injected to produce adequate immunity against the disease. A few years later, it was found that the live virus vaccine, developed by Sabin and others, was safe when taken by mouth. Killed pathogens or their extracts are used to vaccinate against whooping cough (pertussis), typhoid fever, paratyphoid fever, cholera, plague, Rocky Mountain spotted fever, and many respiratory diseases including influenza. The use of such vaccines shows us a very important and practical application of the principles of microbiology.

Another type of vaccine used to prevent tetanus and diphtheria, called a *toxoid* vaccine, is prepared from exotoxins that have been inactivated or made nontoxic by heat or chemicals. These toxoids can be injected safely to cause the formation of antibodies that neutralize the exotoxins of the pathogens, such as those that cause tetanus and diphtheria. Antiserum containing antibodies against toxoids prepared in this way is called *antitoxin*.

As microbiologists made further studies of the characteristics of vaccines, they found that it was practical to vaccinate against several diseases by combining the specific vaccines in a single injection. Thus, diphtheria-pertussis-tetanus (DPT) vaccine contains toxoids for diphtheria and tetanus and killed organisms for whooping cough (pertussis). Sometimes, the Salk poliovirus vaccine is added to form the "quad" vaccine (*quad* = four). A second example is the measles, mumps, rubella (MMR) vaccine that is recommended for all children.

An *autogenous vaccine* is one prepared from a localized infection, such as a staphylococcal boil. The pathogens are killed, then injected into the same person to induce production of more antibodies.

Passive Acquired Immunity   Passive immunity differs from active immunity in that antibodies formed in one person are transferred to another to protect the latter from an infection to which he has been exposed. Because the person receiving the antibodies did not produce them, the immunity thus derived is temporary, lasting about 3 to 6 weeks. The antibodies of passive immunity may be transferred naturally or artificially.

In *naturally acquired passive immunity*, small antibodies (IgG described later in this chapter) present in the mother's blood cross the placenta to reach the fetus while it is in the uterus. Also, the milk or colostrum (secreted for a few days after delivery) contains maternal antibodies to protect the infant during the early months of life.

Artificially acquired passive immunity is accomplished by transferring antibodies from an immune person to a susceptible person. After a patient has been exposed to a disease, the length of the incubation period usually does not allow sufficient time for vaccination to be an effective preventive measure. This is because a span of at least 2 weeks is needed before sufficient antibodies are formed to protect the exposed person. To provide temporary protection in these situations, the patient is given "pooled" immune serum globulin (ISG), that is, antibodies taken from the blood of many immune people. Thus, the patient receives some antibodies to all of the diseases to which the donors are immune. The ISG may be given to provide temporary protection against measles, mumps, polio, diphtheria, and hepatitis in people, especially infants, who are not immune and have been exposed to these diseases.

Hyperimmune serum globulin has been prepared from the serum of people with high antibody levels (titer) against certain diseases. For example, hepatitis B immune globulin (HBIG) is given to protect those who have been, or are apt to be, exposed to hepatitis; tetanus immune globulin (TIG) is used for nonimmunized patients with deep, dirty wounds; and rabies immune globulin (RIG) may be given following a bite by a rabid animal. In botulism, food-poisoning cases, antitoxin antibodies are used to neutralize the toxic effects of the botulin toxin. Remember that passive immunity is always temporary because the antibodies are not produced by the lymphocytes of the protected person.

Immunology

Immunology is the scientific study of immune responses. In this book, only the basic fundamentals of immunology can be presented. The topics briefly discussed in this chapter include active and passive immunity to infectious agents, processes involved in antibody production, cell-mediated immune responses, allergies and other types of hypersensitivities, autoimmunity, and serologic testing for antibodies and antigens.

An *antigen* can be any *foreign* organic substance that is large enough to stimulate the production of antibodies; in other words, it is *immunogenic*. Antigens (or immunogens) may be proteins of more than 10,000 daltons molecular weight, or polysaccharides larger than 60,000, large molecules of DNA or RNA, or any combination of biochemical molecules (*e.g.*, glycoproteins, lipoproteins, nucleoproteins) that make up cells of either microorganisms or macroorganisms. Foreign proteins are the best antigens. An antigen must have one or more antigenic sites, known as determinants (or epitopes), to which antibodies or lymphocytes can bind. The important point is that antigens must be *foreign* materials that the human body does not recognize as *self* antigens, and they must be large enough to be acknowledged by a macrophage. Certainly, all microorganisms fall into this category. Some small molecules called *haptens* may act as antigens if they are coupled with a large carrier molecule such as a protein. Then the antibodies formed against that antigenic determinant combine with the haptens when they are no longer coupled with the carrier protein. As an example, penicillin and other low-molecular-weight chemical molecules may act as haptens, causing some sensitive people to become allergic to them.

Antibodies are glycoproteins produced by lymphocytes in response to the presence of an antigen; and they bind specifically with that antigen. (Actually, the antibody-producing cells are a type of lymphocyte called B cells, which usually work in coordination with T-cell lymphocytes and macrophages, as described later.) A bacterial cell has numerous antigenic determinant sites on its cell membrane, cell wall, capsule, or flagella that stimulate the production of many antibodies. Usually, those antibodies are considered to be "specific" for a particular group of identical bacterial cells. Occasionally, similar antigenic sites (heterophile antigens) are found on other microorganisms or even on tissue cells, and those antibodies that can bind to these similar antigenic sites are referred to as cross-reacting antibodies.

All antibodies are also called *immunoglobulins* (Ig) because they are the globular glycoproteins in the serum that participate in the immune reaction. We usually use the term antibodies to refer to immunoglobulins with particular specificity for an antigen, whereas the term *immunoglobulin* represents all the antibodies a person possesses. Immunoglobulins are also found in lymph, tears, saliva, and colostrum (Fig. 9–7). Colostrum is the clear fluid secreted by the mother's mammary gland after the birth of an infant. This fluid contains a large number of antibodies and some lymphocytes from the mother that serve to protect the newborn during the first few months of life.

The amount and the type of antibodies produced by a given antigenic stimulation depends on the nature of the antigen, the site of antigenic stimulus, the amount of antigen, and the number of times the person is exposed to the antigen. Figure 9–8 shows that after the first exposure to the antigen (such as a vaccine), there is a delayed primary response in the production of antibodies. This delayed response is called the *lag phase*. During this time, the antigen must be processed by macrophages and T lymphocytes. These cells stimulate the small B lymphocytes to develop into large B lymphocytes (plasma cells) that are capable of producing antibodies by protein synthesis, usually in the presence of helper T lymphocytes.

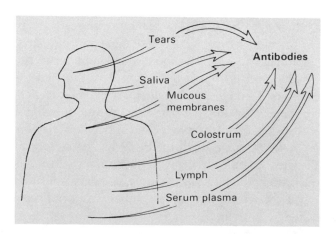

Figure 9–7. Body structures and sites in which antibodies are produced.

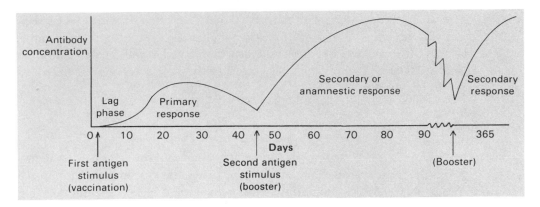

Figure 9-8. Antibody production following exposure to antigen.

This initial immune response is the *primary response*. When the antigen is used up, the number of antibodies in the serum declines as the plasma cells die off. Other antigen-stimulated B lymphocytes become "memory" cells, which are small lymphocytes that can be stimulated to produce antibodies quickly when later exposed to the same antigens. This increased production of antibodies following the second exposure to the antigen (*e.g.*, a booster shot) is the *secondary response*, or the *anamnestic* or *memory response*. A second booster shot of antigen many months later returns the antibody concentration to the level of the secondary response. This is the reason for the immunization of infants and for booster shots given during their first year, before they attend school, and at specific intervals throughout life if the person is continually exposed to those pathogens, as in the case of tetanus.

Some persons are born without the ability to produce protective antibodies. Because they are unable to produce antibodies, they have no gamma globulin in their blood. This abnormality is called *agammaglobulinemia*. These persons are very susceptible to infections by even the least virulent microorganisms in their environment. One treatment of agammaglobulinemia that is often successful consists of a bone marrow transplant, which involves the transfer of precursor white blood cells from a closely related person. Some of these cells become lymphocytes. These lymphocytes may be implanted in the lymph nodes and become immunocompetent, that is, capable of being stimulated by antigens to produce antibodies.

Persons who produce an insufficient amount of antibodies are said to have *hypogammaglobulinemia*. Their resistance to infection is lower than normal, so they usually do not recover from infectious diseases as readily as most other persons.

Some patients are immunosuppressed (unable to make antibodies) after the administration of immunosuppressive drugs or agents, such as antilymphocytic serum before organ transplant surgery. Others are infected with a virus (HIV virus, that causes AIDS), which destroys helper T_H lymphocytes that induce plasma cells to make antibodies and are also involved in cell-mediated immune responses. These patients usually succumb to secondary infections for which they have little resistance.

The Immune System

The immune system encompasses the whole body, but the lymphatic system is the site and source of most immune activity. The cells involved in the immune responses originate in bone marrow (from which most blood cells develop; Fig. 9–9). Three lines of lymphocytes, B cells, T cells, and NK (natural killer) cells, de-

Figure 9–9. Differentiation of blood and lymph cells from bone marrow cells; development of cell-mediated immunity and antibody production.

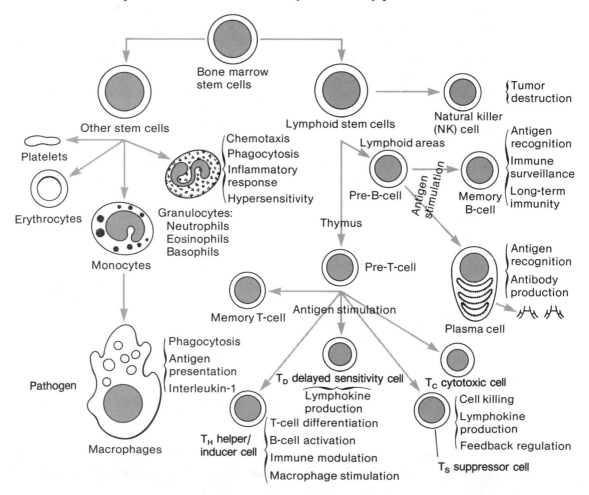

rive from the lymphoid stem cells of bone marrow. About half of these stem cells migrate to the thymus gland where they differentiate into T cells (T for thymus) of the helper, suppressor, or cytotoxic type. Thymus processing of T cells begins shortly before birth. T cells are small lymphocytes found in the blood, lymph, and lymphoid tissues. They do not produce humoral antibodies but do aid in the control of antibody production and are involved in the cell-mediated immune responses (*e.g.*, tissue transplant rejection; cellular immunity to mycobacteria, fungi, and viruses; cytotoxicity of viral-infected cells and tumor cells).

Other lymphocytic stem cells differentiate in the liver and intestinal lymphoid areas into B cells (named for the bursa lymphoid area in birds). B cells migrate to the lymphoid tissues where they produce antibodies that circulate through lymph and blood to protect the individual (humoral immunity). Thousands of B cells exist in the body even though these cells live only about 1 to 2 weeks. When stimulated by an antigen, each B cell is capable of producing hundreds of specific antibodies per second.

The Immune Response

Many chemicals, cells, and reactions are involved in immune responses. Some chemicals and complexes are nonspecific and yet depend on the antigen-antibody complex for activation, as does complement. The specific humoral response always depends on the presence of specific antibodies for each antigen or antigenic determinant. Although some types of cell-mediated responses occur in the presence of antibodies, others do not involve the antigen-antibody complex, as summarized in Figure 9–9.

Humoral Immunity

For antibodies to be produced, a complex series of events must occur, some of which are not completely understood. It is known that macrophages, T cells, and B cells are involved in a cooperative effort.

When bacteria invade, they are first processed by macrophages. It appears that macrophages prepare and present bacterial antigens to the helper T cells (T_H); these antigens appear on the surface of the macrophage. T_H cells serve to stimulate the production of antibody by the B cells but do not manufacture antibodies themselves. T cells are sensitized or primed by the antigen on the macrophage. *Helper T_H cells* induce the B plasma cells to synthesize more antibody, and *suppressor T cells* (T_S) inhibit antibody production in B plasma cells. In this way, the level of antibodies is neither excessive nor insufficient if the control mechanism is working properly. When the antigen is presented to the T cells by the macrophages, some B cells are activated and stimulated to enlarge, differentiate, and divide into clones of antibody-producing *plasma cells* (large B lymphocytes). Antibodies are expelled in gunfire fashion for several days until the plasma cell dies.

Each plasma cell clone makes only one type of antibody: the one that will bind with the antigen responsible for activating the B cell. This specificity is probably determined by the IgD-type antibodies on the surface of the B cell. Those activated B cells that did not become plasma cells, and some primed T cells, remain as memory cells, to respond more quickly when the antigen appears again at a later date.

When the antigen-antibody complex is formed, complement may be activated to destroy the bacterial cell, increase phagocytosis, and neutralize bacterial toxins. Thus, antibody-mediated immunity (AMI) almost entirely controls acute extracellular bacterial infections.

Cell-Mediated Immunity   Antibodies cannot enter cells containing intracellular pathogens; however, the macrophage – T cell-mediated immunity (CMI) serves the body by controlling chronic infections of intracellular parasites (bacteria, protozoa, fungi, viruses). For example, in cytolytic viral infections (*e.g.*, herpes), the virus moves in the body fluids from a lysed cell to an intact cell, during which time the virus can be neutralized and destroyed by the antibody – complement complex, and viral infections can thus be prevented in this manner. However, when the virus is established within the body cells, the cell-mediated immune response (macrophages, T-cytotoxic cells) can destroy many virus-infected cells and damaged tissues but may not completely destroy the virus especially if it becomes latent in nerve ganglion cells as in *Herpes* infections.

Cell-mediated immunity results from several types of antigen-stimulated T lymphocytes. The helper T cells (T_H) cooperate with B cells to initiate the antibody-mediated response; suppressor T cells (T_S) reduce the intensity of antibody-mediated response and moderate the activities of cytotoxic T killer cells (T_C), ensuring that normally the immune response is effective but not destructive.

The T_C cells and NK cells kill infected host cells when the pathogens are established inside the cells. Thus, infected liver cells are destroyed in hepatitis infections during the body's battle against the disease. The AIDS virus that targets T_H cells is particularly destructive because it destroys the very cells that would have helped fight the infection. The lack of T_H cells impairs both humoral and cell-mediated immunity; thus, patients with AIDS are very susceptible to many opportunistic infections and malignancies.

Another T cell (T_D) is involved in delayed hypersensitivity reactions. Its action is delayed because it is formed following antigen sensitization and reacts to produce lymphokines after a subsequent antigen stimulation. This response is discussed later in this chapter.

Nonspecific NK Cells   Some specialized lymphocytes (neither T nor B cells) become nonspecific *natural killer cells* (NK cells). These cells leave the lymphoid area and migrate to the inflammatory site of microbial invasion or area of tumor growth. There they attach to and destroy abnormal cells, including those infected with intracellular agents such as chlamydias and rickettsias, transplanted cells, and tumor or malignant cells, whereas cytotoxic T_C cells target and destroy antigen-bearing virus infected cells. Note that NK cells are not macrophage- or antigen- or antibody-dependent; they strive to rid the body of abnormal or foreign cells. Both NK and T_C cells function by secreting lethal cytotoxic proteins.

Antibody Structure and Function

Antibodies are Y-shaped glycoprotein immunoglobulins (Ig) formed by B lymphocytes in response to stimulation by foreign antigens. Antibodies found in the serum are called humoral or circulating antibodies.

Studies of the gamma globulin component of serum have revealed five classes of antibodies exist. These antibodies, called immunoglobulins, have been designated IgG, IgM, IgA, IgD, and IgE. Each may consist of several subclasses. The functions of each of these classes are listed in Table 9–2.

Immunoglobulin G (IgG) is the most abundant (80%) of the serum antibodies. It binds (attaches) to antigens in the serum as well as the lymph and intercellular fluids. Invading bacteria (antigens) are more easily destroyed by phagocytes or lysed by complement when antibodies are attached to them because the antibodies also may attach to the phagocytes or complement (Fig. 9–10).

Immunoglobulin G is the smallest of the antibodies. It can cross the placenta

Table 9–2. Immunoglobulin Classes and Functions

Ig Class	Molecular Weight	% in Serum (Approx.)	Functions
IgG	150,000	75.000	Protects against disease; attaches to phagocytes and tissues; fixes complement; crosses placental barrier; causes certain immunological diseases; found in serum and lymph
IgM	900,000	10.000	Protects against early infection; bactericidal to gram-negative bacteria; fixes complement; found in serum and lymph
IgA	400,000 or 170,000	15.000	Protects the mucous membranes and internal cavities against infection; found as secretory antibodies in tears, saliva, colostrum, and other secretions
IgE	190,000	0.002	Causes allergies, drug sensitivity, anaphylaxis, and immediate hypersensitivity; combats parasitic diseases
IgD	185,000	0.100	Fetal antigen receptor; conrols antigen stimulation of B cells; found in serum and on lymphocytes

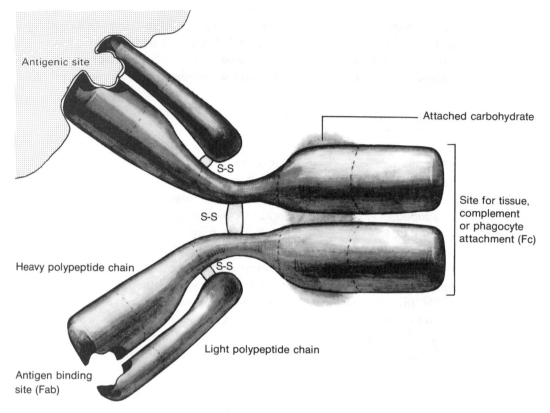

Antigenic site

Attached carbohydrate

S-S

Site for tissue,
complement
or phagocyte
attachment (Fc)

S-S

Heavy polypeptide chain

S-S

Light polypeptide chain

Antigen binding
site (Fab)

Figure 9–10. Basic Structure of immunoglobulin IgG.

and move freely in intercellular fluids and blood. It consists of four polypeptides (amino acid chains): two identical short (light) chains and two longer (heavy) chains held together by disulfide (—S—S—) bonds with attached carbohydrate. (Fig. 9–10). This antibody molecule is bivalent, that is, it has two ends that bind specifically to the antigen that stimulated its production. The middle section of this macromolecule can bind nonspecifically to complement, phagocytes, or tissue cells.

Immunoglobulin M (IgM) is the largest of the gamma globulins. This immunoglobulin consists of five IgG-type molecules held together by disulfide bonds. Because it is star shaped, it usually binds with only five identical antigens. The IgM antibodies are the first antibodies formed in response to infections, especially those caused by gram-negative bacteria. IgM agglutinates bacteria, activates complement, and enhances phagocytosis. Red blood agglutinin antibodies and heterophile antibodies are also IgM antibodies.

Immunoglobulin A (IgA) is designated the secretory antibody, so-called because these immunoglobulins are found in saliva, tears, colostrum, and other body secretions, as well as in the bloodstream and the intestine. IgA molecules usually consist of two IgG-sized antibodies held together by a secretory piece, and they serve to protect the external openings and mucous membranes from invasion by pathogens. Others, IgA molecules, each consisting of one IgG-sized molecule, are found in internal body cavity secretions.

The IgA in colostrum and breast milk helps protect nursing newborns. In the intestine, IgA attaches to viruses, bacteria, and protozoal parasites, such as *Entamoeba histolytica*, and prevents the pathogens from adhering to mucosal surfaces, thus preventing invasion.

Immunoglobublin E (IgE) is also called P-K antibody (in honor of two scientists, Prausnitz and Küstner, who first identified it). These antibodies are more abundant in persons with allergy, drug sensitivity, or anaphylactic shock. Most often, these antibodies are bound to target cells (basophils and mast cells) in tissues and cause the rash or hives seen in various allergies, the "runny nose and eyes" of hay fever and asthma, the local reaction in immediate hypersensitivity skin tests, and shock reaction of anaphylaxis.

Immunoglobulin D (IgD) is a serum antibody, similar to IgG, that may function as a control mechanism for the immune response. The function of this antibody is not clearly understood, but it is probably involved in the determination of which plasma cell produces which antibody (IgG type) because it is found on the surface of B lymphocytes.

Monoclonal Antibodies   Purified monoclonal antibodies against specific antigens have been produced by an innovative technique in which a single plasma cell that produces only one specific type of antibody is fused with a rapidly dividing tumor cell. The new long-lived, antibody-producing cell is called a *hybridoma*. These hybridomas are capable of producing large amounts of specific antibodies called monoclonal antibodies. These antibodies are widely used, especially in developing new diagnostic serologic tests. Because they are uniform, highly specific, and can be produced in large quantities, they can be used routinely to bind with the antigens of particular pathogens in laboratory tests and in allergy and disease testing. Many new procedures are being developed; they may even be used for passive immunization to protect against certain diseases or to neutralize the toxins of botulism, tetanus, and perhaps snake and insect bites.

Hypersensitivity

Hypersensitivity is the defensive immune response gone awry. Sometimes, instead of protecting a person, the antibodies irritate and damage certain cells in the body. This can be compared to the person who builds a fire in the living room to warm the house and burns it down.

There are several different types of hypersensitivity reactions; some involve various antibodies and others do not. All depend on the presence of antigen and T cells sensitized to that antigen.

Hypersensitivity reactions are divided into two general categories, immediate and delayed, depending on the nature of the immune reaction and the time required for an observable reaction to occur. An *immediate reaction* occurs from within a few minutes to 24 hours. There are several types of immediate reactions; type I includes the classic allergic responses of hay fever, asthma, and hives from food; allergic responses to insect stings; drug allergies; and anaphylactic shock. These reactions involve IgE antibodies, mast cells, and basophils. Type II is the cytotoxic hypersensitivity seen in blood transfusion and Rh incompatibility reactions, and in myasthenia gravis, involving IgG or IgM antibodies and complement. Type III is the immune complex reaction of serum sickness and autoimmune diseases (systemic lupus erythematosus [SLE], rheumatoid arthritis), involving IgG or IgM antibodies, complement, and neutrophils. *Delayed hypersensitivity*, which is usually observed after 24 hours, is designated type IV. It is also referred to as cell-mediated immunity, such as occurs in tuberculin and fungal skin tests, contact dermatitis, and transplantation rejection. Delayed hypersensitivity does not involve antibodies but does depend on sensitized or primed T cells that secrete lymphokines in response to a second exposure to the sensitizing antigen (Fig. 9–11).

The Allergic Response   Immediate hypersensitivity (type I) is probably the most commonly observed type of hypersensitivity because approximately 80% of the American population is allergic to something. People who are prone to allergies produce IgE (sometimes called reagin) antibodies that become cell bound when they are exposed to allergens, the antigens that cause allergic reactions. The type and severity of an allergic reaction depend on a combination of factors, including the nature of the antigen, the amount of antigen entering the body, the route by which it enters, the length of time between exposures to the antigen, the person's ability to produce IgE antibodies, and the site of IgE attachment (Fig. 9–12).

The allergic reaction results from the presence of IgE antibodies bound to basophils in the blood or to mast cells in connective tissues, following the person's first exposure to the allergen. When the cell-bound IgE binds with the allergen during the second or later exposure, the sensitized cells respond by producing and releasing irritating and damaging substances. These mediators of the allergic response include histamine, prostaglandins, serotonin, bradykinin, slow-reacting

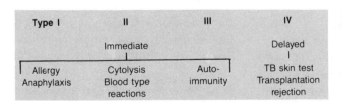

Figure 9–11. Types of hypersensitivity immune responses.

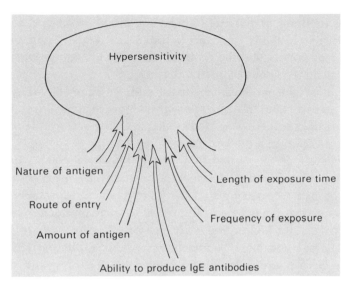

Figure 9–12. Factors in development of hypersensitivity.

substance of anaphylaxis (SRS-A), leukotrines, and other mediating chemicals that attract eosinophils.

Localized anaphylaxis   Hay fever, asthma, and hives are localized allergic anaphylactic diseases. The symptoms depend on how the antigen enters the body and the site of IgE attachment. If the antigen (pollens, dust, fungal spores) is inhaled and deposits on the mucous membranes of the respiratory tract, IgE antibodies are formed and attach to the mast cells in that area. Subsequent exposure to those inhaled antigens allows the allergens to bind to the attached IgE, causing the mast cells to release large amounts of histamine. This substance initiates the classic symptoms of hay fever. Antihistamines are quite useful in treating hay fever because they neutralize histamine. Antihistamines are not as effective in treating asthma, however, because the mediators of this lower respiratory allergy include the leukotrines in addition to histamine. Allergens entering through the digestive tract (food and drugs) can also sensitize the host, causing hives, vomiting, and diarrhea.

Systemic anaphylactic shock   The severe allergic reaction called systemic anaphylactic shock occurs after injection of an allergen to which the host has been sensitized. Frequently, these allergens are drugs or insect venom and, occasionally, certain foods. With penicillin, the drug serves as a hapten, binding to host serum proteins, sensitizing mast cells and circulating basophils. Subsequent injections of large doses of penicillin into the sensitized host may cause the release of large amounts of histamine and other mediators of allergy into the circulatory system.

The shock reaction usually occurs immediately (within 20 minutes) after reexposure to the allergen. The first symptoms are flushing of the skin with itching, headache, facial swelling, and difficulty in breathing; this is followed by falling blood pressure, nausea, vomiting, abdominal cramps, and urination (caused by smooth muscle contractions). In many cases, acute respiratory distress, unconsciousness, and death may follow shortly. Swift treatment with epinephrine (adrenaline) and antihistamine usually stops the reaction.

Health professionals must take particular care to ask patients if they have any allergies or sensitivities. In particular, those people with allergies to penicillin and other drugs and to insect stings should wear Medic-Alert tags so that they do not receive improper treatment during a medical crisis.

Anaphylactic reactions can be prevented by avoiding known allergens. In some cases, skin tests are used to identify the offending allergens. Then, desensitization may be accomplished by injecting small doses of allergen, repeatedly, several days apart. This treatment may be effective by causing the production of increased amounts of circulating IgG antibody instead of IgE. Thus, the IgG should bind with the allergen and block its attachment to the cell-bound IgE. These circulating IgG molecules are called *blocking antibodies*. This preventive measure usually works better for inhaled allergens than for allergens that are ingested or injected.

Autoimmune Diseases   An autoimmune disease is a type III hypersensitivity response that may occur when a person's immune system no longer recognizes certain body tissues as "self" and attempts to destroy those tissues as being "nonself", or "foreign." This may occur with certain tissues that are not exposed to the immune system during fetal development so that they are not recognized as self. Such tissues may include the lens of the eye, the brain and spinal cord, and sperm. Subsequent exposure to this tissue (by surgery or injury) may allow antibodies (IgG or IgM) to be formed, which together with complement (C') could cause destruction of these tissues, resulting in blindness, allergic encephalitis, or sterility.

In some cases, immune complexes may cause destruction of heart or kidney tissues. It is believed that antibodies (IgG and IgM) formed against group A, β-hemolytic streptococci, may bind with streptococcal antigens deposited in heart tissues or glomeruli of the kidney. When the immune complex (strep antigen + IgG + C') is formed, some heart or kidney cells might also be lysed (bystander lysis). This would explain the progressive tissue damage that occurs during recurrent streptococcal sore throat infections with rheumatic fever or glomerulonephritis complications.

Serum sickness is also a cross-reacting antibody immune reaction in which antibodies formed to globular proteins in horse serum (used for antitoxin treatments) may also bind with similar proteins in the patient's serum. The formation of these immune complexes (antigen + antibody + complement) causes the symptoms of fever, rash, kidney malfunction, and joint lesions of serum sickness.

It is believed that certain drugs and viruses may alter the antigens on host cells, thus inducing the formation of autoantibodies or sensitized T cells to react against these altered tissue cells. This may be the underlying basis of multiple sclerosis, kuru, Hashimoto's thyroiditis, rheumatoid arthritis, SLE, and other autoimmune diseases.

Cell-mediated Hypersensitivity The delayed hypersensitivity of type IV is characterized by sensitized T cells that secrete active substances in the absence of antibodies. As an example, when antigens enter and bind with tissue cells (as in tuberculosis), they may be phagocytized by macrophages and then the antigens sensitize T cells. When these primed T cells are subsequently exposed to the antigen complex, they secrete a group of chemicals called *lymphokines*. The lymphokines then destroy the antigen directly, attract additional lymphocytes and macrophages to the area, and increase phagocytic activity. Finally, the inflamed area is walled off by scar tissue, and the tubercule of tuberculosis is formed. The action of T cells, lymphokines, and macrophages causes the localized reaction seen in tuberculosis and fungal skin tests. The beginning of the reaction may be seen after a few hours, and the inflammation, fever, redness, and swelling remain for several days. A similar reaction occurs in contact dermatitis (poison oak and poison ivy).

The rejection of transplanted tissues containing foreign histological (tissue) antigens appears to occur in a similar manner, except that lymphokines as well as antibodies cause the rejection of the transplant.

Immunodiagnostic Procedures

By means of various clinical and research experiments it has become possible to identify the presence of various antibodies to specific antigens.

The antigens may be living microorganisms, or parts of bacteria such as flagella, capsules, or toxins. The study of antigen-antibody reactions is called *serology*. Serologic techniques are used to type blood for blood banks and transfusions, to diagnose diseases, to identify microorganisms, to type tissue for transplantation, and to detect allergy or hypersensitivity. The most common *in vitro* (in the laboratory) serologic tests are *agglutination, precipitin, complement fixation and lysis, fluorescent antibody technique, radioimmunoassay, and enzyme-immunoassays*. Sometimes it is necessary to use *opsonization, capsular swelling,* or *immobilization* to detect specific antibodies.

These tests are all performed in the artificial environment of the laboratory, using the patient's serum to determine if the patient has antibodies to certain antigens. The presence of specific antibodies in the patient's serum could indicate that the patient has the disease, is immune to the disease, or is allergic to the antigen. Other tests are performed *in vivo* (in living animal), such as the skin tests, in which the antigens are injected into the skin (subcutaneously) to detect the presence of antibodies. Reddening at the site of injection would indicate that the patient either has the disease or is immune or allergic to it. Each of these serological tests is summarized in Table 9–3 and a description of them follows.

Table 9–3. Serological Tests to Detect Antibodies

Reaction In vitro	Reagents			Results	
	Antigen	Antibody	Other	+	−
Agglutination	Red blood cells or bacteria	Patient's serum		Clumping	No clumping
Precipitin	Toxins, hormones, proteins	Patient's serum	Agar or solution	Precipitate	No precipitate
Lysis by Complement	Cells, bacteria	Patient's serum	Complement	Lysis	No lysis
Complement Fixation	Viruses, Toxins Foreign proteins	Patient's serum	Complement	C Fixation	No C fixation
				No free C	Free C
Add indicator system	Sheep red blood (SRB) cells	Antisheep red blood cell antiserum		No lysis of SRB cells	Lysis of SRB cells by C

Table 9–3. Serological Tests to Detect Antibodies (*continued*)

Reaction In vitro	Reagents			Results	
	Antigen	Antibody	Other	+	−
Fluorescent Antibody Technique	Pathogen	Patient's serum	Fluorescein	Fluorescent pathogen	No fluorescence
Opsonization	Bacteria	Patient's serum	Phagocytes	More bacteria in phagocytes	Fewer bacteria in phagocytes
Capsular Swelling (Quellung Reaction)	Encapsulated bacteria	Patient's serum		Capsule swells	No swelling
Immobilization	Motile bacteria	Patient's serum		No motility	Motility
Radio-immunoassay	Patient's serum	Rabbit antiserum	Radioactive antigen	Low radioactivity	High radioactivity
Enzyme-linked assay	Test microbe	Patient's serum	Enzyme linked antibody +Substrate	Color change	No color change

Agglutination   Agglutination tests are used to detect the presence and amount of humoral (serum) antibodies to particulate antigens, such as those on red blood cells or bacteria. As the word suggests, particulate antigens are antigenic sites on particles, such as cells or latex particles.

The agglutination technique is used in the Venereal Disease Research Laboratory (VDRL) and rapid plasma reagin (RPR) tests for syphilis, the Widal test for typhoid fever, the Weil-Felix test for rickettsial diseases, and tests for pregnancy. It also has many other applications.

Hemagglutination (the agglutination of red blood cells) often is caused by viruses. Antibodies to these viruses would inhibit the hemagglutination reaction and could be used to positively identify the virus. This adaptation of the agglutination technique is called *hemagglutination inhibition* and is frequently used to identify influenza viruses.

Precipitin   In the precipitin test, the patient's serum is used to demonstrate antibodies to soluble proteins or polysaccharide antigens, such as exotoxins or serum proteins. The antigens and antibodies are suspended in agar to allow diffusion to take place to ensure that the correct concentration of the antigen and antibody is reached. At this point (the zone of optimal proportions), a precipitate is formed and may be seen as a white line in the agar (Fig. 9–13). This would indicate that the patient has antibodies to that specific antigen. The precipitin test is useful in detecting antibodies to the exotoxins of tetanus, diphtheria, and scarlet fever. It is also used to identify various serum proteins in blood. An interesting application is its use in the criminology laboratory as a means to determine whether a particular blood stain is from animal or human blood. Here the serum proteins are extracted and identified by the antibodies that bind specifically with them.

Other precipitation-type tests (*i.e.,* immunoelectrophoresis) are performed by separating the proteins in human serum (electrophoresis), adding known antibodies, and observing the precipitin lines (Fig. 9–14). This powerful test is often used to determine complement and antibody deficiencies in individuals.

Lysis by Complement   When the IgG and IgM antibodies are bound to antigens, the antibodies become activated and react with complement (C). This reaction in turn activates the complement. If the antigens are on cells, such as red blood cells, or on pathogens, such as *Vibrio cholerae*, the activated complement will lyse (destroy) the cells. An application of this reaction is in the indicator system in the complement fixation test, to be described shortly. Another use is to identify the presence of specific antibodies to a pathogen in a patient's serum, as in cholera.

Complement Fixation   Complement is bound (fixed) when antigens bind with antibodies, even if the antigens are not on a red blood cell or bacterial cell. Antigens, such as viruses or toxins, cause fixation (or binding) of complement when the specific antibodies to them are present (reaction I). Because this reaction can-

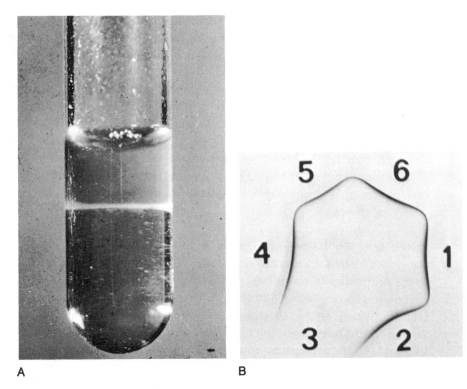

A   B

Figure 9-13. Precipitin ring test. (A) A line of precipitation forms where the antigen and antiserum meet. (Volk WA, Wheeler MF: Basic Microbiology, 3rd ed. Philadelphia, JB Lippincott, 1973) (B) Wells 1 through 6 contain different antigenic fractions of *Yersinia pestis*. (Courtesy of Dr. Tornebene)

Figure 9-14. Immunoelectrophoresis: whole human serum was placed in the well (*circle*) and subjected to electrophoresis. After 2 hours, the electric current was turned off and anti-whole human serum was placed in a trough along the length of the slide. The precipitin lines were formed where the antibodies and the antigens (separated components of whole human serum) diffused together in optimal proportions. (Volk WA, et al: Essentials of Medical Microbiology. 5th ed. Philadelphia, JB Lippincott, 1991)

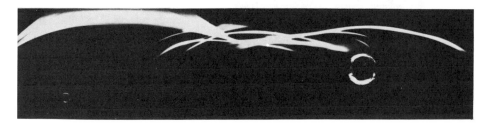

not be detected visually, sheep red blood cells and antisheep red blood cell antibodies (the indicator system) are added to the serum (reaction II). If all the complement is bound in reaction I, there is no unbound or free complement present to lyse the sheep red blood cells in reaction II; thus, the test results are positive because the specific antibodies to the virus or toxin were present in the patient's serum. If there were no antibodies present (if the patient were not immune) to the virus or toxin, there would be *no* antigen-antibody-complement binding in reaction I; consequently, there would be free complement present to bind and lyse the sheep red blood cells in reaction II. Therefore, the test results would be negative.

This complex reaction is used to identify certain virus infections, such as smallpox, influenza, and poliomyelitis, as well as fungal, rickettsial, chlamydial, and protozoal diseases.

Fluorescent Antibody Technique   Fluorescent dyes (called fluorochromes), which are easily seen glowing under the ultraviolet microscope, can be attached to the antibodies from the patient's serum, which will adhere to the pathogen. The pathogen might be *Treponema pallidum* (syphilis) or *Streptococcus pyogenes* ("strep" throat). Thus, the pathogen is beautifully outlined by the fluorescent dye when it is examined with the ultraviolet microscope if the patient's serum contains the specific antibodies for those pathogens. More often, the fluorescent dye is attached to rabbit antibodies to human gamma globulin, which will then outline the pathogen on the slide if the patient's gamma globulin contains antibodies to that pathogen. This test is often used for positive identification of β-hemolytic and group A *Streptococcus pyogenes* (Fig. 9–15), *Treponema pallidum, Neisseria meningitis, Salmonella typhi, Haemophilis influenzae,* rabies virus and many other pathogens.

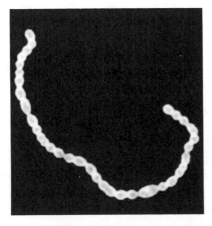

Figure 9–15. *Streptococcus pyogenes* stained with fluorescent antibody (original magnification $\times$ 200). (Volk WA, Wheeler MF: Basic Microbiology, 4th ed. Philadelphia, JB Lippincott, 1984)

Radioimmunoassay   Radioimmunoassay (RIA) is a sensitive, versatile technique, using radioactively labeled antigen or antibody. It is frequently used to determine small amounts of drugs, hormones, or antigens, such as hepatitis B antigen in blood donor serum.

Enzyme-linked Immunosorbent Assays (ELISA)   These enzyme-linked assays (ELA) are sensitive techniques that use an enzyme-antibody-antigen combination adsorbed onto the sides of a test well. If the patient has antibodies or antigens for the disease agent, the linkage is formed; when the substrate for the enzyme is added, a color change develops, which indicates a positive test result. If the patient does not have the serum antigen or the antibody sought, the enzyme is not linked and no color change is seen. These techniques are commonly used to test for AIDS, rubella (German measles), and certain drugs present in serum.

Opsonization   The opsonization test is based on the fact that phagocytes can engulf more bacteria if the specific antibodies for those bacteria are present. A control slide with bacteria and phagocytes is observed, and the number of bacteria inside each phagocyte is counted. This number is compared with the number of bacteria engulfed by phagocytes in the presence of serum from a patient with antibodies to the bacteria. This test is seldom used in a clinical laboratory; its value is as a confirming test for bacterial diseases.

Capsular Swelling (Quellung Reaction)   When serum containing antibodies to encapsulated bacteria is added to those bacteria and observed microscopically, the capsule appears to swell. The swelling is frequently referred to as the Quellung reaction (see Figure 7–4). Various capsular types of *Streptococcus pneumoniae* and other encapsulated bacteria can be identified by this test.

Immobilization   If the pathogen is motile (flagellated), the immobilization test can be used. When a patient's serum is added to motile bacteria, the bacteria is immobilized if specific antibodies to the bacterial flagella are present. Identification of cholera, salmonella, and shigella infections is more reliable using this technique; however, it is rarely used in clinical laboratories because other tests are more readily available.

Toxin Neutralization   The neutralization of toxins usually is demonstrated by *in vivo* tests. These demonstrate that specific antitoxins (antibodies) neutralize the effect of a toxin.
The animal test for diphtheria   A mouse injected with the toxin of diphtheria will die. But if the toxin is mixed with the serum of a patient who is immune to diphtheria and then the combined toxin and serum is injected into a mouse, the mouse will live.
The Schick test   Diphtheria toxin is injected under the skin (subcutaneously).

The site becomes reddened if the person is susceptible to diphtheria, but no redness is seen if the person is immune, because antibodies are present.

The Dick test   The scarlet fever exotoxin is injected subcutaneously; redness occurs at the site in the susceptible person but not in one who is immune.

The Schultz-Charlton test   The rash of scarlet fever can be positively identified by means of the Schultz-Charlton test. The antitoxin (antibodies) to the scarlet fever toxin is injected into an area of rash. If the rash clears, the patient has scarlet fever, but if it does not clear, the rash is due to other causes.

Use of Serological Tests   Serologic reactions can provide information that is useful in the diagnosis of many infectious diseases. Most of them are extremely valuable because they can be performed quickly and easily with a high degree of specificity and sensitivity. However, some of the newer techniques may not be widely used, because of their cost.

Summary

The nonspecific defenses of the human body are those general mechanisms that serve to protect it from harmful foreign substances. The first line of defense is the mechanical and chemical barrier against foreign invaders provided by the skin, the mucous linings of the body openings, and the defenses in the digestive, respiratory, and urogenital systems. The chemical and physical processes involved in inflammation and phagocytosis make up the second line of defense.

The human body's third line of defense against the invasion of foreign microorganisms is the immune response. Immunology is the science of the immune responses in the body.

An antigen is any high-molecular-weight foreign protein or polysaccharide that causes an antibody to be formed and that binds specifically with that antibody. An antibody is a protein produced by lymphocytes in the lymphoid areas in response to a foreign antigen, and it usually attaches only to that antigen.

There are several types of acquired immunity, active acquired immunity, and passive acquired immunity.

All antibodies have specific structures and functions. There are five classes of antibodies or immunoglobulins: IgG, IgM, IgA, IgD, and IgE. Immunoglobulin G (IgG) protects against disease, attaches to phagocytes and tissues, fixes complement, crosses the placental barrier, and causes certain immunological diseases. Immunoglobulin M (IgM) protects against early infection and bacteriocidal gram-negative bacteria and fixes complement. Immunoglobulin A (IgA), the secretory antibodies in tears, saliva, colostrum, and other secretions, protects the mucous membranes against infections. Immunoglobulin E (IgE) comprises the tissue-bound antibodies of allergy, drug sensitivity, anaphylaxis, and hypersensitivity. The IgD is found in serum and may be an antibody control mechanism.

An individual may also develop hypersensitivity in which the defense immune response has gone awry, and, instead of protecting the individual, the antibodies irritate certain cells in the body. There are two types of hypersensitivity: immediate and delayed.

The formation of antibodies against antigens of one's own tissues and the destruction of these tissues is called the autoimmune response. An example of this type of response is rheumatoid arthritis.

Clinical and research tests have been designed to indicate the presence of various antibodies to specific antigens. This study of antigen-antibody reactions is called serology. These tests include agglutination, precipitation, lysis by complement, complement fixation, fluorescent antibody technique, opsonization, capsular swelling, immobilization, and toxin neutralization.

Study Outline

I. First line of defense: mechanical and chemical barriers
   A. Skin
   B. Mucous membranes of body openings
      1. Mucous traps
      2. Flushing action
      3. Ciliary action
      4. Lysosomes
      5. Digestive enzyme
      6. Normal flora

II. Second line of defense
   A. Interferon
   B. Interleukins
   C. Complement
   D. Properdin
   E. Prostaglandins
   F. Phagocytosis
   G. Inflammation

III. Immunity, third line of defense
   A. Innate (nonspecific) resistance
   B. Acquired immunity
      1. Active
      2. Passive

IV. Immunology
   A. Antigens
   B. Antibodies, immunoglobulins

V. The immune system

VI. The immune response
   A. Antibody production
   B. Antibody structure and function
   C. Hypersensitivity and cell-mediated immune responses
      1. Immediate
      2. Delayed: cell-mediated immunity

VII. Immunodiagnostic procedures

Problems and Questions

1. What factors contribute to natural resistance to disease?
2. List the nonspecific defenses of the skin, respiratory system, digestive system, and urogenital tract.
3. List some serum proteins that aid in the destruction of invading microorganisms.
4. Describe the process of phagocytosis.

5. What are the four main symptoms of inflammation?
6. What are the causes of the symptoms of inflammation?
7. What is the immune response? Is it always a protective mechanism?
8. What types of substances are effective antigens?
9. Where in the body are antibodies formed?
10. When are antibodies formed?
11. What is the anamnestic response?
12. What is the main difference between active and passive acquired immunity?
13. How are antibodies transferred in passive immunity?
14. List five classes of immunoglobulins. Where are each of these found?
15. What are the main differences among the four types of hypersensitivity?
16. What is an allergen? Give some examples.
17. Give an example of the delayed hypersensitivity reaction.
18. Describe an example of an autoimmune disease.
19. List seven *in vitro* antigen-antibody reactions and when they are used.
20. List four *in vivo* antigen-antibody tests and when they are used.

Self Test

After you have read Chapter 9, examined the objectives, studied the new words, reviewed the study outline, and answered the questions at the end of the chapter, complete the following self test.

Matching Exercises

Complete each statement from the list of words provided.

Resistance Against Pathogens

bile   interferon   species
complement   lysozyme   specific
digestive enzymes   nonspecific
innate   indigenous microflora

1. Complement, interferon, and phagocytes are some of the body's
   _____ defenses.
2. The _____ is secreted by the liver, stored in the
   gallbladder, and released into the small intestine, where it lowers the
   surface tension of particles, such as bacteria, to make them more digestible.
3. An enzyme found in nasal secretions that lyses the cell walls of certain
   bacteria is _____.
4. When antibodies are formed that bind with the specific antigens that
   caused their formation, the body is activating its _____
   resistance against foreign substances.

5. The usually harmless microorganisms that reside on the skin and in the mucous membranes of many body systems are the _____.

6. _____ is a protein that is secreted by cells infected by viruses and serves to prevent the surrounding cells from producing viruses.

7. A certain species of animals resistant to a disease found in other species is said to have _____ resistance.

8. The digestive tract contains many _____, which frequently digest certain bacteria in the acid or basic areas.

9. The natural, inherited defense mechanisms that give certain individuals or species some resistance to certain diseases are _____ resistance.

10. A complex group of proteins found in serum that aids in the inactivation and destruction of bacteria is _____.

Immunology

agammaglobulinemia   antitoxins   IgM
allergen   complement   immunocompetent
anamnestic response   hypogammaglobulinemia   immunoglobulins
anaphylactic response   IgA   plasma
antibodies   IgE   primary response
antigen   IgG   serum

1. The fluid that remains when the clots and blood cells are removed from blood is _____.

2. When a person is not able to produce antibodies, he has an abnormality known as _____.

3. The smallest but most abundant of the antibodies found in the serum is _____.

4. Any foreign material that can stimulate the production of antibodies is an _____.

5. Lymphocytes that can be stimulated to produce antibodies are _____.

6. _____ is the antibody found in allergic diseases that is usually bound to cells or tissues.

7. An antigen that causes an allergic reaction is an _____.

8. The antibodies that are formed in response to toxin or toxoid antigens are _____.

9. When small lymphocytes are initially stimulated by antigens (such as vaccines) to develop into plasma cells to produce antibodies, this process is the _____ _____.

10. The fluid that remains from blood when only the blood cells are removed is _____.

11. The largest serum antibody and the first to be formed against pathogens is _____.

12. If an individual produces less than the normal amount of antibodies, the abnormality is _____.

13. A group of serum proteins that are activated by specific antigen-antibody combinations is _____.

14. When memory lymphocytes are restimulated by antigens to produce the same antibodies again (as when a booster vaccine is given), the _____ _____ has occurred.

15. The secretory antibody found in tears, saliva, and colostrum is _____.

16. The protein molecules that are produced by B lymphocytes in response to the presence of antigens are _____.

17. When the anamnestic response occurs as a serious allergic shock reaction, it is the _____ _____.

Immune Response

allergy
artificially acquired active
   immunity
immediate

delayed
autoimmune
artificially acquired passive
   immunity

naturally acquired active
   immunity
naturally acquired passive
   immunity

1. Hayfever, asthma, and anaphylactic shock are all examples of _____ hypersensitivity.

2. _____ _____ _____ _____ results when a person normally produces antibodies to a disease.

3. Skin rashes caused by _____ are examples of _____ hypersensitivity.

4. When people are vaccinated so that they produce antibodies to the antigens in the vaccine, they develop _____ _____ _____ _____.

5. The rejection of an organ transplant, such as a kidney transplant, is an example of _____ hypersensitivity.

6. When antitoxin is given to a person who has tetanus, the individual has been given _____ _____ _____ _____.

7. When people's bodies form antibodies against their own tissues and destroy their own organs, such as the heart, kidney, or thyroid, we say that they have an _____ disease.

8. A newborn has temporary material antibodies to protect him from

disease; we say he has _____ _____
_____ _____.

Antigen-Antibody Reactions

agglutination   complement fixation   opsonization
precipitation   fluorescent antibody   capsular swelling
lysis by complement   toxin neutralization   immobilization

1. When complement is activated by antibodies attached to cellular antigens, the cells break because of _____
   _____ _____.

2. Whenever complement is present when the specific antibodies bind with their antigens, _____ _____ occurs.

3. When antibodies inactivate an exotoxin, _____
   _____ occurs.

4. The Schick and Dick tests are examples of _____
   _____ reactions.

5. Blood typing is a good example of an _____ test.

6. The _____ test can only be used with motile pathogens.

7. The Quellung test or _____ _____ can only be used on pathogens with capsules.

8. The VDRL and RPR tests for syphilis are _____ tests.

9. _____ is used to indicate the presence of antibodies to soluble antigens, proteins, or toxins.

10. An increase in phagocytosis due to the presence of specific antibodies to certain pathogens is a test called _____.

11. Pathogens such as streptococci are often identified by attaching a fluorescent dye to the specific antibody that will bind with them; this is called the _____ _____ technique.

True or False (T or F)

____ 1. Phagocytes can digest all types of bacteria.

____ 2. The symptoms of inflammation are heat, swelling, redness, pain, and sometimes loss of function.

____ 3. The main purpose of the inflammatory response is to destroy bacteria.

____ 4. The ciliated epithelial cells lining the postnasal membranes engulf and digest bacteria.

____ 5. There are indigenous microflora in the healthy bladder.

____ 6. The continual flushing of urine through the urethra prevents pathogens from invading the urinary system.

_____ 7. Interferon defends the body by lysing the cell wall of gram-negative bacteria.

_____ 8. Most phagocytes are also leukocytes.

_____ 9. The reticuloendothelial system is a system of tissues found in the spleen, liver, lymph nodes, blood vessels, and intestines.

_____ 10. Antigens may be proteins or polysaccharides or both.

_____ 11. Foreign proteins are stronger antigens that foreign polysaccharides.

_____ 12. An effective vaccine must always contain living pathogens.

_____ 13. A good vaccine must contain sufficient antigens to cause antibodies to form to protect the person from the disease.

_____ 14. Attenuated microorganisms are living, weakened mutated pathogens that no longer cause disease but cause the production of antibodies that can protect against that disease.

_____ 15. Colostrum is a good source of antibodies to protect newborns.

_____ 16. Passive immunity is always temporary.

_____ 17. The TB skin test reaction is an example of immediate hypersensitivity.

_____ 18. Rheumatic fever is an autoimmune disease that may follow β-hemolytic streptococcal infections.

_____ 19. *In vitro* means the tests are performed in the living animal.

_____ 20. The precipitins, opsonins, and agglutinins are all antibodies.

_____ 21. An electron microscope must be used to observe the fluorescent antibodies attached to a pathogen.

_____ 22. Antibodies and antibiotics are two words for the same thing.

_____ 23. A series of antigen-antibody (*in vitro*) tests on a sick person that show an increasing antibody titer indicates that the patient's body is fighting the infection.

_____ 24. An exotoxin is liberated only after the cell is destroyed or dead.

_____ 25. Antitoxins are often used in the treatment of diphtheria, botulism, and tetanus.

_____ 26. If the complement fixation test is positive (no hemolysis of sheep red blood cells), the patient's serum does *not* contain antibodies specific for the antigen.

_____ 27. Anaphylactic shock kills humans, chiefly, by severe spasms of the smooth muscles of the body.

Multiple Choice

1. First line of body defense is?
    a. unbroken skin
    b. antibody molecules
    c. antigen molecules
    d. T cells
    e. phagocytic cells

2. What stimulates the leukocytes to migrate to an injured area of the body?
    a. phagocytosis
    b. chemotaxis
    c. they just do it

d. leukocytes do not migrate to an injured area

e. prostaglandins

3. Interferon, an antiviral substance, has the following properties:

a. is cell-specific, not virus-specific

b. it is a small protein molecule

c. it can inhibit certain viral infections

d. all of the above

e. none of the above

4. The reticuloendothelial system functions as follows:

a. removes bacteria and other particulate matter from circulating fluid

b. cells migrate to the areas of injury and engulf foreign substances

c. in inflammatory response, contributes fibrin

d. all of the above

e. none of the above

5. Mechanical and chemical defenses against infection include

a. intact skin and mucous membranes

b. fatty acids secreted by the sebaceous glands

c. lysozyme in tears and other secretion

d. ciliary action in respiratory tract

e. all of the above

6. Phagocytes function by

a. destroying all bacteria they encounter

b. producing complement

c. engulfing foreign material

d. providing the first line of defense

7. Normal urine drawn during a catheterization should contain

a. erythrocytes

b. *Enterobacter aerogenes*

c. *Candida albicans*

d. none of the above

8. Pyogenic bacteria, such as *Pseudomonas*, cause

a. greater heat in the area of inflammation than other bacteria

b. pus formation

c. vasoconstriction

d. destruction of phagocytes

9. The humoral response is

a. a nonspecific defense

b. initiated by mast cells

c. the production of antibodies

d. possible only against bacteria

10. Antibodies are produced by

a. blood cells

b. B lymphocytes

c. antigens

d. complement

11. Immunity to gonorrhea is

a. temporary naturally acquired passive immunity

b. permanent artificially acquired active immunity

c. permanent naturally acquired passive immunity

d. temporary naturally acquired active immunity

12. Naturally acquired passive immunity would result from

a. subclinical disease

b. colostrum

c. injection of antitoxin

d. all of the above

13. The vaccines for typhus, measles, and mumps are

a. toxoids

b. killed pathogens

c. extracts of pathogens

d. attenuated living organisms

14. The newborn's antibodies are

a. IgG
b. IgA
c. IgM
d. there are no antibodies present at birth

15. Botulism would be treated with
    a. hyperimmune gammaglobulin
    b. botulism toxoid
    c. antitoxin
    d. autogenous vaccine

16. The Schultz-Charlton test involves
    a. the injection of antitoxin into a test animal
    b. the injection of antitoxin into the patient
    c. the injection of toxin into the patient
    d. the combining of patient serum with toxin and complement

17. The normal adult human being can respond immunologically to
    a. protein antigens only
    b. polysaccharide antigens only
    c. most substances recognized as self
    d. nonhuman substances only
    e. many thousands of different antigenic determinants

Major Diseases of the Body System

Objectives

After studying this chapter, you should be able to

1. Name the major organs that might become infected in each body system
2. List the most common normal microbial flora usually found in the various body systems
3. Outline the causative agent, reservoir, mode of transmission, pathogenesis, treatment, and control measures for the major infectious disease of each system
4. For each body system, list some examples of diseases that are caused by bacteria, viruses, fungi, or protozoa

New Words

Choleragin (kal'-er-ah-gin). The exotoxin produced by *Vibrio cholerae*, that causes cholea

Cystitis (sis-ti'-tis). An infection of the urinary bladder

Cytotoxins (sigh-tow-tok'-sins). Toxic substances that injure certain cells

Dermatophytes (der-mah'-toe-fites). Fungi capable of growing on the skin surface, causing ringworm or tinea diseases

Enterotoxin (en'-ter-oh-tok'-sin). An exotoxin causing damage to intestinal cells, producing diarrhea

Exudate (eks'-oo'-date). A viscous secretion containing blood cells and cellular debris from site of inflammation

Gingivitis (gin-je-vi'-tis). An inflammation of the gingiva (gums)

Immunoglobulins (im'-you-no-glob'-you-lyns). The globulin proteins of the serum and other body secretions, including the humoral antibodies

Immunosuppression (im'-you-no-sue-presh'-un). Depression of the immune response

Malaise (mal-az'). A general feeling of illness and discomfort

Necrotoxin (neck'-row-tox'-sin). An exotoxin that destroys certain cells

Neurotoxin (new'-row-tox'-sin). An exotoxin that damages nerve tissue and interferes with nerve impulses

Oncogenic (on'-ko-jin'-ick). Capable of producing tumors

Prophylactic agent (pro'-fi-lack'-tick). An agent to ward off disease

Sebum (see'-bum). The secretion of the sebaceous (oil) glands of the skin

Tetanospasmin (tet'-ah-no-spaz'-min). The neurotoxic exotoxin produced by *Clostridium tetani*, that causes tetanus

Urethritis (you'-re-thri'-tis). An inflammation of the urethra of the urinary system

In the previous chapters you have studied the disease process, how pathogens cause disease, modes of transmission, how the body attempts to defend itself, and the chemotherapeutic agents and vaccines used to cure and prevent certain diseases. This chapter summarizes the major infectious diseases of normal skin and skin lesions, the eyes, the ears, the oral cavity, the respiratory system, the gastrointestinal tract, the urogenital areas, the cardiovascular system, and the nervous system. Many of these infections involve several body systems, or in other types of infection, the pathogen may move from one area to another. The source of the disease-causing microbe may be opportunistic normal flora, but usually the causative agent is transmitted to the recipient from a reservoir of infection (see Chapter 7).

The early signs and symptoms of many diseases are influenzalike; usually the patient develops slight fever, headache, fatigue, malaise, gastrointestinal upset, or sneezing and coughing. Only specific signs and symptoms, characteristic of the major diseases are mentioned here.

Diseases of the Skin

Normal Skin

As seen in Figure 10–1, the structure of skin is not simple. Normal healthy, intact skin serves as a formidable protective barrier for the underlying tissues. Vast numbers of microbes survive on and within the epidermal layers, in pores, and in hair follicles (see Table 6–1). Their growth is controlled by the (1) amount of moisture present, (2) pH, (3) temperature, (4) salinity of perspiration, (5) chemical wastes such as urea and fatty acids, and (6) other microbes present that secrete fatty acids and antimicrobic substances. Proper hygienic cleanliness and washing serves to flush away dead epithelial cells, many transient and resident microbes,

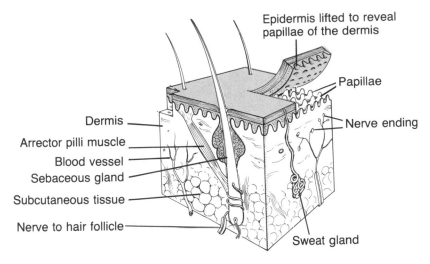

Figure 10–1. Cross-section of the skin. (Lindberg JB, Hunter ML, Kruszewski AZ: Introduction to Person-Centered Nursing. Philadelphia, JB Lippincott, 1988)

and the odorous organic materials present in perspiration, sebum, and microbial secretions.

Once the skin barrier is broken (wounds, surgery, or burns), the opportunists may infect the underlying tissues, invade capillaries and lymph, and be carried by phagocytes to many regions of the body.

Opportunistic Normal Flora

Most microbes that colonize the skin are harmless, but several genera of aerobes and anaerobes may cause infections when the ecological balance of the skin environment changes chemically, physically, or microbiologically (Fig. 10–2).

Major Microbial Opportunists

Gram-positive cocci Staphylococcus epidermis, Staphylocccus aureus, Micrococcus species, and Streptococcus species are facultative anaerobes that may invade through breaks in skin to cause local, deep, or systemic infections. Many of them produce invasive enzymes and damaging exotoxins capable of causing serious diseases, such as the toxic shock syndrome caused by S. aureus.

Gram-positive bacilli These pleomorphic rods, frequently referred to as diphtheroids, include Corynebacterium, Brevibacterium, and Propionibacterium species, which frequently cause hair follicle and sweat gland infections.

Gram-negative bacilli In moist areas, armpits, perineum, and between toes, Pseudomonas and some enteric rods may be found. Microbes can grow profusely on the organic compounds in perspiration and sebum, producing malodorous

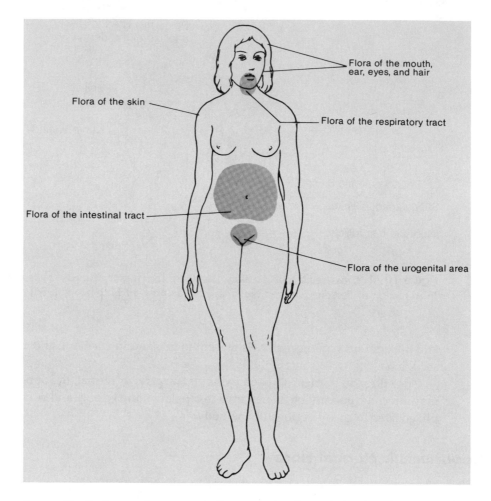

Figure 10–2. Areas where most indigenous microflora reside: skin, hair, mouth, ears, eyes, throat, nose, intestinal tract, and urogenital tract.

fatty acids. Many deodorants contain antimicrobial agents that inhibit the growth of these bacteria.

Viral Infections of the Skin

Chickenpox, Varicella, Shingles

Characteristics   Chickenpox is a respiratory infection and generalized viremia with local vesicular lesions on the skin of the face, thorax, and back that become encrusted. Vesicles also form in mucous membranes. Usually a mild, self-limiting disease, but it can be severely damaging to fetus in pregnancy. Reye's syndrome (a severe encephalomyelitis with liver damage) may follow clinical chickenpox if aspirin is given to children under 16 years of age. Secondary bacterial infections (pneumonia, otitis media, bacteremia) frequently occur. Shingles is a reactivation of varicella provirus in adults; it is an inflammation of sensory ganglia of cutaneous sensory nerves, producing rash and pain.

Pathogens   Varicella-zoster virus or herpes-zoster virus.

Reservoir   Humans.

Transmission   Inhalation of virus via contaminated droplets or direct contact with vesicles, or contaminated articles.

Incubation period   13–17 days. Contagious: 1 to 2 days before onset of rash and 5 days after first crop of vesicles.

Epidemiology   Usually occurs in winter and early spring. Two million cases each year are estimated. Long lasting immunity usually follows childhood disease.

Control   Isolation for 1 week after eruption of vesicles.

Usual treatment   No vaccine yet available. Live, attenuated varicella vaccine. Varicella-Zoster Immune Globulin (VCIG) is effective if given within 96 hrs. after exposure. Antiviral chemotherapy (acyclovir or vidarabine) may be effective. Antibiotics to prevent secondary bacterial infections.

Measles, Rubeola

Characteristics   Upper respiratory infection, high fever, coughing, light sensitivity, Koplik's spots in mouth, maculopapular skin rash. Complications include bronchitis, pneumonia, otitis media. Autoimmune subacute sclerosing panencephalitis (SSPE) may follow a latent period.

Pathogen   Measles virus; a paramyxovirus.

Reservoir   Humans.

Transmission   Inhalation of droplets during contact with children.

Incubation period   8–13 days.

Epidemiology   In 1990, 26,520 cases reported in the United States to the Centers for Disease Control (CDC). Measles cases dropped 99% in the United States and Canada after immunization programs were initiated.

Control   Immunization with live, attenuated measles virus in measles, mumps, rubella (MMR) vaccine.

Usual treatment   Bed rest, fluids, preventive nursing care to prevent complications and secondary infections. Antiviral chemotherapy and antibiotics to prevent bacterial infections may be helpful.

German Measles, Rubella

Characteristics   Rash, flat pink spots spreading from face, with tender lymph nodes, low-grade fever. A milder disease than rubeola; it may be subclinical. During first trimester of pregnancy may cause congenital rubella syndrome in fetus. Encephalitis is a rare complication.

Pathogen   Rubella virus; a togavirus (Fig. 10–3).

Reservoir   Humans.

Transmission   Inhalation of droplets during direct contact with infected individuals; occasionally via contaminated articles.

Incubation period   14–21 days.

Epidemiology   In 1990, 1,093 cases in United States reported to CDC. Endemic worldwide, fewer epidemics in immunized communities.

Control   Immunization with live, attenuated rubella virus in MMR vaccine, especially for young women before pregnancy, and serological testing for immunity. Isolation for 7 days after onset of rash.

Usual treatment   No chemotherapy available.

Figure 10–3. Development of rubella virus in the surface and cytoplasmic membranes of infected cell cultures. (*A*) Viral particles budding from cytoplasmic membranes into vacuoles and into the cytoplasm. Numerous mature virions are present within vacuoles (original magnification × 60,000). (*B*) Viral particles budding from the surface of an infected cell (original magnification × 60,000). (Oshiro LS et al: J Gen Virol 5:205)

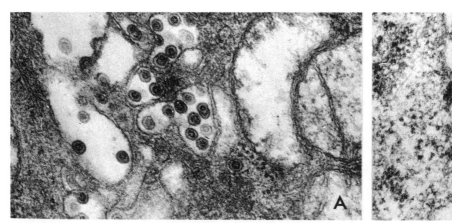

Warts (Condyloma Acuminata)

Characteristics   Fibrous superficial papules of the skin (see Fig. 10–19), and mucous membranes including genitalia.

Pathogen   Human papillomavirus, of papovavirus group.

Reservoir   Humans.

Transmission   Direct contact and sexual intercourse, fomites; spread by scratching.

Incubation period   1–20 months.

Epidemiology   Worldwide occurrence.

Control   Destroyed by freezing, acids, electrosurgery, or laser therapy.

Usual treatment   Podophyllum chemotherapy for persistent epidermal warts or idoxuridine for venereal warts. Interferon may prove to be effective for genital and laryngeal warts.

Bacterial Infections of the Skin

Impetigo, Pyoderma

Characteristics   Skin lesions forming pustules, then amber crusts (Fig. 10–4), itching, peeling of skin.

Pathogens   *Staphylococcus aureus* or *Streptococcus pyogenes* or both. Identified by culture and serologic techniques.

Pathogenicity   Spread through skin by producing hyaluronidase. Staphylococcal toxins cause scalded skin syndrome and peeling.

Reservoir   Humans.

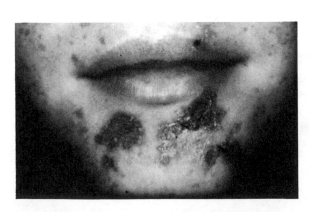

Figure 10–4. Impetigo. (Dobson RL, Abele DC: The Practice of Dermatology. Philadelphia, JB Lippincott, 1985)

Transmission   By direct contact, through broken skin, scratching.

Incubation period   4–10 days.

Control   Disinfectant skin lotions.

Usual treatment   Topical disinfectants and antibiotics, such as penicillin, erythromycin cephalosporin, clindamycin, vancomycin.

Scarlet Fever, Scarlatina, Erysipelas

Characteristics   Skin rash.

Pathogen   *Streptococcus pyogenes* (see Fig. 9–15) β-hemolytic, group A, gram-positive, cocci that form chains. Identified by culture and serologic techniques.

Pathogenicity   Erythrogenic toxins; secondary complication of "strep" throat (pharyngitis) in susceptible individuals.

Reservoir   Humans.

Transmission   Person-to-person, by secretions and close contact.

Incubation period   1–3 days.

Control   Isolation until after 24 hours of antibiotic therapy.

Usual treatment   Penicillin, erythromycin, cephalosporins, clindamycin.

Folliculitis, Hair Follicle Infections, Furuncles (Boils), Carbuncles

Characteristics   Hair follicle pustules, small or large.

Pathogens   *Staphylococcus aureus*; gram-positive cocci in clusters. *Pseudomonas aeruginosa*; gram-negative bacilli.

Reservoir   Humans, especially the skin, and contaminated hot pools.

Transmission   Direct contact, water or fomites, poor personal hygiene, skin abrasions, cuts, contaminated hot tubs and swimming pools, *Staphylococcus aureus* may become systemic and cause recurring boils and carbuncles.

Incubation period   Variable, usually 4–10 days.

Control   Good personal hygiene, properly treated hot tubs and pools.

Usual treatment   Topical bacitracin or polymyxin B for *aureus*; gentamicin or carbenicillin systematically for *Pseudomonas*.

Acne

Characteristics   Inflammatory pustules, cysts, and papules; infections of sebaceous glands in hair follicles on face, chest, and back.

Pathogens   Interaction of *Propionibacterium acnes*, *Staphylococcus aureus*, and *Corynebacterium* spp.

Reservoir   Humans.

Transmission   Direct contact with susceptible individuals. Usually occurs during puberty because of hormonal changes.

Incubation period   Variable, usually 4–10 days.

Control   Cleanliness, good personal hygiene

Usual treatment   Locally applied benzoyl peroxide, salicylic acid, or sulfur. Systemic antibiotics such as tetracycline, minocycline (minocin), and, Cleacin-T or drug therapy with isotretinoin (Accutane) for severe cases, and Retin A for moderate control.

Anthrax, Woolsorter's Disease

Characteristics   Cutaneous blackened lesions called eschars caused by necrotoxin. Pneumonia and/or systemic infection may develop.

Pathogen   *Bacillus anthracis*, a gram-positive, aerobic, endospore-forming bacillus.

Pathogenesis   Endospore germinates; bacteria produces necrotic toxins.

Reservoir   Spores in soil and on hides and skins of infected animals.

Transmission   From animal hair, wool, and hides by (1) direct contact, endospores into skin abrasions; (2) inhalation of endospores; (3) ingestion of endospores.

Incubation period   3–5 days.

Epidemiology   No cases reported in United States in 1990.

Control   Avoid contact with infected animals and soils contaminated by spores from infected animals. Vaccination of animals and humans who work with animals and animal products.

Usual treatment   Penicillin, tetracycline, erythromycin, chloramphenicol.

Leprosy, Hansen's Disease

Characteristics   (1) Neural, tuberculoid form: lesions on skin and peripheral nerves, loss of sensation. (2) Cutaneous, lepromatous form: progressive disfiguring nodules in skin; invades throughout body.

Pathogen   *Mycobacterium leprae*, an acid-fast bacillus, cultured only in armadillos, monkeys, and mouse footpads.

Reservoir   Humans and perhaps infected armadillos.

Transmission   (1) Prolonged exposure through skin or mucous membranes; (2) via droplets to respiratory tract.

Epidemiology   203 cases in United States reported to CDC in 1990. Worldwide prevalence.

Control   Early detection and isolation until treatment is effective.

Usual treatment   Prolonged treatment with rifampin or with dapsone and clofazimine.

Fungal Infections of the Skin

Many fungi cause skin lesions and may enter the body through the skin, such as *Sporothrix* and *Candida*, but the most common are the dermatophytes that cause ringworm or superficial fungal infections of the skin, hair, and nails. The cell-mediated immune responses to fungi result in inflammation and limitation of the spread of the fungus.

Dermatomycosis, Tinea, Ringworm, Dermatophytosis

Characteristics   Fungal lesions on skin (tinea corporis), scalp (tinea capitis), groin (tinea cruris or "jock itch"), foot (tinea pedis or "athele's foot"), and nails (tinea unguium).

Pathogens   Various species of *Microsporum*, *Epidermophyton*, and *Trichophyton*; filamentous fungi.

Reservoir   Humans, animals, and soil.

Transmission   Direct or indirect contact with fungal spores from lesions or fomites, such as shower stalls, toilet articles, and athletic supporters. Spores enter through breaks in skin and moist areas, and germinate into filamentous growths.

Incubation period   4–14 days.

Control   Keep susceptible areas clean and dry.

Usual treatment   Topical application of miconazole (Lotrimin), clotrimazole, and other antifungal agents. Oral griseofulvin for scalp and nail infections.

Burn and Wound Infections

When the skin barrier is broken by burns, wounds, and surgical procedures, many normal flora and environmental bacteria can invade and cause local or deep-tissue infections. They may also become systemic and produce exotoxins, causing severe damage to the individual.

Burns

Many patients die after being burned severely because of loss of body fluids and the presence of toxic microbial invaders, including *Staphylococcus aureus*, *Streptococcus pyogenes*, *Pseudomonas aeruginosa*, and many fungi. These organisms usually grow aerobically in the burned area. They can produce many exotoxins (cytotoxins, necrotoxins, and neurotoxins) and perhaps cause death to the patient.

Burn victims must be treated in an aseptic environment in which the health care personnel are gloved, gowned, and masked. The burns may be left open to the air to speed healing or covered with artificial skin or film to reduce contamination and loss of fluids. Some antimicrobial topical agents (silver sulfadiazine, for example) may be used to reduce the possibility of infections during the prolonged healing period.

Wound and Surgical Infections

Most gunshot, stab, puncture, bite, and abrasive wounds are contaminated during the wounding process. The microbes introduced are frequently anaerobes from dust and normal flora that grow rapidly deep within the wound; other facultative aerobes flourish on the surface of the wound, secreting enzymes to invade the blood and lymph. Bacterial and fungal spores may also be introduced, causing local and deep-seated infections.

Any traumatic injury must be opened and thoroughly cleansed to remove debris and to inhibit the growth of microbes; then it is usually covered lightly to prevent further contamination.

Staphylococcus (see Figs. 1–8 and 1–9) and *Streptococcus* (see Fig. 9–15) species are the most frequent bacteria that cause focal infections. They may invade by secreting hyaluronidase and other spreading factors to cause severe toxic systemic infections of many areas, including the brain, spinal cord, and bone. *Pseudomonas aeruginosa*, from soil and feces, is notorious for causing deep, antibiotic-resistant infections. This gram-negative bacillus produces protease enzymes that enable it to move through tissues and an exotoxin that inhibits protein synthesis. Antibiotic sensitivity tests are essential to ensure that the appropriate antibiotic is administered.

The anaerobic *Clostridium* species are of grave concern in puncture wounds. Endospores of *Clostridium tetani* (see Fig. 10–28) may be introduced from soil and fecal contamination. When these spores germinate into vegetative bacteria, neurotoxins are produced that cause involuntary muscle spasms and respiratory failure. The availability of vaccines and antitoxins has greatly reduced deaths from tetanus in developed countries.

Clostridium perfringens, the major causative agent of gas gangrene, is not only of concern in accidental wounds but in surgical sites as well. The contaminating spores germinate, and the vegetative pathogens produce many invasive enzymes and exotoxins, resulting in necrotic areas with gas present.

Fungal infections, such as sporotrichosis, are caused by the introduction of soil fungi and spores that invade cutaneous and lymphatic tissues through wounds that are sometimes as small as a thorn prick. This slowly progressing disease is usually localized and self-limiting, but severe cases may be treated with amphotericin or potassium iodide.

Bites

Human, insect, and animal bites introduce oral microflora into the wound. Because the organisms from human bites are adapted to humans, they are more likely to produce infections than those of animal sources. Every bite should be thoroughly cleansed, disinfected, and left open to the air to prevent microbial growth. Bite wounds should not be closed tightly with stitches and bandages because this procedure would encourage the growth and anaerobic bacteria.

Human Bites   Severe infections may result from anaerobic growth of *Bacteroides* and *Actinomyces*, as well as the facultative *Streptococcus* and *Staphylococcus* species and many other oral microbes. There is even some concern about the oral introduction of some viruses such as, human immunodeficiency virus (HIV), into the bloodstream through bites by infected individuals.

Animal Bites   In general, bites of animals may introduce microbes, such as staphylococci and streptococci, which cause local infections in humans. The bacteria, *Pasteurella multocida* and *P. haemolytica*, are frequently found in dog- and cat-bite wounds and may cause severe local infections and pasteurellosis. Rat-bite fever, caused by *Streptobacillus moniliformis* or *Spirillum minor*, is naturally carried by rats, mice, cats, squirrels, and weasles. The rabies virus is transmitted by the bites of infected dogs, foxes, coyotes, wolves, cats, bats, skunks, raccoons, and other rabid animals. Many other disease-causing microbes are introduced through the skin to the circulatory or nervous systems by bites of arthropod vectors (ticks, fleas, lice, mites, and mosquitoes); these diseases include encephalitis, Colorado tick fever, Rocky Mountain spotted fever, typhus, plague, tularemia, malaria, and Lyme disease and are discussed elsewhere in this chapter.

Diseases of the Eye

The eye consists of tissues similar to and contiguous with the skin. The anatomy and structure of the eye are illustrated in Figure 10–5.

The external surface of the eye is lubricated, cleansed, and protected by tears, mucus, and sebum. Thus, continual production of tears and the presence of lysozyme and other antimicrobial substances found in tears greatly reduce the numbers of normal flora organisms found on the eye surfaces.

Infections of the eye caused by bacteria, chlamydias, and viruses should be differentiated from allergic and conjunctivitis by microscopic examination of the exudate, culture of pathogens, or antigen-antibody laboratory tests (fluorescent antibody or enzyme-linked immunosorbent assay, ELISA).

Viral Conjunctivitis, Acute Hemorrhagic Conjunctivitis (AHC), Herpes Conjunctivitis

Characteristics   Viral invasion of eyelids, conjunctiva, and cornea; usually self-limiting in 1–3 weeks.

Subconjunctival hemorrhages caused by adenovirus or enterovirus. Herpes lesions and occasional blindness from herpesvirus infections.

Figure 10–5. Anatomy of the eye. (Wolf KP: Eyewise. Philadelphia, Harper & Row, 1982)

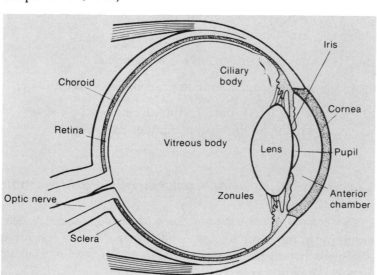

Pathogens   Picornaviruses (enterovirus 70), coxsackievirus, adenoviruses, herpes simplex, types 1 and 2.

Reservoir   Humans.

Transmission   Person-to-person, direct or indirect contact with infected eye secretions. Herpes is transmitted through saliva or genital secretions.

Incubation period   Herpes, 2–12 days; others, 1–3 days.

Control   Personal hygiene, drainage/secretion precautions. Strict asepsis in eye clinics.

Usual treatment   Herpes lesions may be treated with idoxuridine or adenine arabinoside (vidarabine; Vira-A or Ara-A) ophthalmic ointments. No recommended treatment for other self-limiting viral eye infections.

Bacterial Eye Infections

Bacterial Conjunctivitis, Pink Eye

Characteristics   Irritation, reddening of conjunctiva, edema of eyelids, mucopurulent discharge, sensitivity to light. Highly contagious.

Pathogens   *Haemophilus aegyptius, Streptococcus pneumoniae,* other streptococci, staphylococci, *Haemophilus influenzae, Moraxella lacunata, Pseudomonas aeruginosa, Coorynebacterium diphtheriae* may be causative agents.

Reservoir   Humans.

Transmission   Human-to-human, through eye and respiratory discharges, fingers, clothing, eye makeup, eye medications, ophthalmic instruments, and contact lens-wetting and lens-cleaning agents.

Incubation period   1–3 days, depending on causative agent.

Control   Personal hygiene. Drainage/secretion precautions, sterilization of fomites.

Usual treatment   Ophthalmic tetracycline, erythromycin, gentamicin, or sulfonamide, depending on the susceptibility of pathogen.

Chlamydial Conjunctivitis, Inclusion Conjunctivitis, Paratrachoma

Characteristics   In neonates, acute conjunctivitis with mucopurulent discharge; may result in mild scarring of conjunctivae and cornea. May be concurrent with chlamydial nasopharyngitis or pneumonia. In adults, may be concurrent with nongonococcal urethritis or cervicitis.

Pathogens *Chlamydia trachomatis*, immunotypes B and D through K.

Reservoir Humans.

Transmission Nasopharynx, rectal and genital secretions to eye, by fingers, sexual contact; to newborns, by infected birth canal; nonchlorinated swimming pools, by genitourinary exudates. Spread by flies to eyes.

Control Identification and treatment of chlamydial genital infections of expectant parents.
Drainage/secretion precautions. Chlorination of swimming pools. Erythromycin or tetracycline ophthalmic ointments in eyes of newborns (Chlamydias are not susceptible to silver nitrate or penicillin.)

Usual treatment Erythromycin orally for infected pregnant women and infected neonates. Topical tetracycline, erythromycin, or sulfonamide for eye infections.

Trachoma, Chlamydia Keratoconjunctivitis

Characteristics Highly contagious, acute or chronic conjunctival inflammation, resulting in scarring of cornea and conjunctiva, deformation of eyelids, and blindness.

Pathogens *Chlamydia trachomatis*, immunotypes C, A, and B.

Reservoir Humans.

Transmission Direct contact with infected ocular or nasal secretions or contaminated articles. Venereal transmission by infected cervix or urethra; to newborns through the birth canal. Spread by flies.

Incubation period 5–12 days.

Control Personal hygiene, improved sanitation and living conditions. Drainage/secretion precautions of hospitalized patients.

Usual treatment Topical ophthalmic tetracycline or erythromycin, oral tetracycline or erythromycin.

Gonococcal Conjunctivitis, Ophthalmia Neonatorum

Characteristics Acute redness and swelling of conjunctiva, purulent discharge (Fig. 10–6). Corneal ulcers, perforation, and blindness, if untreated.

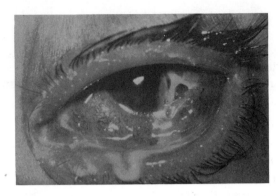

Figure 10–6. Purulent conjunctivitis caused by gonorrhea. (Moffett HL: Clinical Microbiology, 2nd ed. Philadelphia, JB Lippincott, 1980)

Pathogens *Neisseria gonorrhoeae*; gram-negative, kidney bean-shaped diplococci. Identified by Gram-stained smears, culture, and serologic tests.

Reservoir Humans.

Transmission Infection of cervix, birth canal, and secretions. To newborn, during passage through infected birth canal. To adults, through infected genital secretions.

Incubation period 1–5 days.

Control Instill 1% silver nitrate solution in eyes at birth. Ophthalmic erythromycin or tetracycline may be used to prevent chlamydial, as well as gonococcal eye infections.

Usual treatment Penicillin, or oral cefotaxime for penicillin-resistant gonococci (penicillinase-producing *N. gonorrhoeae*, PPNG).

Diseases of the Mouth

The oral cavity is a complex ecosystem suitable for growth and interrelationships of many types of microorganisms. The actual normal microbiota living in the mouth vary greatly from person to person.

When the anatomy of the mouth (Fig. 10–7) is studied, it is obvious that there are many areas where bacteria can attach, colonize, and proliferate, even in the presence of the normal defenses. In the healthy mouth, the saliva secreted by salivary and mucous glands, helps control the growth of opportunistic normal flora. Saliva contains enzymes, immunoglobulins (IgA), and buffers to control the near-neutral pH and continually flushes microbes and food particles through the mouth. Other antimicrobial secretions and phagocytes are found in the mucus that coats the oral surfaces. The hard, complex, calcium tooth enamel, bathed in protective saliva, usually resists damage by oral microbes; however, if the ecological balance is upset or is not properly maintained, oral disease may result.

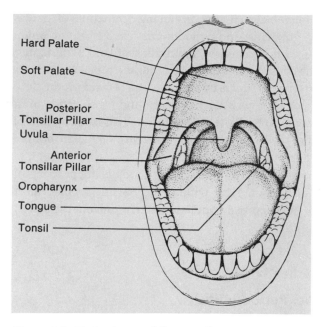

Figure 10-7. Anatomy of the mouth.

Indigenous Microflora and Oral Disease

The indigenous microflora of the mouth has been shown recently to include more than 1, 000 different strains of bacteria, both aerobes and anaerobes. Only a fraction of these oral microbes have been identified. Some of them are beneficial because they produce secretions that are antagonistic to other bacteria. Although several species of *Streptococcus* (*salivarius, mitis, sanguis,* and *mutans*) and *Actinomyces* species often interact to protect the oral surfaces, in other circumstances, they are involved in oral disease.

The anaerobic condition produced by the oxidation-reduction interactions of the oral flora organisms allow certain genera of anaerobic bacteria (*Bacteroides, Fusobacterium, Lactobacillus, Actinobacillus,* and *Treponema*) to become involved in the production of oral diseases. The coating that forms on unclean teeth, called dental plaque, is a coaggregation of bacteria and their products. Many of these microorganisms produce a slime layer or glycocalyx that enables them to attach firmly and cause damage to the tooth enamel. Certain carbohydrates are metabolized by streptococci (especially *S. mutans*) and lactobacilli, producing lactic acid, which encourages other bacteria to grow and become involved in the decay process. Calculus, a calcium phosphate material produced by some bacteria (*e.g., Actinomyces*), is a hard plaque deposit. Calcium phosphate may derive from the enamel dissolved by lactic acid-producing bacteria.

The progressive microbial activities involving formation of dental plaque, dental caries (decay), gingivitis, and periodontitis result from the unique microbial population, reduced host defenses, improper diet, and poor dental hygiene. These diseases are the consequence of at least four microbial activities, including (1) formation of dextran from sugars by streptococci, (2) acid production by lactobacilli, (3) deposition of calculus by *Actinomyces*, and (4) secretion of inflammatory substances (endotoxin) by *Bacteroides* species. This combination of circumstances damages the teeth, soft tissues (gingiva), alveolar bone, and the periodontal fibers attaching teeth to bone.

Oral disease can be prevented by maintaining good health, proper oral hygiene (brushing, flossing), an adequate diet without sugars, and regular fluoride treatments to help control the microbial population and to prevent the damaging bacterial interactions.

Bacterial Infections of the Oral Cavity

Dental Caries, Gingivitis, Periodontitis

Characteristics Damage to teeth, gums, and alveolar bone, resulting from complex interaction of bacteria with dietary sugars.

Pathogens *Streptococcus mutans, S. mitis* (Fig. 10–8), *S. salivarius*, and *S. sanguis, Actinomyces naeslundii, A. viscosus, Lactobacillus, Bacteroides, Actinobacillus, Fusobacterium, Capnocytophaga*.

Pathogenicity Lactic acid and endotoxin production.

Reservoir Human oral cavity.

Transmission Direct contact.

Incubation period Variable.

Control Good oral hygiene, adequate diet without sucrose, fluoride in water, toothpaste, other preparations, and perhaps a vaccine.

Usual treatment Cleaning, filling decayed tooth areas, fluoride paste, and other treatments by dentists.

Acute Necrotizing Ulcerative Gingivitis (ANUG), Vincent's Infection, Trench Mouth

Characteristics A noncontagious peridontitis with gingival ulcers, associated with lack of oral hygiene, nutritional deficiency, debilitating disease, stress, at least two synergistic microorganisms.

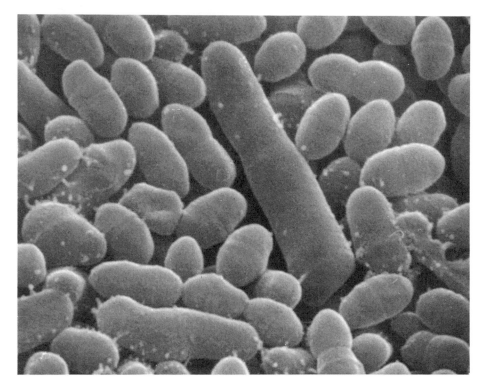

Figure 10–8. Electron micrograph of *Streptococcus mutans* in dental plaque. (Photo by Joan Foster)

Pathogens *Bacteroides* and *Fusobacterium* spp., anaerobic gram-negative bacilli. *Borrelia* and *Treponema* spp., anaerobic gram-variable spiral-shaped bacteria. Sometimes *Capnocytophaga*, *Eikenella*, and other bacteria may occur in lesions.

Pathogenicity Lactic acid and endotoxin production.

Reservoir Human mouth.

Transmission Food, direct contact, lack of oral hygiene.

Incubation period Variable.

Control Gentle local debridement, oral hygiene, adequate nutrition, high fluid intake and rest.

Usual treatment Penicillin, erythromycin, tetracycline, or metronidazole.

Diseases of the Ear

When the anatomy of the ear (Fig. 10–9) is studied, one observes that there are only three pathways for pathogens to enter: (1) through the eustachian tube, from the throat and nasopharynx; (2) from the external ear; and (3) through the blood or lymph. Usually, the bacteria are tapped in the middle ear when a bacterial infection in the throat and nasopharynx causes the eustachian tube to close. The result is an anaerobic condition in the middle ear, allowing anaerobes to grow and cause pressure on the tympanum (eardrum). Swollen lymphoid (adenoid) tissues, viral infections, and allergies may also close the auditory tube, especially in young children.

Figure 10–9. Anatomy of the ear. (Chaffee EE, Lytle IM: Basic Physiology and Anatomy, 4th ed. Philadelphia, JB Lippincott, 1980)

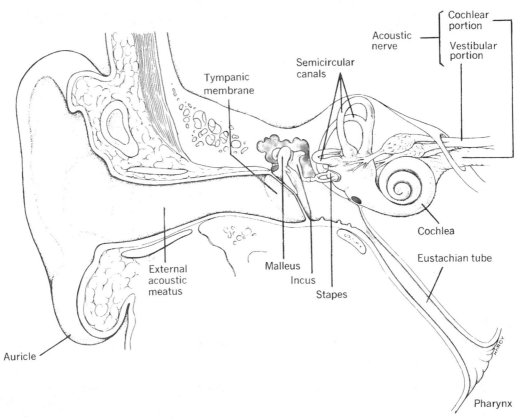

Ear Infections

Otitis Media, Middle Ear Infection

Characteristics Pressure in middle ear, flattening of tympanum, pain, fever, production of exudate, perforation and scarring of eardrum, and if untreated loss of hearing. Most common under age 8.

Pathogens Bacteria: *Haemophilus influenzae, Streptococcus pneumoniae, Streptococcus pyogenes, Staphylococcus aureus.*
Viral: Measles virus, parainfluenza virus, and respiratory syncytial virus (RSV).

Pathogenicity Bacterial exotoxins and viral destruction of cells.

Reservoir Human respiratory nasopharynx.

Transmission Complication following colds, nose and throat infections, direct contact.

Incubation period Variable.

Control For *H. influenzae*, vaccinate to prevent meningitis. Rifampin prophylaxis is also used for prevention of meningitis. For streptococci, search for and treat carriers.

Usual treatment Ampicillin for *H. influenzae*, amoxicillin or penicillin for streptococci, erythromycin for penicillin-resistant strains. Enhance body defenses for viral infections. Insertion of tympanum tubes by physician to relieve pressure and the anaerobic condition.

External Otitis, External Ear Infections, Swimmer's Ear

Characteristics Infection of ear canal with itching, pain, discharge, tenderness, redness, swelling, loss of hearing.

Pathogens *Escherichia coli, Pseudomonas aeruginosa, Proteus vulgaris, Staphylococcus aureus*; rarely by a fungus, such as *Aspergillus.*

Reservoir Contaminated water trapped in ear canal; also normal opportunistic flora.

Transmission Swimming pool or bath water. Articles inserted in ear canal for cleaning out debris and wax.

Incubation period 1–3 days.

Control Prevent contaminated water from entering and being trapped by wax in external ear canal. Allow physician to clean wax and debris from ears.

Usual treatment Remove infected debris. Topical treatment with neomycin and polymyxin B for gram-negative rods; 1% hydrocortisone for swelling.

Diseases of the Respiratory System

To simplify discussion of the functions, defenses, and diseases of the area, the respiratory system (Fig. 10–10) is often separated into the upper respiratory tract (URT), consisting of the nose and pharynx (throat), and the lower respiratory tract (LRT), including the larynx, trachea, bronchial tubes, and alveoli. The most common diseases are those of the upper respiratory tract (*e.g.*, colds and sore throats), which may predispose the patient to more serious infections, such as sinusitis, otitis media, bronchitis, and pneumonia.

Typical indigenous microflora found in the mucosa of the nose and throat include bacterial species of *Streptococcus*, *Staphylococcus*, *Haemophilus*, *Corynebacterium*, *Neisseria*, *Bacteroides*, *Branhamella*, *Fusobacterium*, and *Actinomyces*. Many of these microorganisms may cause opportunistic diseases of the respiratory tract.

Figure 10–10. The respiratory system. (Chaffee EE, Lytle IM: Basic Physiology and Anatomy, 4th ed. Philadelphia, JB Lippincott, 1980)

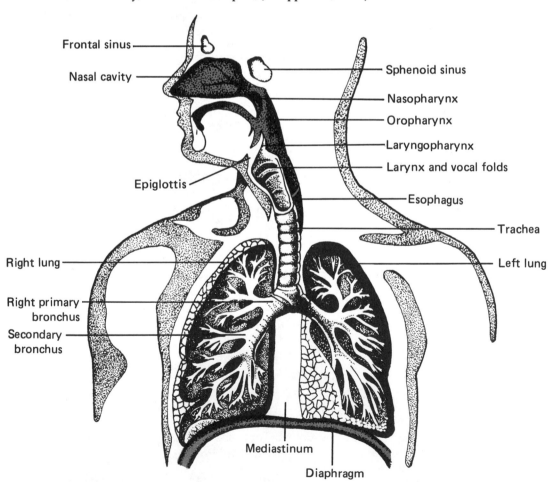

Nonspecific Respiratory Infections

Pneumonia

Characteristics An acute nonspecific infection of the alveolar spaces and tissue of the lung, with fever, cough, acute chest pain, and respiratory distress; identified by chest x-rays. Pneumonia is usually a secondary infection.

Pathogens May be caused by gram-positive or gram-negative bacteria, mycoplasmas, viruses, fungi, or protozoa. The bacteria causing pneumonia include *Streptococcus pneumoniae* (see Fig. 7–4), other streptococci, *Staphylococcus aureus* (see Figs. 1–8 and 1–9), *Haemophilus influenzae*, *Neisseria meningitidis*, *Pseudomonas aeruginosa*, *Yersinia pestis*, *Klebsiella pneumonia*, and other gram-negative enteric bacilli. *Rickettsia*, *Chlamydia*, and *Mycoplasma* spp. may also be causative agents. Many viral respiratory infections may result in pneumonia. Especially in susceptible and immunocompromised individuals, the fungi *Histoplasma*, *Coccidioides*, *Candida*, *Cryptococcus*, *Blastomyces* and the protozoan *Pneumocystis carinii* may be etiologic agents.

Reservoir Humans.

Transmission Direct contact, respiratory secretions, hands, and fomites.

Incubation period Depends on pathogen involved.

Control Depends on pathogen involved.

Usual treatment Antibiotic therapy depends on the causal agent identified in sputum or other LRT specimens.

Vial Respiratory Infections

Common Cold, Acute Viral Rhinitis, Acute Coryza, Upper Respiratory Infection (URI)

Characteristics Coryza (profuse discharge from nostrils), sneezing, sore throat, bronchiolitis, bronchitis. Secondary bacterial infections frequently follow.

Pathogens Many (>100) types of rhinovirus, adenovirus (Fig. 10–11), coronavirus, (RSV), influenza, parainfluenza, and other viruses.

Reservoir Human respiratory system.

Transmission Respiratory secretions by way of hands, direct contact, airborne droplets, soiled articles.

Incubation period 1–3 days.

Epidemiology Most common in fall, winter, and spring.

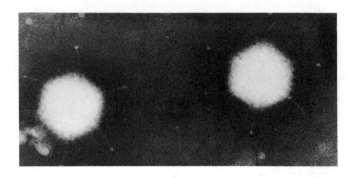

Figure 10-11.
Electromicrograph of purified type 5 adenovirus particles embedded in sodium silicotungstate (original magnification × 350,000). (Valentine RC, Pereira HG: J Mol Biol 13:13, 1965)

Control   Sanitary disposal of oral and nasal discharges. Disinfect eating and drinking utensils. Avoid contact with infected individuals. Oral live adenovirus vaccine is effective in the military for specific adenovirus epidemics.

Usual treatment   New antiviral agents. Antibiotics should be reserved for bacterial complications (sinusitis, otitis media, tonsillitis, bronchitis, pneumonia).

Croup, Acute Laryngotracheobronchitis

Characteristics   Acute viral inflammation of respiratory tract with subglottic swelling, respiratory distress with a high-pitched sound during inspiration.

Pathogens   Usually parainfluenza virus, less often RSV, influenza A or B, or other viruses and *Mycoplasma pneumoniae* (a bacterium)

Reservoir   Humans.

Transmission   Direct oral contact, droplets, fomites.

Incubation period   Variable.

Epidemiology   Usually seen in susceptible children 3 months to 3 years old. Symptoms are most dramatic at night, lasting 3-4 days.

Control   Usually self-limiting and not contagious.

Usual treatment   Vaporizers, humidifiers, hot shower steam may relieve symptoms. Hospitalization with oxygenation may be necessary in severe cases. Antibiotics are rarely indicated, but amantadine or other antiviral agents may help.

Influenza, "Flu"

Characteristics   A specific acute viral respiratory infection with fever, chills, headache, cough, nasal drainage; sometimes causing bronchitis, pneumonia, and death in severe cases. Rare nausea, vomiting, and diarrhea.

Pathogens   Influenza virus, types A, B, and C. Usually type A is associated with pandemics and widespread epidemics.

Reservoir   Humans.

Transmission   Respiratory secretions, direct contact, fomites, hands.

Incubation period   24–72 hours.

Epidemiology   Pandemics occurred in 1889, 1918, 1947, 1957, 1968. Type A epidemics occur every 1–3 years and type B every 3–4 years.

Control   Yearly immunization; prophylactic amantadine or rimantadine may be used against type A for high-risk patients. Good personal hygiene and avoiding crowds during epidemics may prevent infection.

Usual treatment   Amantadine reduces symptoms if given early in type A disease.

Bacterial Respiratory Infections

Diphtheria

Characteristics   An acute contagious respiratory disease, with fibrinous pharyngeal pseudomembrane, causing myocardial and neural tissue damage.

Pathogens   *Corynebacterium diphtheriae*, pleomorphic, gram-negative bacilli that group in palisade arrangements. Toxigenic strains are infected with a corynebacteriophage, resulting in exotoxin production that causes the heart and nerve damage. Identified by culture and serologic techniques.

Reservoir   Humans.

Transmission   Airborne droplets, direct contact, contaminated fomites, raw milk.

Incubation period   2–5 days.

Epidemiology   Four cases in United States in 1990 were reported to CDC. Diphtheria occurs during colder months among unimmunized children and adults. Disease has disappeared in areas with effective immunization programs.

Control   Community program of immunization of all infants and children with diphtheria-pertussis-tetanus (DPT) vaccine. Give diphtheria-tetanus booster vaccines at appropriate intervals. Patient isolation, quarantine, and disinfection of all fomites.

Usual treatment   Administer antitoxin in suspected cases with erythromycin or penicillin in confirmed cases. Treat carriers with erythromycin or penicillin.

Legionellosis, Legionnaires' Disease, Pontiac Fever

Characteristics An acute bacterial pneumonia with headache, high fever, dry cough, chills, diarrhea, pleural and abdominal pain.

Pathogens *Legionella pneumophilia*, a gram-negative bacillus, requiring special medium to grow *in vitro* (see Fig. 8–2). Additional species are being identified. Identification by culture, fluorescent antibody, and ELISA tests.

Reservoir Soil, dust, and environmental water sources; lakes, creeks, hot-water and air-conditioning systems, shower heads, ultrasonic nebulizers, tap water and distilling water systems.

Transmission Airborne from water or dust; not person-to-person.

Incubation period 2–10 days.

Epidemiology In 1990, in the United States, 1,284 cases were reported.

Control Search for environmental sources of infection, periodic superchlorination or superheating of water supply.

Usual treatment Erythromycin with rifampin.

Strep Throat, Streptococcal Pharyngitis

Characteristics An acute bacterial infection of the throat with fever, pain; inflammation of pharynx and tonsils; white patches of pus on pharyngeal epithelium. Rheumatic fever and glomerulonephritis complication may result in heart and kidney damage because of hypersensitivity reactions.

Pathogens *Streptococcus pyogenes* (see Fig. 9–15), β-hemolytic, gram-positive cocci, catalase-negative (Fig. 10–12). The strain that produces an erythrogenic toxin causes scarlet fever rash. Identified by throat culture on blood agar plate, by susceptibility to bacitracin disks, and by fluorescent antibody serologic techniques.

Reservoir Humans.

Transmission Human-to-human, by direct contact, usually hands, aerosol droplets, secretions from patients, and carriers.

Incubation period 1–3 days.

Epidemiology Over 200,000 cases/year in United States, mostly among children (5–14 years); 3% develop rheumatic fever.

Control Throat cultures followed by antibiotic treatment; personal hygiene and cleanliness. No protective immunity following recovery; no effective vaccines.

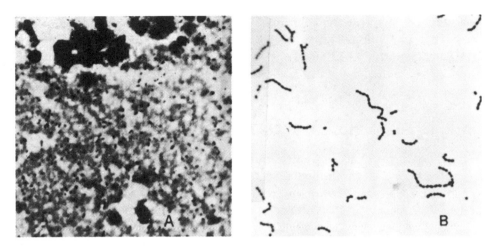

Figure 10–12. (*A*) Group A *β*-hemolytic streptococci in pneumonic lesion (rat) (original magnification × 600). (*B*) Chain formation characteristics of usual growth of streptococci in artificial media. Smear made from 24-hr culture in serum broth (original magnification × 1000). (*A*) (Glaser RJ, Wood WB Jr.: Arch Pathol 52:244, 1951. (*B*) (Davis BD, et al: Microbiology, 4th ed. Philadelphia, Harper & Row, 1990)

Usual treatment   Penicillin, erythromycin to prevent ear infections, rheumatic fever, glomerulonephritis, and other complications.

Tuberculosis

Characteristics   An acute or chronic mycobacterial infection of the pulmonary tract; may invade lymph nodes to cause systemic disease. Infected patients show a positive hypersensitivity skin test and pulmonary tubercles may be seen on chest x-rays.

Pathogens   Primarily *Mycobacterium tuberculosis*; occasionally other *Mycobacterium* spp.; an acid-fast, nonmotile bacillus. Identified by culture techniques.

Reservoir   Humans; rarely, in diseased cattle.

Transmission   Airborne droplets, prolonged direct contact, milk, and contact with infected cattle.

Incubation period   4–12 weeks

Epidemiology   In the United States, more than 20,000 new cases a year; in 1990, there were 23,720 new cases reported to CDC.

Control   Tuberculin testing of humans and cattle. Chest x-ray of TB skin-test–positive people and prompt treatment. Vaccination or preventive treatment of close contacts of infected individuals.

Usual treatment   A combination of antimicrobial drugs such as isoniazid (IHN) with rifampin (RIF), streptomycin (SM), ethambutol (EMB), or parazinamide (PZA) is given for 9–12 months.

Insight: Tuberculosis (TB) Elimination and AIDS

The Centers for Disease Control published a plan in April, 1989, which established a goal to eliminate TB (*i.e.*, a case rate of 0.1 cases per 100,000 people) by the year 2010, with an interim goal to be reached (*i.e.*, a case rate of 3.5 cases per 100,000 people) by the year 2000.

An expected decline in the number of cases prior to 1989 was offset by an increase of cases in the 25-to-44-years age group and among the racial/ethnic minorities during the 1985–1988 period. Increases occurred among both males and females. The trend for race/ethnicity primarily reflect the increasing occurrence of TB in persons infected with human immunodeficiency virus (HIV). HIV infection is an important risk factor for developing clinically apparent TB among persons already infected with *Mycobacterium tuberculosis*. The CDC recommends that all HIV-infected persons be screened for TB and, if infected, be offered curative or preventive therapy. Similarly, persons with TB and positive tuberculin tests should be evaluated for HIV infection to ensure that appropriate counseling and treatment are started.

Reports indicate that noncompliance with prescribed therapy is the greatest remaining obstacle to the elimination of TB. Ideally, 90% of patients should complete therapy within 12 months. The strategies that may be effective to counteract noncompliance include the use of outreach workers to administer and observe therapy and provide incentive for compliance, education programs for health professionals, studies of compliance predictors and enhancers, and research targeted toward reducing the duration of therapy and the number of drug doses required. Careful monitoring of all patients for compliance and the widespread use of compliance-enhancing strategies is essential for eliminating TB. (From *Morbidity and Mortality Weekly Report*, 1990; 39(33). U.S. Department of Health and Human Services, Centers for Disease Control, Atlanta, Georgia.)

Whooping Cough, Pertussis

Characteristics An acute bacterial childhood infection. The initial catarrhal stage produces mild symptoms resembling the common cold. The second paroxysmal stage is marked by uncontrollable sieges of coughing in an attempt to expel the thick mucus in the trachea and bronchi. Pneumonia may be a complication.

Pathogens *Bordetella pertussis*, a small, encapsulated, nonmotile, gram-negative coccobacillus that produces endotoxins and exotoxins. Identified by fluorescent antibody serologic techniques.

Reservoir Human respiratory tract.

Transmission Airborne via droplets from coughing.

Incubation period 7–10 days usually; up to 21 days.

Epidemiology In 1990, in the United States, 4,188 cases were reported to the CDC.

Control Vaccination of all young children with DPT (P for pertussis) containing killed *B. pertussis*.

Usual treatment Erythromycin, tetracycline, or chloramphenicol.

Protozoan Respiratory Infections

Pneumocystosis, Pneumocystis Pneumonia, Interstitial Plasma-cell Pneumonia

Characteristics A subacute pulmonary protozoan disease found in chronically ill children, immunosuppressed patients, and persons with acquired immunodeficiency syndrome (AIDS). Asymptomatic in immunocompetent people; most common cause of death in AIDS patients. Patients show respiratory insufficiency with cyanosis; pulmonary infiltration of intra-alveolar tissue with frothy exudate. Usually fatal in untreated patients.

Pathogen *Pneumocystis carinii* (Fig. 10–13), a protozoan in cyst and sporozoite form, a sporozoan.

Reservoir Humans.

Transmission Direct contact, transfer of pulmonary secretions from infected to susceptible persons. Perhaps airborne.

Incubation period 1–2 months or longer.

Control Prophylaxis treatment of immunosuppressed patients with co-trimoxazole. Careful disinfection of respiratory therapy equipment.

Usual treatment Co-trimoxazole or pentamidine.

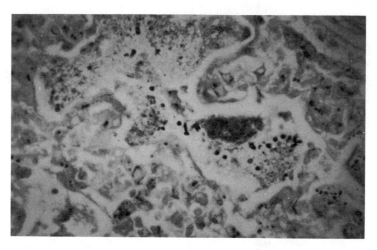

Figure 10–13. *Pneumocystis carinii* appears as dark oval bodies when stained with special silver stain. Foamy material is also seen throughout the several alveoli in this section of the lung (original magnification × 250). (Moffett HL: Clinical Microbiology, 2nd ed. Philadelphia, JB Lippincott, 1980)

Diseases of the Gastrointestinal Tract

The digestive tract consists of a long tube with many expanded areas designed for the digestion of food, the absorption of nutrients, and the elimination of undigested materials (Fig. 10–14). A continuous stream of transient and resident microbiota enter and leave the gastrointestinal tract. Most of the microorganisms ingested with food are destroyed in the stomach and duodenum and are inhibited from growing in the lower intestines by the resident microflora. They are then flushed from the colon during defecation, along with large numbers of indigenous microbes.

The largest number of resident microorganisms are found in the lower small intestine and colon. There, the availability of nutrients and moisture at a constant 37°C allows many facultative and obligate anaerobes to thrive. Most of these intestinal microbiota are obligate anaerobic *Bacteroides* and *Fusobacterium* species, with fewer *Clostridium* and *Veillonella* species. Facultative anaerobic bacteria occur less abundantly but are better understood because they are easier to isolate and cultivate. Included in this group are the coliforms, the indicator organisms of fecal contamination of water supplies. These enterobacteria usually include *Escherichia, Enterobacter, Proteus,* and *Klebsiella* species.

Also found in fecal material are many viruses, most of which are harmless; however, some can cause gastroenteritis under certain conditions. Some may be ingested with contaminated food, such as hepatitis A virus in contaminated raw oysters.

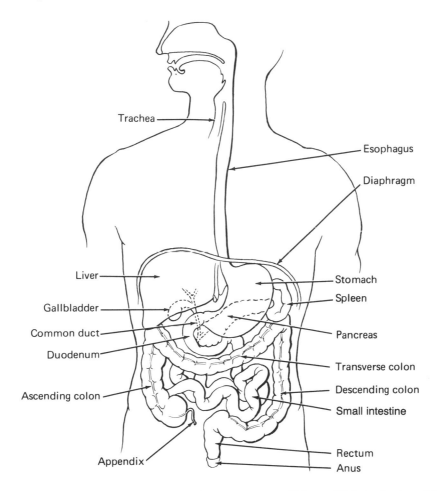

Figure 10–14. Anatomy of the digestive system. (Scherer JC: Introductory Medical-Surgical Nursing, 5th ed. Philadelphia, JB Lippincott, 1991)

Viral Gastrointestinal Infections

Viral Gastroenteritis, Viral Diarrhea, Epidemic Acute Infectious Nonbacterial Gastroenteropathy, "24–Hour Flu"

Characteristics   A self-limiting viral infection of the lining of the gastrointestinal tract with nausea, vomiting, diarrhea, abdominal pain, headache, malaise, and low-grade fever.

Pathogens   Norwalk virus, adenoviruses, echoviruses, rotavirus, coxsackieviruses, poliovirus, and others. Identified by serologic techniques.

Reservoir   Humans.

Transmission   Fecal-oral route, fecal contamination of food, water, and hands.

Incubation period   24–48 hours.

Control   Isolation of patient, enteric precautions.

Usual treatment   Replacement of fluids and electrolytes. Amantadine occasionally reduces symptoms.

Viral Hepatitis

Viral hepatitis includes a group of diseases involving inflammation of the liver caused by several viruses: type A (HAV), type B (HBV), non-A, non-B (NANB), sometimes called type C (HCV), and delta-type (HDV) virus.

Viral Hepatitis A (HA), Type A Hepatitis, Infectious Hepatitis, Epidemic Hepatitis

Characteristics   Liver inflammation with fever, nausea, abdominal discomfort, usually jaundice. Prolonged convalescence.

Pathogen   Hepatitis A virus (HAV), a picornavirus, similar to an enterovirus; the non-A, non-B hepatitis viruses may cause similar hepatitis symptoms. Serologic and radioimmunologic identification techniques.

Reservoir   Humans.

Transmission   Fecal-oral route, person-to-person. Fecal contamination of water, food, milk, undercooked shell fish.

Incubation period   15–50 days, average 28–30 days.

Epidemiology   In 1990, in the United States, 28,919 cases were reported to CDC.

Control   Good sanitation practices, personal hygiene. Passive immunization of exposed individuals with hyperimmune gamma globulin. Vaccination for high-risk persons. Isolation of infected patients, enteric precautions.

Usual treatment   None. Immune serum may reduce symptoms and speed recovery.

Viral Hepatitis B (HB), Type B Hepatitis, Serum Hepatitis, Australia Antigen Hepatitis

Characteristics   Viral infection and liver damage with anorexia, rash, and jaundice. May lead to chronic hepatitis or cirrhosis of liver in immunodeficient patients.

Pathogen   Hepatitis B virus (HBV), a DNA virus with several major antigenic subtypes. May also involve coinfection with delta hepatitis virus, an RNA virus. A non-A, non-B hepatitis viruses causes similar blood-liver infections when transferred via transfusions. Identified by serologic tests.

Reservoir Humans.

Transmission Person-to-person, by saliva, semen, and other body fluids; parenteral route, through contaminated syringes, needles, dialysis, and other equipment serving as vectors.

Incubation period 45–108 days, average 60–90 days.

Epidemiology In the United States, 19,939 cases were reported to CDC in 1990.

Control Vaccination against HBV. Active and passive immunization of exposed individuals. Isolation of infected persons with blood and body fluid precautions. Sterilization of all equipment.

Usual treatment Immune globulin (IG), hyperimmune gamma globulin (HBIG), or antiviral chemotherapy when available.

Bacterial Gastrointestinal Infections

Campylobacter Gastroenteritis

Characteristics An acute enteric disease with diarrhea, nausea, vomiting, fever, malaise, abdominal pain, usually self-limiting, lasting 1–4 days.

Pathogens *Campylobacter jejuni* and *C. coli* of many serotypes. Rigid, helical spirilla. Identified by cultural and serologic techniques.

Reservoir Animals, including cattle, sheep, swine, poultry, other birds, rodents, cats, dogs, other pets.

Transmission Ingestion of bacteria in food, milk, water; contact with infected pets, wild animals, and infected infants.

Incubation period 1–10 days, average 3–5 days.

Control Thorough cooking of foods, especially poultry; pasteurize milk; chlorinate water supplies. Hand-washing after animal contact. Isolation of hospitalized patients, enteric precautions.

Usual treatment Replacement of fluids and electrolytes. Antibiotic therapy; erythromycin, tetracycline, or aminoglycosides.

Cholera

Characteristics An acute enteric diarrheal disease with watery stools, vomiting, rapid dehydration, loss of blood volume, shock. Death frequently results if untreated.

Pathogens *Vibrio cholerae* type 01, El Tor strain of *V. cholerae*, or other serotypes. A gram-negative curved rod, C- or S-shaped that secretes an enterotoxin, called choleragin. Identified by culture analysis, morphologic characteristics, and serologic techniques.

Reservoir Humans and environmental reservoirs.

Transmission Fecal-oral route; vomitus and feces-contaminated water and foods; soiled hands; flies. Raw or undercooked seafoods from contaminated waters. Sometimes carriers.

Incubation period 1–5 days.

Epidemiology Occurs worldwide. In 1990, only nine cases were reported in the United States. These cases involved people who ingested oysters from the coastal areas of the Gulf of Mexico, and seafood in Central and South America.

Control Isolation of hospitalized patients, enteric precautions. Concurrent disinfection of feces, vomitus, hands, linen, and fomites. Adequate sewage processing and water treatment. Fly control. Vaccination in some countries. Prophylactic tetracycline for exposed families, doxycycline, or furazolidone treatment.

Usual treatment Prompt fluid and electrolyte replacement therapy; tetracycline, co-trimoxazole, furazolidone, and other chemotherapy to shorten duration of disease.

Enteropathogenic *Escherichia coli* Diarrhea, "Traveler's Diarrhea"

Characteristics Watery diarrhea with, or without, mucus or blood, vomiting, abdominal cramping.

Pathogens *E. coli*, three types; invasive, enterotoxigenic, and enteropathogenic. Gram-negative rods; some produce enterotoxin, others invade colon mucosa. Identified by cultural and serologic tests (see Fig. 2–9).

Reservoir Infected humans, carriers.

Transmission Fecal-oral route, fecal contaminated water, food, hands, fomites, or direct contact.

Incubation period 12–72 hours.

Control Proper sewage disposal, water treatment, hand-washing practices. Enteric precautions for hospitalized cases.

Usual treatment Fluid and electrolyte replacement therapy; ampicillin or co-trimoxazole treatment for severe cases and carriers.

Salmonellosis and Typhoid Fever

Characteristics A gastroenteritis, inflammation of stomach and intestines with abdominal pain, headache, nausea, usually vomiting and diarrhea. Typhoid fever, the most severe form, is a bacteremia, characterized by constipation, intestinal hemorrhage, enlarged spleen and lymph nodes, rose spots on trunk, sustained fever.

Pathogens *Salmonella typhi* causes typhoid fever; *S. cholerae-suis, S. typhimurium,* and many other serologic types of *S. enteritidis* cause salmonellosis. Motile gram-negative bacilli with endotoxins. *Salmonella typhi* produces exotoxins and endotoxins. Identified by cultural and serologic techniques.

Reservoir Humans, animals, wild and domestic cattle, poultry, pigs, dogs, cats, turtles, fish, and many others.

Transmission Fecal-oral route; uncooked and undercooked feces-contaminated meat, eggs, and milk products; sewage, polluted water; hands and fingers of infected persons and carriers; flies and other flying insects.

Incubation period 1–3 weeks for typhoid fever; 1–3 days for salmonellosis.

Epidemiology In United States, only 503 cases of typhoid fever were reported in 1990.

Control Isolation of hospitalized patients with enteric precautions. Water purification; effective sewage disposal; pasteurization of milk; thorough cooking of foods of animal and egg origin; proper hand-washing techniques; control of flies; clean food preparation area; and treatment of carriers and infected pets. Eliminate food preparation by infected persons and carriers.

Usual treatment Fluid and electrolyte replacement therapy. Ampicillin or amoxicillin with co-trimoxazole or chloramphenicol for resistant strains, quinolones, and cephalosporins.

Shigellosis, Bacillary Dysentery

Characteristics An acute bacterial infection of lining of small and large intestine; diarrhea with blood, mucus, and pus; nausea, vomiting, cramps, fever, sometimes toxemia and convulsions.

Pathogens Several serotypes of *Shigella dysenteriae, S. flexneri, S. boydii,* and *S. sonei.* Gram-negative bacilli, nonmotile. Plasmid associated with toxin production and virulence. Identified by cultural and biochemical techniques.

Reservoir Humans, some primates.

Transmission   Fecal-oral route from patients or carriers. Feces-contaminated hands and fingernails, contaminated food and milk, sewage-polluted water. Flies and cockroach vectors.

Incubation period   1–7 days, average 1–3 days.

Control   Eliminate fecal contamination of food, milk, and water. Proper hand-washing and fomite cleaning. Enteric precautions with patients. Infected individuals should neither prepare nor serve food.

Usual treatment   Fluid and electrolyte replacement therapy. Co-trimoxazole ampicillin, tetracyclines, or naldixic acid antibiotic therapy. Chloramphenicol for resistant strains.

Bacterial Foodborne Intoxications, Food Poisoning

Foodborne intoxication or food poisoning refers to diseases resulting from the ingestion of food or water contaminated with bacterial exotoxins produced by such bacteria as *Vibrio cholerae*, enterotoxigenic *E. coli*, *Clostridium botulinum*, *C. perfringens*, and *Staphylococcus aureus*.

Botulism

Characteristics   A neuromuscular disease caused by ingestion of food contaminated by *C. botulinum* spores, containing neurotoxins secreted by the pathogen. Infant botulism and wound botulism are produced by living exotoxin-producing bacteria in the gastrointestinal tract or wounds, respectively. Neurotoxins may cause nerve damage, visual difficulty, respiratory failure, flaccid paralysis of voluntary muscles, brain damage, coma, and death within a week, if untreated.

Pathogen   *Clostridium botulinum*, a spore-forming gram-positive, anaerobic bacillus that produces several exotoxins.

Reservoir   Dust, soil, dirty foods, honey, improperly canned foods, neutral *p*H foods, lightly cured foods.

Transmission   Ingestion of foods in which the pathogen has produced exotoxin; improperly cooked foods with near-neutral *p*H.

Incubation period   12–36 hours.

Epidemiology   Only 86 cases in United States reported in 1990.

Control   Careful washing, canning, processing, and cooking of food. Thorough cleaning of wounds. Never add raw honey to babies' milk or foods.

Usual treatment   Antitoxin and treatment of respiratory failure.

Clostridium perfringens Food Poisoning

Characteristics   A gastrointestinal toxemia with colic, diarrhea, nausea, rarely vomiting. Usually a mild disease of short duration, <24 hours, rarely fatal.

Pathogen   *Clostridium perfringens*, a gram-positive, spore-forming, enterotoxin-producing, anaerobic, thermophilic bacillus.

Reservoir   Spores in soil, gastrointestinal tract of humans and animals.

Transmission   Ingestion of food, contaminated by dirt or fecal material, kept at moderate temperatures allowing bacterial growth and exotoxin production.

Incubation period   6–24 hours.

Control   Cook food well, serve hot or cold. Train food processors in proper hand-washing and food-handling techniques.

Usual treatment   None. Usually a self-limiting disease.

Staphylococcal Food Poisoning

Characteristics   A gastroenteritis toxemia with acute onset of cramps, vomiting, nausea, occasional diarrhea, subnormal temperature and blood pressure resulting from ingested enterotoxins in foods.

Pathogens   *Staphylococcus aureus* growing in foods produces exotoxins.

Reservoir   Humans: skin, abscesses, nasal secretions; bovine-contaminated milk.

Transmission   Ingestion of *S. aureus*-contaminated foods containing staphylococcal enterotoxin; particularly starchy foods and meats.

Incubation period   1–7 hours.

Control   Training food preparers in proper personal hygiene, in cleanliness in kitchen areas, and in the need for refrigeration of starchy foods and meats. Prevent infected persons from preparing food.

Usual treatment   Fluid replacement if needed.

Protozoan Gastrointestinal Diseases

Amebiasis, Amebic Dysentery

Characteristics   A protozoan intestinal disease with dysentery, fever, chills, bloody or mucoid diarrhea or constipation, and colitis; may progress to liver, lungs, pericardium, or brain.

Pathogen *Entamoeba histolytica*, a protozoan of class Sarcodina; occurs in two stages: cysts (the infective stage) and the motile, reproducing trophozoite. The ameba may embed in mucous membranes of the colon, forming abscesses, or may pass with the fluid diarrhea.

Reservoir Humans, usually asymptomatic carriers.

Transmission Feces-contaminated warm water and vegetables, flies on food; soiled hands of infected food handles; oral-anal sexual contact.

Incubation period Variable days to months.

Control Sanitary sewage disposal. Protection and treatment of water supplies. Personal hygiene and hand-washing before preparing and eating food. Eliminate fertilization of crops with human fecal material. Control flies around foods. Enteric precautions with hospitalized patients.

Usual treatment Metronidazole (Flagyl) with iodoquinol. Fluid and electrolyte replacement.

Giardiasis, Giardial Enteritis

Characteristics A protozoan infection of the small intestine, with nausea, gas, abdominal pain, acute malodorous diarrhea, malabsorption, and damage to mucosal membranes; may be asymptomatic.

Pathogen *Giardia lamblia* (see Fig. 2–20), a flagellate protozoan; trophozoites attach to mucosal membranes; cysts and sometimes trophozoites are expelled in feces.

Reservoir Humans; possibly beaver; other wild and domestic animals.

Transmission Fecal-oral route; ingestion of cysts in fecal-contaminated cold water or foods; person-to-person by soiled hands to mouth.

Incubation period 5–25 days or longer.

Control Proper filtration of public water supplies (chlorine does not destroy cysts); sanitary disposal of feces; boil all emergency water supplies.

Usual treatment Quinacrine (Atabrine) or metronidazole (Flagyl)

Diseases of the Urogenital Tract

When the male and female urinary and reproductive systems are studied, it is easy to observe many areas in which infections may occur. The urinary tract is nor-

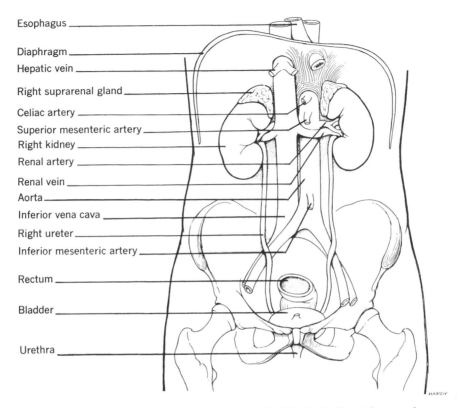

Esophagus

Diaphragm

Hepatic vein

Right suprarenal gland

Celiac artery

Superior mesenteric artery

Right kidney

Renal artery

Renal vein

Aorta

Inferior vena cava

Right ureter

Inferior mesenteric artery

Rectum

Bladder

Urethra

Figure 10–15. Urinary tract. (Chaffee EE, Lytle IM: Basic Physiology and Anatomy, 3rd ed. Philadelphia, JB Lippincott, 1973)

mally protected from pathogens by the frequent flushing action of urination (Fig. 10–15). The acidity of normal urine also discourages the growth of many microorganisms. Only at the opening (meatus) of the urethra are indigenous microflora found in the male urogenital tract and in the female urinary system. These urethral bacteria include *Bacteroides, Streptococcus, Mycobacterium, Lactobacillus,* and *Neisseria,* as well as some gram-negative enteric bacteria. However, the female genital area supports the growth of many additional microflora organisms. In the adult vagina, there are many species of *Staphylococcus, Streptococcus, Lactobacillus, Neisseria, Clostridium, Actinomyces, Bacteroides,* diphtheroids, enterobacteria, and *Candida* yeasts. The balance among these microbes depends on the estrogen levels and pH of the site. The rest of the reproductive systems of both sexes should remain free of microbial life (Fig. 10–16). When any of these and other microorganisms invade further, many nonspecific infections may occur.

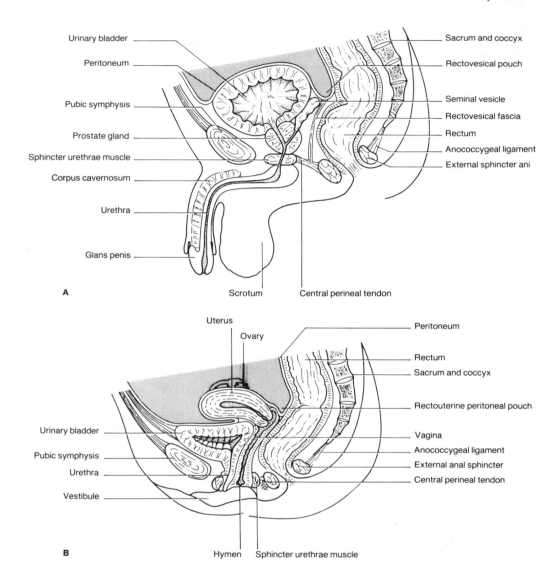

Figure 10–16. Reproductive systems. (*A*) Male; (*B*) Female. (Akesson EJ, Loeb JA, Wilson-Pauwels L: Thompson's: Core Textbook of Anatomy, 3rd 3d. Philadelphia, JB Lippincott, 1990)

Sexually Transmitted Diseases

The term sexually transmitted disease (STD), formerly called venereal disease (VD), includes any of the infections transmitted by sexual activities. They are diseases of not only the reproductive and urinary tracts, but also of the skin, mucous membranes, blood, lymphatic and digestive systems, and many other body areas. The (AIDS) and chlamydial infections are the epidemic STDs of the 1990s. Because the AIDS virus (HIV) primarily causes damage to the helper (T_H) lymphocytes and thus inhibits antibody production, it is discussed later with diseases of the circulatory systems. Hepatitis B, amebiasis, and giardiasis can also be considered sexually transmitted diseases.

Urinary Tract Infections

Urethritis, Cystitis, Ureteritis, Prostatitis

Characteristics Inflammatory infections of the urethra (urethritis), the urinary bladder (cystitis), the ureters (ureteritis), or the prostate (prostatitis). May lead to kidney infections (pyelonephritis) and damage.

Pathogens Any of the normal flora introduced by poor personal hygiene, sexual intercourse, insertion of catheters, and so forth. Most common pathogens include *E. coli*, *Proteus* spp., *Pseudomonas* spp., and fecal streptococci (enterococci). Nosocomial infections caused by *Serratia*, *Pseudomonas*, and *Klebsiella* spp. are common. Nonspecific urethritis is frequently caused by species of *Chlamydia*, *Ureaplasma*, and *Mycoplasma*, usually introduced by sexual contact. The gonococci may also invade the urinary tract as well as the reproductive system.

Reservoir Humans.

Transmission Poor personal hygiene; sexual intercourse; introduction of catheters and other instruments.

Incubation period Variable, 1–15 days.

Control Personal cleanliness, particularly before intercourse; use of condoms. Sterilization of catheters, cystoscopes, and other instruments and proper disinfection of the urethral area before use of these instruments.

Usual treatment Appropriate antibiotic or chemotherapeutic agent for the identified pathogen.

Viral Urogenital Infections

Genital Herpes, Venereal Herpes

Characteristics A herpesvirus infection of the reproductive system, producing herpetic lesions externally and/or internally with fever, headache, malaise; may become latent in nerve ganglia and asymptomatic. Progression of lesion: papule, vesicle, pustule, ulcer, crusting, healing.

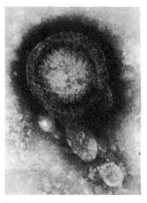 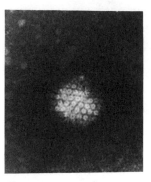

A   B

Figure 10–17. Herpes simplex virus particles
embedded in phosphotungstate. (*A*) Enveloped full
particle showing the thick envelope surrounding the
nucleocapsid. (*B*) Naked full particle; the structure
of the capsomers is plainly visible (original
magnification × 200,000). (Watson DH, et al:
Virology 19:250, 1963)

Pathogen   Herpes simplex virus (HSV), type 2 usually; type 1 occasionally (Fig. 10–17).

Reservoir   Humans.

Transmission   Direct sexual contact; oral-genital, or oral-anal contact, during
presence of lesions (Fig. 10–18). Mother-to-neonate during pregnancy and
birth, or autoinoculation from another lesion.

Incubation period   2–28 days or longer, may remain as latent infection indefinitely.

Control   Refrain from intercourse with person with herpetic lesions; use of condoms.
Cesarean delivery of infected mothers before membranes rupture.
Prophylactic oral acyclovir for women of reproductive age.

Usual treatment   Acyclovir; intravenous, oral, or topical.

Genital Warts, Papilloma Venereum, Condyloma Acuminata

Characteristics   Viral disease with skin and mucous membrane lesions that are
smooth or filiform, cauliflowerlike, fleshy or flat growths in genital areas,
internally or externally (Fig. 10–19). In babies of infected mothers, laryngeal
papillomas. Some infections become malignant.

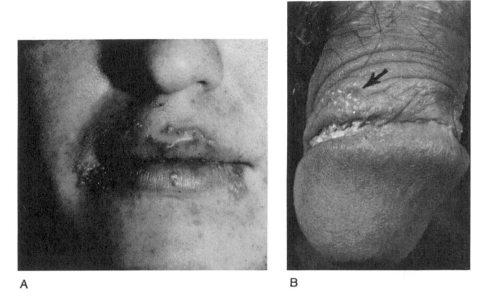

A   B

Figure 10–18. (A) Recurrent herpes simplex of the lip. (B) Recurrent herpes progenitalis. (Dobson RL, Abele DC: The Practice of Dermatology. Philadelphia, JB Lippincott, 1985)

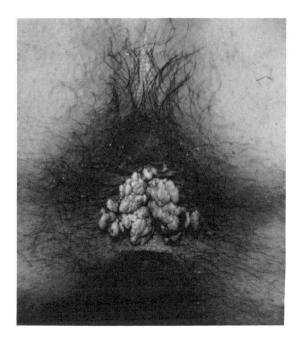

Figure 10–19. Anogenital warts (condylomata accuminata or moist warts). (Dobson RL, Abele DC: The Practice of Dermatology. Philadelphia, JB Lippincott, 1985)

Pathogen   Human papilloma virus (HPV) of genotypes 6, 11, 16, or 18. The latter two are more often involved in malignancies.

Reservoir   Humans.

Transmission   Direct contact, usually sexual; through breaks in skin or mucous membranes. From mother to neonate during birth.

Incubation period   1–8 months or longer.

Control   Avoid direct contact with lesions; use of condoms. Cesarean section delivery for infected mothers.

Usual treatment   Local treatment with 25% podophyllin, 5-fluorouracil (5-FU), or other cytotoxic agents, but not in pregnant women. Cryosurgery with liquid nitrogen. Surgical removal, laser therapy, or electrocautery. Treatment repeated with recurrence.

Bacterial Urogenital Infections

Chlamydial Infections, Genital Chlamydiasis

Characteristics   The most frequent cause of nonspecific (NSU) and nongonococcal urethritis (NGU), cervicitis, vaginitis, salpingitis, epididymitis, and newborn conjunctivitis and pneumonia. Many asymptomatic carriers.

Pathogen   *Chlamydia trachomatis* serotypes D–K; tiny obligately intracellular, gram-negative bacteria in two forms, elementary body and reticulate body. Concomitant infectious agents may include *Ureaplasma ureolyticum*, *Mycoplasma hominis*, and other sexually transmitted pathogens in 50% of cases. Identified by cell culture, staining, and serologic techniques.

Reservoir   Humans.

Transmission   Direct sexual contact or mother-to-neonate during birth.

Incubation period   2–3 weeks, may be latent.

Control   Personal cleanliness, sex education, use of condom. Prophylactic treatment of contacts and pregnant women with infection.

Usual treatment   Tetracycline or doxycycline. Erythromycin for pregnant women and resistant cases.

Gonorrhea

Characteristics   A very common acute infectious disease of urethra, anus, vagina, cervix, fallopian tubes (salpingitis), and other reproductive organs. Causes pelvic inflammatory disease (PID), a yellow purulent urethral discharge (most commonly seen in men). Frequently asymptomatic. Also, may result in rectal gonorrhea, proctitis, conjunctivitis (see Fig. 10–6), and disseminated infections.

Pathogen   *Neisseria gonorrhoeae*, gram-negative diplococcus. Some strains have plasmids for β-lactamases (penicillinase-producing *Neisseria gonorrhoeae*, or PPNG, strains). Identified microscopically, culturally, and serologically.

Reservoir   Humans.

Transmission   Direct mucous-to-mucous membrane or sexual contact; adult-to-child (may indicate sexual abuse); mother-to-neonate during birth.

Incubation period   2–7 days, or longer. Frequently asymptomatic.

Epidemiology   In United States, 672,738 new cases reported to CDC in 1990.

Control   Refrain from intercourse with infected partners. Use of condoms. Culture tests on pregnant women.

Usual treatment   Ceftriaxone, doxycycline, ciprofloxacin. Erythromycin for pregnant women.

Syphilis, Venereal Syphilis

Characteristics   An acute and chronic treponemal disease in three stages: a primary chancre lesion (Fig. 10–20A), secondary skin rash with fever and mucous membrane lesions (Fig. 10–20B), long latent period, and tertiary stage with

Figure 10–20. Syphilis. (*A*) Primary, showing a chancre of the lip with unilateral adenopathy (*arrow*). (*B*) Secondary, with mucous patches on the tongue. (Dobson RL, Abele DC: The Practice of Dermatology. Philadelphia, JB Lippincott, 1985)

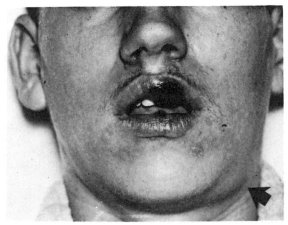

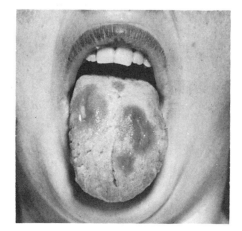

A   B

damage to central nervous system, cardiovascular system, visceral organs, bones, sense organs, and other sites.

Pathogen *Treponema pallidum*, a gram-variable spirochete. Identified by darkfield microscopy and serologic tests.

Reservoir Humans.

Transmission Direct contact with lesions, body secretions, blood, semen, saliva, vaginal discharges; usually during sexual contact; blood transfusions; mother-to-fetus by placental transfer.

Incubation period 10 days to several weeks.

Epidemiology In United States 48,128 new cases of venereal syphilis and 685 cases of congenital syphilis were reported in 1990 (see Figure 7–7b).

Control VDRL or RPR tests with confirming serology for high-risk persons and pregnant women. Avoid sexual contact with infected persons; use of condoms.

Usual treatment Long-acting penicillin G (benzathine penicillin), or procaine penicillin. Tetracycline or doxycycline for penicillin-sensitive persons.

Protozoan Urogenital Infections

Trichomoniasis

Characteristics A protozoan disease causing vaginitis in women: may cause a profuse, thin, malodorous, yellowish discharge; often asymptomatic. In men, an infection of urethra, prostate, or seminal vesicles; usually asymptomatic.

Pathogen *Trichomonas vaginalis*, a flagellate protozoan. Identified microscopically or immunologically; rarely by culture.

Reservoir Humans.

Transmission Direct mucous contact, sexual intercourse.

Incubation period 4–20 days.

Control Avoid sexual relations with infected persons. Use of condoms. Concurrent treatment of sexual partners.

Usual treatment Metronidazole (Flagyl).

Other Sexually Transmitted Diseases

Many other pathogens may be transmitted by sexual intercourse. Three, seen more often in parts of the world other than in the United States, are chancroid, granuloma inguinale, and lymphogranuloma venereum (LGV). Chancroid is caused by the bacterium *Haemophilus ducreyi* and can be treated with erythromycin or co-trimoxazole SMZ. Granuloma inguinale is a chronic infection caused by a bacterium named *Calymmatobacterium granulomatis (Donovania granulomatis)* and is treatable with tetracycline or TMP–SMZ. LGV is a chlamydial infection that invades the lymph nodes, rectum, and reproductive tract; caused by *Chlamydia trachomatis* types L-1, L-2, and L-3 (see Fig. 2–14); treated with tetracycline, erythromycin, or sulfonamides. It should be noted that many sexually transmitted diseases occur and are transmitted simultaneously.

Diseases of the Circulatory System

The circulatory systems, consisting of the cardiovascular system and lymphatic system (Fig. 10–21), carry blood or lymph throughout the body. Included in these fluids are many cells: erythrocytes, leukocytes, platelets (thrombocytes), and lymphocytes. Most leukocytes function to protect the body from pathogens by phagocytosis and by antibody production.

Normally, the blood is sterile; it contains no resident normal microflora. When microbes invade the bloodstream septicemia results if they are not quickly destroyed. In this septic condition the patient has chills and fever; also, bacteria and their toxic products are found in the bloodstream. The lymph occasionally picks up microorganisms from the intestine, lungs, and other areas, but these transient organisms are usually quicker engulfed by phagocytic cells in the liver and lymph nodes. Frequently, transient bacteremia (temporary bacteria in the blood) results from dental extractions, wounds, bites, and damage to the intestinal, respiratory, or reproductive tract mucosa. However, when pathogenic organisms are capable of resisting or overwhelming the phagocytes and other body defenses — or when the individual is immunosuppressed or is otherwise more susceptible than normal — a systemic disease may occur.

Viruses often invade the circulatory systems and damage certain target cells, an example of which is HIV (AIDS virus), that destroys T_H lymphocytes, causing the immune system to malfunction. Some cardiovascular diseases are the result of toxemia, the production of damaging exotoxins secreted by bacteria and carried to target areas by the bloodstream. Toxic shock syndrome, rheumatic fever, tetanus, and botulism are examples of such diseases. Fungal and protozoan cardiovascular diseases may cause damage by actually clogging the capillaries in various regions of the body.

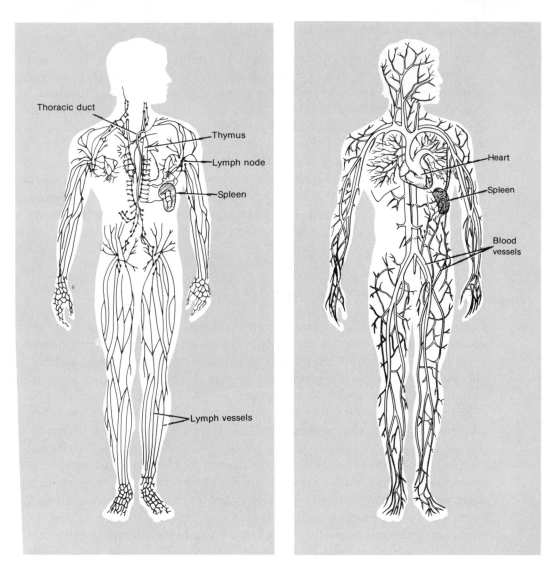

Figure 10–21. (*A*) The cardiovascular system. (*B*) The lymphatic system. (Tortora GJ, Anagnostakos NP: Anatomy and Physiology, 4th ed. Philadelphia, Harper & Row, 1985)

Viral Lymphatic and Cardiovascular Infections

AIDS, Acquired Immunodeficiency Syndrome

Characteristics   A viral infection that destroys T_H lymphocytes (Fig. 10–22) of the immune system causing immunosuppression, allowing secondary infections. Viruses (CMV, herpes), protozoa (*Pneumocystis* and *Toxoplasma*), bacteria (mycobacteria), and fungi (*Candida*) may invade, usually resulting in death.

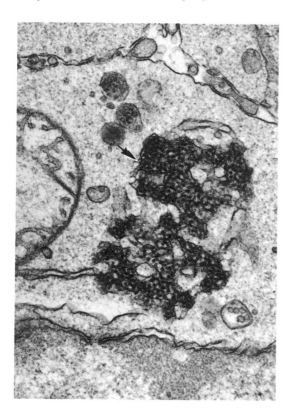

Figure 10–22. A large inclusion (*arrow*) within the cytoplasm of a peripheral blood mononuclear cell from a patient with AIDS (original magnification × 40,000). (DeVita VT, Jr, Hellman S, Rosenberg SA: AIDS. Philadelphia, JB Lippincott, 1985)

Frequent complications include Kaposi's sarcoma. Symptoms include fever, fatigue, diarrhea, weight loss, enlarged lymph nodes, brain and spinal cord damage; may be asymptomatic as AIDS-related complex (ARC) for several years.

Pathogen   Human immunodeficiency virus (HIV) (Fig. 10–23).

Reservoir   Humans.

Transmission   Direct sexual contact, homosexual or heterosexual; contaminated intravenous needles and syringes; blood transfusion with contaminated blood, and blood products. Transplacental and mother-to-child transfer.

Incubation period   6 months to 5 years, or longer.

Epidemiology   Epidemic worldwide. In United States, 41,129 new cases reported in 1990 (see Fig. 7–7A).

Control   Avoid sexual contact with high-risk persons: those having multiple sex partners, homosexual males, bisexuals, and those sharing drug paraphernalia (soak needles in 10% Clorox). Use of condoms. For hospitalized patients: take precautionary measures for handling blood and body fluids.

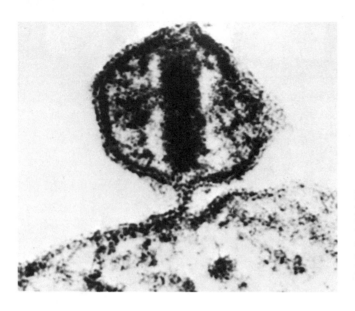

Figure 10–23. Extracellular HIV retrovirus particle from a lymphocyte of a patient with ARC. Note the dense cylindrical core. (DeVita VT, Jr, Hellman S, Rosenberg SA: AIDS. Philadelphia, JB Lippincott, 1985)

Usual treatment   Azidothymidine (AZT), other derived nucleotides such as dideoxycytidine; treatment of secondary infections.

Colorado Tick Fever

Characteristics   An acute viral infection with fever, headache, fatigue, aching, and occasionally encephalitis or myocarditis, following tick bite. In western North America. Usually self-limiting.

Pathogen   An arbovirus.

Reservoir   Tick-infested small mammals.

Transmission   Bite of virus-infected tick to humans, from infected small mammals, ground squirrels, porcupines, or chipmunks.

Incubation period   4–5 days.

Control   Control of ticks and infected rodent hosts. Blood and body fluid precautions for hospitalized patients.

Usual treatment   None, but rest and nutritious diet.

Infectious Mononucleosis

Characteristics   An acute viral disease of B lymphocytes, spleen, and liver with high fever, sore throat, fatigue, weakness, and generalized lymphadenopathy;

showing transformed B lymphocytes. Usually self-limiting, may be asymptomatic and latent.

Pathogen   Epstein-Barr virus (EBV), a human herpes virus type 4 that may be oncogenic. Identified by heterophile antibody and immunofluorescent antibody (IFA) tests.

Reservoir   Humans.

Transmission   Person-to-person, by direct contact and by exchange of saliva and other body fluids.

Incubation period   4–6 weeks.

Control   Limit kissing contacts. Disinfect articles contaminated with nose and throat discharges.

Usual treatment   None, but rest and nutritious diet.

Mumps, Infectious Parotitis

Characteristics   An acute viral infection of salivary glands, usually the parotid gland. Deafness, meningoencephalitis, mastitis, nephritis, thyroiditis, and pericarditis complications may occur; in adults, orchitis (inflammation of testes) or oophoritis (ovary infection).

Pathogen   Mumps virus, a paramyxovirus. Identified by serologic techniques.

Reservoir   Humans.

Transmission   Direct contact and fomites via respiratory secretions, aerosol droplets, saliva.

Incubation period   2–3 weeks, usually 18 days.

Epidemiology   In 1990, in United States, 5,075 cases were reported to CDC.

Control   Live-attenuated vaccine MMR, (measles, mumps, rubella), for children and nonimmune adults. For hospitalized patients, respiratory isolation.

Treatment   No specific chemotherapy.

Rickettsial Cardiovascular Infections

Rocky Mountain Spotted Fever, Tickborne Typhus Fever

Characteristics   The most common rickettsial spotted fever. An infection of the vascular endothelial cells, with high fever, muscle pain, headache, chills, and maculopapular rash on extremities after third day; if untreated, may result in death.

Pathogen   *Rickettsia rickettsii*, a gram-negative bacteria; obligate intracellular parasite. Identified by immunofluorescent (IF) antibody (IFA) and nonspecific Weil-Felix reaction.

Reservoir   Infected ticks on dogs, rodents, and other animals.

Transmission   Bite of infected tick, from animals to humans; tick parts or feces into break in skin.

Incubation period   2–14 days after tick bite.

Epidemiology   In United States, 654 cases reported in 1990.

Control   Avoid tick-infested areas. Search for ticks on self and dogs after being in tick-infested areas. Avoid crushing ticks during removal.

Usual treatment   Tetracycline or chloramphenicol.

Endemic Murine Typhus Fever, Fleaborne Typhus

Characteristics   An acute febrile disease (similar to, but milder than, epidemic typhus) with fever, headache, and rash on body trunk.

Pathogen   *Rickettsia typhi.*

Reservoir   Infected rats with infective rat fleas.

Transmission   Rats to fleas that defecate rickettsia into bite site and skin wounds of humans.
Rat→flea→human.

Incubation period   1–2 weeks.

Control   Apply insecticide to rat-infested areas, then use rodent control measures. Avoid contact with rats.

Usual treatment   Tetracycline, doxycycline, or chloramphenicol.

Epidemic Typhus Fever, Louseborne Typhus

Characteristics   An acute rickettsial disease with very high prolonged fever, severe headache, rash appearing on trunk by sixth day. Toxemia may involve kidneys, heart, spleen, and nerves.

Pathogen   *Rickettsia prowazekii*, a gram-negative bacteria, identified by IFA tests.

Reservoir   Humans.

Transmission   Humans to body lice (Fig. 10–24) to humans.

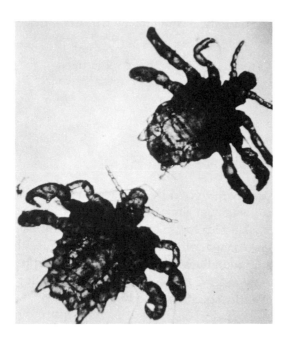

Figure 10-24. Pubic louse or *Phthirus pubis* as seen with × 7.5 lens of microscope. Infected lice may transmit typhus. (Sauer GC: Manual of Skin Diseases, 6th ed. Philadelphia, JB Lippincott, 1991)

Incubation period   1–2 weeks.

Control   Use of insecticide to kill body lice. Improve personal cleanliness practices. Immunization of susceptible people.

Usual treatment   Chloramphenicol or tetracycline.

Bacterial Cardiovascular Infections

Subacute Bacterial Endocarditis (SBE)

Characteristics   A bacterial infection of heart valves damaged by rheumatic fever, syphilis, atherosclerosis, congenital heart deformities. Bacterial masses with fibrin break away to form clots that clog small blood vessels in brain, heart, kidney, spleen, liver, or other organs; resulting in death.

Pathogens   Most often species of non-group A streptococci, gram-positive cocci of low virulence. Identified by serologic techniques.

Reservoir   Humans.

Transmission   (1) Parenteral; (2) mechanical invasion of blood vessels; (3) surgery, catheterization, minor trauma, dental work.

Incubation period   Variable.

Control   Personal hygiene; sterile and aseptic techniques by dentists, physicians, and nurses.

Treatment   Bactericidal antibiotics specific for the pathogen identified.

Lyme Disease

Characteristics   A tick-borne disease characterized by 3 stages: 1) Early local stage, distinctive large skin lesions (usually at site of tick bite) 2) Early disseminated systemic stage, skin blotches, malaise, fatigue, arthritis, carditis, meningitis, encephalitis. 3) prolonged arthritis, debilitating fatigue, chronic encephalomyelitis, neuropathy (numbness, loss of memory), facial palsy. Isolates from skin lesions grow at 33 C on Barbour, Stoenner, Kelley (BSK) medium and may be identified by specific antibody tests.

Pathogen   A spirochete, *Borrelia burgdorferi.*

Reservoir   Carried by ticks that feed on mice, dogs, horses, cattle, deer, and humans. The deer tick, *Ixodes dammini,* serves as the vector in Northeast and upper Midwest United States; *Ixodes pacificus* is the vector in Western U.S., *I. ricinis* in Europe, and *I. persulatus* in Asia.

Transmission   Large animals or rodents to ticks which bite humans and transmit the spirochetes during several hours of feeding. Congenital transmission is rare. No person to person transmission has been observed.

Incubation period   From 3 to 33 days after tick bite. The first early local stage may be almost asymptomatic.

Epidemiology   In 1990, 7997 cases were reported. The disease first became nationally reportable January, 1991.

Control   Avoid tick infested areas and animals. Wear light colored clothing covering legs and arms, closed tightly at feet and hands. Use tick repellant [diethyltoluamide (DEET) or permethrin] on pantlegs and sleeves. Check total body surface for ticks every 4 hours and remove attached ticks including mouth parts with tweezers. A vaccine is available for dogs but is not yet available for humans.

Usual treatment   For adults, treat with tetracycline, doxycycline, or cephalosporin for 10–30 days. For children <8 yrs. treat with amoxicillin for 10–30 days. Erythromycin or ceftriaxone may be used for those allergic to penicillin or tetracycline.

Plague, Bubonic Plague (Black Death), Septicemic Plague, Pneumonic Plague

Characteristics An acute or severe infection involving the lymph nodes (enlarging to buboes) or lungs or disseminated throughout the body; resulting in death if untreated. Pneumonic plague is very contagious and usually fatal.

Pathogen *Yersinia pestis*, a gram-negative, pleomorphic, nonmotile bacillus. Identified by bipolar staining of organism; culture of bubo aspirate or sputum or CSF; by IFA or ELISA tests.

Reservoir Wild rodents and fleas on rodents.

Transmission Wild rodents to fleas to humans; from rodents directly to humans (bubonic plague); or respiratory pathway from person to person, (pneumonic plague).

Incubation period 2–6 days.

Epidemiology In United States, only 2 human cases reported in 1990.

Control Avoid contact with rodents and fleas from rodents. Strict isolation of pneumonic patients.

Usual treatment Steptomycin, tetracycline, or chloramphenicol.

Tularemia, Rabbit Fever

Characteristics An acute infection with primary local ulcer, lymph node, swelling. May be systemic, pneumonic, or gastrointestinal disease.

Pathogen *Francisella tularensis*, a small, gram-negative pleomorphic bacillus. Identified by IFA and heterophil antibody tests.

Reservoir Wild animals, such as rabbits, muskrats, beaver; some domestic animals; hard ticks.

Transmission By handling or ingestion of contaminated meat; by drinking contaminated water; or by bites of infected animals, flies, and ticks.

Incubation period 2–10 days.

Epidemiology In United States, only 137 human cases reported in 1990.

Control Use impervious gloves when handling and dressing rabbits, cook wild meat well, avoid bites of insects and ticks in infected areas. Vaccinate high-risk persons.

Usual treatment Streptomycin, gentamicin, or tobramycin.

Protozoan Cardiovascular Infections

Malaria

Characteristics   A systemic protozoan infection with fever, chills, sweats, headache, asymptomatic periods, rarely progressing to shock, renal and liver failure, and coma.

Pathogens   The sporozoans: *Plasmodium vivax, P. malariae, P. falciparum*, and *P. ovale*, that have a complex life cycle through the mosquito to the liver and erythrocytes of humans. Identified in blood smears.

Reservoir   Humans.

Transmission   Bite of infective female *Anopheles* mosquito; also by transfusion or contaminated syringes.

Incubation period   12–30 days or longer.

Epidemiology   In United States, 1,185 cases were reported in 1990.

Control   Insecticides and draining of breeding areas to destroy anopheline mosquitoes. Use of chemosuppressive drugs: chloroquine, primaquine, Fansidar or Maloprim (pyrimethamine and dapsone). Use of diethyltoluamide insect repellent on skin.

Usual treatment   Chloroquine, Fansidar, mefloquine or primaquine (for chloroquine-resistant cases), quinine.

Toxoplasmosis

Characteristics   A systemic protozoan disease with fever, lymphadenopathy, lymphocytosis, rarely with central nervous system symptoms, pneumonia, myocarditis, rash, and death. Primary infection may be asymptomatic. Often complicates AIDS.

Pathogen   *Toxoplasma gondii*, an obligate intracellular sporozoan.

Reservoir   Rodents, cattle, sheep, pigs, goats, chickens, birds. Cats shed oocysts in fecal material.

Transmission   Humans eat infected meats, usually pork or mutton, and ingest oocysts in contaminated food and water, or inhale dust contaminated with oocysts from cat feces. Children may inhale or ingest oocysts from sandboxes containing cat feces. Transplacental infection occurs during primary infection in mother; may cause severe damage to fetus.

Incubation period   5–23 days.

Epidemiology   Estimated over 2 million people per year infected.

Control   Cook meats thoroughly. Dispose of kitty litter feces daily into toilet or bury. Pregnant women should avoid cat litter pans and cat feces-contaminated soil. Vaccinate pet cats.

Usual treatment   Pyrimethamine and sulfadiazine with folinic acid.

Trypanosomiasis, Chagas' Disease, American Trypanosomiasis

Characteristics   A systemic protozoan disease with chancre at site of tsetse fly or reduviid bug bite; then intense headache, lymphadenopathy, insomnia, anemia, and rash. Late stages involve central nervous system; (CNS); "sleeping sickness," or heart failure, and frequently death.

Pathogen   *Trypanosoma gambiense, T. rhodesiense* (African) and *T. cruzi* (American) flagellate protozoa.

Reservoir   Humans and wild animals.

Transmission   To humans by bite of tsetse fly or reduviid bugs that have ingested blood of infected humans or animals.

Incubation period   3–21 days or longer.

Control   Control of tsetse fly and reduviid bugs. Treatment of infected humans.

Usual treatment   Suramin, pentamidine, or melarsoprol; none for Chagas' disease.

Diseases of the Nervous System

The central nervous system (CNS) is well protected; it is encased in bone, covered with the membranous three-layered meninges, bathed and cushioned in cerebro-spinal fluid (CSF), and nourished by capillaries. These capillaries make up the blood-brain barrier, supplying nutrients but not allowing larger particles, such as microorganisms and most antibiotics, to pass from the blood into the brain.

There are no indigenous normal microflora of the nervous system. The microbes must gain access to the CNS through trauma (fracture or medical procedure), via the blood and lymph to the CSF, or along the peripheral nerves (Fig. 10–25).

An infection of the meninges is called meningitis, and encephalitis is an infection of the brain itself. Several viruses may produce viral or aseptic meningitis and encephalitis. The most common are enteroviruses, coxsackieviruses, echoviruses, and mumps viruses; others include arboviruses, polioviruses, adenoviruses, measles, herpes, and varicella viruses. The arboviruses (arthropodborne viruses) are introduced by mosquito vectors and cause several forms of viral encephalitis.

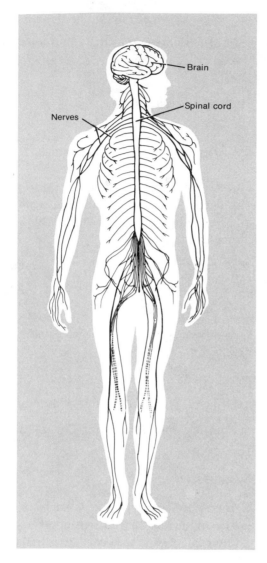

Figure 10–25. The nervous
system. (Tortora GJ,
Anagnostakos NP: Anatomy and
Physiology, 4th ed. Philadelphia,
JB Lippincott, 1984)

The bacteria that cause almost all bacterial meningitis are *Haemophilus influenzae*, *Neisseria meningitidis*, and *Streptococcus pneumoniae* (see Fig. 7–4). Less commonly, other *Streptococcus* species, *Staphylococcus aureus*, *Listeria monocytogenes*, *Escherichia coli*, *Pseudomonas aeruginosa*, *Salmonella*, *Klebsiella*, and other enterobacteria are found. Some free-living amebae that may cause meningoencephalitis are of the genera *Naegleria* and *Acanthamoeba*. Other protozoa that may invade the meninges are the *Toxoplasma* and *Trypanosoma*. Occasionally fungal pathogens, especially *Cryptococcus neoformans*, are seen in meningitis patients.

Early symptoms of meningitis are similar to those of colds. Later, fever, severe headache, pain, and stiffness of neck and back develop. Then neurological symptoms of dizziness, convulsions, minor paralysis, coma, and death within a few hours may occur.

Diagnosis is usually by symptoms, examination, and culture of the cerebrospinal fluid obtained by a lumbar puncture (spinal tap). The treatment of meningitis is supportive, and chemotherapeutic agents may be administered, depending on the causal agent involved.

Several central nervous system diseases are caused by toxins. Some examples of bacterial neurotoxins are botulin, the exotoxin of botulism; neurotoxins of *Staphylococcus aureus* in toxic shock syndrome, and the tetanospasmin of tetanus. Fungal toxins include ergot from grain molds and mushroom poisoning. *Gonyaulax* is an alga found in algal blooms; it produces neurotoxins, which may concentrate in bivalve shell fish and cause paralytic symptoms after ingestion of the contaminated shall fish.

Viral Nervous System Infections

Poliomyelitis, Infantile Paralysis

Characteristics An acute viral infection of the medulla, spinal cord, and nerves, with fever, headache, nausea, vomiting, sore throat, muscle pain and spasms, neck and back stiffness, with or without paralysis. Usually asymptomatic, or mild disease similar to influenza. Most often infects young children, occasionally further damage occurs many years later.

Pathogen Poliovirus types 1, 2, and 3; small RNA enteroviruses (Fig. 10–26). Type 1 (wild type) most often causes paralysis. Types 2 and 3 are frequently vaccine-associated. Identified by tissue culture, cytopathic effects, and neutralizing antibody tests.

Reservoir Human gastrointestinal tract.

Transmission By direct contact or fecal-oral route in areas with poor sanitation. Virus is inhaled or ingested, carried by lymph to lymph nodes, to blood, to CNS, damaging motor nerve impulses to muscles. During infection and after vaccination with attenuated live vaccine, viruses are transmitted by pharyngeal secretions and fecal material.

Incubation period 3–35 days, usually 7–14 days.

Epidemiology In United States, only 6 paralytic polio cases were reported in 1990.

Control Immunize all infants and children with a series of Salk inactivated polio vaccine (IPV) or Sabin oral attenuated live poliovirus vaccine (OPV). In hospitalized patients, isolate with enteric precautions. Adequate sewage and water treatment precautions. Adequate sewage and water treatment.

Usual treatment None. Provide therapy and assistance for paralytic patient.

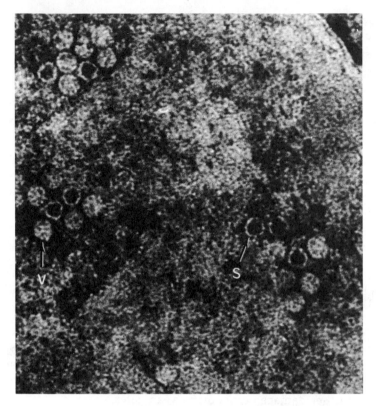

Figure 10–26. Development of poliovirus particles in pieces of cytoplasmic matrix of artificially disrupted cells. Particles in various stages of assembly from empty shells (*s*) to complete virions (*v*) can be seen (original magnification × 200,000). (Horne RW, Nagington J: J Mol Biol 1:333, 1959. Copyright by Academic Press, Inc., Ltd.)

Rabies

Characteristics   A fatal acute viral encephalomyelitis (CNS infection) of mammals, with depression, headache, fever, malaise, paralysis, hydrophobia (fear of water), salivation, spasms of throat muscles, convulsions, and death caused by respiratory failure.

Pathogen   Rabies virus (Fig. 10–27), a rhabdovirus; a large, complex, enveloped RNA virus. Identified by virus isolation and IFA antibody tests to confirm direct observation of Negri inclusion bodies in animal brain tissue.

Reservoir   Many wild and domestic mammals: dogs, foxes, coyotes, cats, skunks, raccoons, and bats.

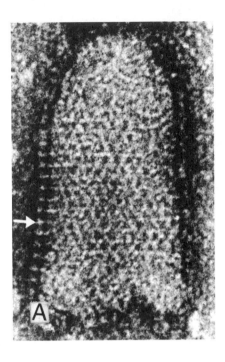

Figure 10–27. Intact rabies virus particle embedded in phosphotungstate and viewed in negative contrast. On the left are well-resolved surface projections 6–7 nm long (*arrow*) (original magnification × 400,000). (Hummeler K, et al: J Virol 1:152, 1967)

Transmission   Rabid animal bites introducing virus-laden saliva; airborne transmission from bats in caves; person-to-person by saliva.

Incubation period   2–8 weeks or longer.

Epidemiology   In United States, only one human case, but 4,219 animal cases reported in 1990.

Control   Vaccinate all pets (dogs, cats, raccoons, skunks, monkeys). Avoid all sick, aggressive, or friendly, wild animals. Prophylactic immunization of high-risk persons with human diploid cell rabies vaccine (HDCV). Isolation of hospitalized patients.

Usual treatment   Prompt treatment of bite wounds with soap and water and local infusion of rabies immune globulin (RIG) antiserum. Vaccinate patient with HDCV.

Bacterial Nervous System Infections

Tetanus

Characteristics   An acute infectious neuromuscular disease induced by the exotoxin, tetanospasmin, with convulsions and intermittent spasms of the voluntary

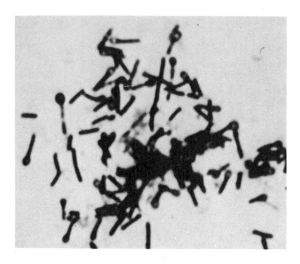

Figure 10–28. Cells of *Clostridium tetani* after 24 hours on a cooked meat—glucose medium. Note spherical terminal endospores (original magnification × 4,500). (Volk WA, et al: Essentials of Medical Microbiology, 4th ed. Philadelphia, JB Lippincott, 1991)

muscles, especially masseter and neck; exhaustion, respiratory failure, and death may result.

Pathogen   *Clostridium tetani* (Fig. 10–28), a motile, gram-positive, anaerobic, spore-forming bacillus that produces a potent neurotoxin, tetanospasmin.

Reservoir   Soil contaminated with feces; intestines of humans and animals.

Transmission   Spores of *C. tetani* are introduced into a puncture wound, burn, or needle prick by contamination with soil, dust, or feces. Spores anaerobically germinate within the wound into vegetative *C. tetani* producing the exotoxin.

Incubation period   3–21 days or longer.

Epidemiology   In United States 60 cases reported in 1990.

Control   Active immunization of all children with DPT, a combined diphtheria-tetanus-pertussis vaccine, containing tetanus toxoid. Boosters of DT should be given at 10-year intervals and after a wound or accident with no booster for 5 years. Unimmunized persons may be given human tetanus immune globulin (TIG) following a puncture wound.

Usual treatment   Dirty wounds should be cleaned and left open, when feasible, to inhibit the anaerobic growth. Administer penicillin to destroy wound organisms, antitoxin (TIG) to neutralize the exotoxin, and vaccinate with DT.

Summary

The major infectious diseases of skin, wounds, eyes, ears, mouth, respiratory system, gastrointestinal tract, urogenital areas, cardiovascular and nervous systems are presented, mostly in outline format. In this way you can discern the characteristics of the disease, the pathogens that may cause the disease, mechanisms of pathogenicity, reservoirs, modes of transmission, incubation period, means of control, and recommended treatment for each disease presented. A brief survey of the anatomy is shown by drawings and the indigenous microflora of each area is discussed because the source of the etiologic agent may be from opportunistic normal microflora in a compromised host whose defenses are impaired.

Many of these infections may move from one area of the body to another, involving several body systems. They are discussed relative to either the site of entry or where they usually cause the most damage.

Study Outline

Major infectious diseases of the body systems

I. Diseases of the skin
   A. Viral infections
   B. Bacterial infections
   C. Fungal infections
   D. Burn and wound infections
II. Diseases of the eye
   A. Viral infections
   B. Bacterial infections
III. Diseases of the mouth
   A. Bacterial infections
IV. Diseases of the ear
   A. Bacterial infections
V. Diseases of the respiratory system
   A. Nonspecific infections
   B. Viral infections
   C. Bacterial infections
   D. Protozoan infections
VI. Diseases of the gastrointestinal tract
   A. Viral infections
   B. Bacterial infections
   C. Foodborne intoxications and food poisoning
   D. Protozoan diseases
VII. Diseases of the urogenital tracts
   A. Sexually transmitted diseases
   B. Urinary tract infections
   C. Viral infections
   D. Bacterial infections
   E. Protozoan infections
   F. Other STDs
VIII. Diseases of the circulatory system
   A. Viral infections
   B. Rickettsial infections
   C. Bacterial infections
   D. Protozoan infections
IX. Diseases of the nervous system
   A. Viral infections
   B. Bacterial infections

Problems and Questions

1. Name six factors that control the number of microbes on the skin. How may opportunists invade through the skin?
2. Which bacteria cause most burn, wound, and bite infections? What types of toxins do they produce?
3. How do oral bacteria interact to cause dental caries? How can you prevent dental caries?
4. By what pathways may microbes invade to cause ear infections? Which bacteria are usually found in ear infections?
5. Why is pneumonia called a nonspecific disease? Name several pathogens that might cause pneumonia.
6. Differentiate between foodborne infections and foodborne intoxications. Name some examples of each.
7. Which protozoa cause gastrointestinal infections? How do they get there?
8. How are urinary tract infections transmitted? Why might *E. coli* be found more often in female cystitis than in male cystitis?
9. How may sexually transmitted infections be prevented? List the genital infections that may cause congenital and neonatal infections. How could transmission to the fetus and newborn be prevented?
10. Differentiate between typhus fever and typhoid fever. How are they transmitted and controlled?
11. By what means might children be exposed to plague, tularemia, toxoplasmosis, and rabies? After exposure, how should the children be treated to prevent or reduce the symptoms of these diseases?
12. List several areas, systems, or organs where there are no indigenous microflora. Why might this be so?
13. What are the usual symptoms of disease in the nervous system? Define meningitis and encephalitis.
14. List several diseases caused by neurotoxins. List several nonspecific diseases discussed in this chapter.

Self Test

After you have read Chapter 10, examined the objectives, studied the new words, reviewed the study outline, and answered the questions at the end of the chapter, complete the following self test.

Matching Exercises

Match each of the diseases under the Column I heads with the appropriate item in Column II. An answer from Column II may be used once or more than once.

Diseases — Types of Etiologic Agents

Column I

_____ 1. Gonorrhea
_____ 2. Trachoma
_____ 3. Tuberculosis
_____ 4. Histoplasmosis
_____ 5. Amebiasis
_____ 6. Candidiasis
_____ 7. Syphilis
_____ 8. AIDS
_____ 9. Common cold
_____10. Streptococcal sore throat
_____11. Legionellosis
_____12. Rocky Mountain spotted fever
_____13. Warts
_____14. Athlete's foot
_____15. Botulism
_____16. Whooping cough
_____17. Measles
_____18. Mumps
_____19. Trichomoniasis
_____20. Hepatitis

Column II

a. Virus
b. Bacteria
c. Fungi
d. Protozoa

Diseases — Synonyms

Column I

____1. Measles
____2. German measles
____3. Chickenpox

Column II

a. Variola
b. Rubeola
c. Varicella
d. Rubella

Diseases — Etiologic Agents

Column I

_____ 1. Primary atypical pneumonia
_____ 2. Pneumococcal pneumonia
_____ 3. Legionellosis
_____ 4. Histoplasmosis
_____ 5. Whooping cough
_____ 6. Diphtheria
_____ 7. Strep throat
_____ 8. Acute rhinitis
_____ 9. Otitis media
_____10. Thrush
_____11. Boils, carbuncles
_____12. Colds

Column II

a. *Bordetella pertussis*
b. *Streptococcus pneumoniae*
c. Influenza virus
d. *Mycoplasma pneumoniae*
e. *Legionella pneumophila*
f. *Histoplasma capsulatum*
g. *Coccidioides immitis*
h. *Candida albicans*
i. *Staphylococcus aureus*
j. Rhinovirus
k. *Corynebacterium diphtheriae*
l. *Streptococcus pyogenes*
m. *Haemophilus influenzae*
n. *Staphylococcus epidermidis*
o. *Streptococcus lactis*
p. Mumps virus

True and False (T or F)

_____   1. Chickenpox can be diagnosed by finding Guarnieri bodies as cytoplasmic inclusions in infected cells.

_____   2. Reye's syndrome is a severe encephalomyelitis and severe liver involvement in adults following a viral infection treated with aspirin.

_____   3. Measles is a mild childhood disease easily controlled by vaccination.

_____   4. Koplik spots are small bluish-yellow spots that occur in the mouth on the buccal mucosa of rubella patients.

_____   5. Infection of a fetus with rubella during the first trimester can cause severe birth defects.

_____   6. Patients most susceptible to *P. aeruginosa* infections are hospitalized burn patients.

_____   7. Trachoma is probably one of the most important conditions of the eyes worldwide, especially where poor hygienic practices exist.

_____   8. Lymphogranuloma venereum is a syndrome with initial symptoms of conjunctivitis.

_____   9. The causative agent of the most common form of pneumonia is *Streptococcus pneumoniae*.

_____ 10. The majority of respiratory tract infections are not bacterial but viral.

_____ 11. A vaccine against colds is possible because of the immunological similarity of the group of viruses that cause colds.

_____ 12. *Corynebacterium diphtheriae* excretes a powerful endotoxin that results in the formation of a pseudomembrane that can block respiratory passages.

_____ 13. Control of diphtheria is based entirely on the mass immunization of children.

_____ 14. Complications following some streptococcal infections include rheumatic fever and acute glomerulonephritis.

_____ 15. A positive tuberculin skin test is interpreted as indicating an active infection.

_____ 16. Typhoid fever is the most serious type of salmonellosis.

_____ 17. Urinary tract infections are almost always caused by strict pathogens.

_____ 18. Catheterization is not performed routinely for the collection of urine samples for microbiological examinations.

_____ 19. *Trichomonas vaginalis* appears to be spread as a venereal disease pathogen.

_____ 20. AIDS is caused by a virus that specifically destroys certain lymphocytes.

_____ 21. Mumps virus infects the sublingual salivary glands.

_____ 22. Rocky Mountain spotted fever (RMSF) is caused by a rickettsial organism, carried by body lice.

_____ 23. Pneumonic plague is almost always fatal and is very contagious.

_____ 24. An infection or inflammation of the membranes enclosing the brain and spinal cord is called meningitis.

_____ 25. Antibiotics are useful in the treatment of rabies.

Multiple Choice

1. Reye's syndrome is sometimes associated with
   a. influenza complications
   b. chickenpox
   c. using aspirin to treat fever during influenza
   d. all of the above

2. The eye is generally protected from damage by
   a. sebum lubricating the eyeball
   b. tears washing the eye
   c. mucous secretions moisten the eye
   d. all of the above

3. *Chlamydia trachomatis* causes
   a. skin infections
   b. secondary infections of burns
   c. cold sores
   d. eye disease

4. *Bacteroides* is of concern in dental disease because it
   a. causes gum infections and loosens teeth
   b. is anaerobic
   c. survives in the gingival sulcus
   d. produces endotoxins
   e. all of the above

5. Saliva functions in oral health by
   a. rinsing teeth, buffering acids
   b. providing IgA to destroy oral flora

c. providing proper anaerobic
    conditions
d. all of the above

6. Otitis media is frequently caused by
    a. bacteria of normal throat
        microflora
    b. *Streptococcus pneumoniae*
    c. *Haemophilus influenzae*
    d. all of the above

7. The most common pathogens of
    the upper respiratory tract are
    a. some bacterial species
    b. a variety of virus groups
    c. protozoa
    d. opportunistic fungi
    e. the indigenous microflora

8. Serum hepatitis is caused by
    a. HAV
    b. HBV
    c. NANB
    d. rotavirus
    e. echovirus

9. Infections of the bladder are
    referred to as
    a. pyelonephritis
    b. glomerulonephritis
    c. cystitis
    d. bladder wall infection (BWI)

10. MMR refers to
     a. mortality and morbidity report
     b. a viral disease
     c. mumps-measles-rhinovirus
     d. mumps-measles-rubella

11. Entertoxin of *Staphylococcus aureus*
     affects the

a. nervous system reflexes
b. produces gastrointestinal tract
    diarrhea
c. induces bouts of repeated
    vomiting
d. all of the above

12. Rabies immune globulin is used in
     which circumstance?
     a. To immunize pets
     b. To immunize humans
     c. Treatment for rabies exposure
     d. All of the above

13. Dermatomycosis refers to
     a. a viral eye disease
     b. a bacterial skin infection
     c. a fungal skin infection
     d. a protozoan

14. Rhinitis refers to
     a. infections of the parotid
         salivary glands
     b. inflamed mucous membranes
         in the nose
     c. inflamed and infected tonsils
     d. inflamed and infected
         membranes of the throat
     e. none of a–d choices

15. The effects of botulism are
     a. double vision, dizziness,
         respiratory paralysis
     b. diarrhea, fluid-electrolyte loss
     c. diarrhea, bloody stools,
         production of mucus
     d. liver cancer
     e. abortion in sheep

Appendix

Classification of Bacteria According to *Bergey's Manual of Systematic Bacteriology*

.

Kingdom Procaryotae

Divided into four divisions:

Division I. Gracilicutes

procaryotes with thin cell walls, implying a gram-negative type of cell wall.

Division II. Firmicutes

procaryotes with thick and strong skin, indicating a gram-positive type of cell wall.

Division III. Tenericutes

procaryotes of a pliable and soft nature, indicating the lack of a rigid cell wall.

Division IV. Mendosicutes

procaryotes with faulty cell walls, suggesting the lack of conventional peptidoglycan.

*Genera that have been placed in more than one volume: *Gardnerella*, *Lachnospira*, and *Butyrivibrio* have thin, gram-positive walls but stain as gram-negatives. *Halobacterium*, *Halococcus*, and *Thermoplasma* are *Archaeobacteria* that are also included among the GRAM-NEGATIVE RODS AND COCCI or THE MYCOPLASMAS.

Genus *Flavobacterium*
Genus *Alcaligenes*
Genus *Serpens*
Genus *Janthinobacterium*
Genus *Brucella*
Genus *Bordetella*
Genus *Francisella*
Genus *Paracoccus*
Genus *Lampropedia*

Section 5
Facultatively Anaerobic
Gram-Negative Rods
Family I. *Enterobacteriaceae*
  Genus I. *Escherichia*
  Genus II. *Shigella*
  Genus III. *Salmonella*
  Genus IV. *Citrobacter*
  Genus V. *Klebsiella*
  Genus VI. *Enterobacter*
  Genus VII. *Erwinia*
  Genus VIII. *Serratia*
  Genus IX. *Hafnia*
  Genus X. *Edwardsiella*
  Genus XI. *Proteus*
  Genus XII. *Providencia*
  Genus XIII. *Morganella*
  Genus XIX. *Yersinia*
Other genera of the family
Enterobacteriaceae:
  Genus *Obesumbacterium*
  Genus *Xenorhabdus*
  Genus *Kluyvera*
  Genus *Rahnella*
  Genus *Cedecea*
  Genus *Tatumella*
Family II. *Vibrionaceae*
  Genus I. *Vibrio*
  Genus II. *Photobacterium*
  Genus III. *Aeromonas*
  Genus IV. *Plesiomonas*
Family III. *Pasteurellaceae*
  Genus I. *Pasteurella*
  Genus II. *Haemophilus*
  Genus III. *Actinobacillus*

Other genera:
  Genus *Zymomonas*
  Genus *Chromobacterium*
  Genus *Cardiobacterium*
  Genus *Calymmatobacterium*
  Genus *Gardnerella**
  Genus *Eikenella*
  Genus *Streptobacillus*

Section 6
Anaerobic Gram-Negative Straight,
Curved, and Helical Rods
Family I. *Bacteroidaceae*
  Genus I. *Bacteroides*
  Genus II. *Fusobacterium*
  Genus III. *Leptotrichia*
  Genus IV. *Butyrivibrio**
  Genus V. *Succinimonas*
  Genus VI. *Succinivibrio*
  Genus VII. *Anaerobiospirillum*
  Genus VIII. *Wolinella*
  Genus IX. *Selenomonas*
  Genus X. *Anaerovibrio*
  Genus XI. *Pectinatus*
  Genus XII. *Acetivibrio*
  Genus XIII. *Lachnospira**

Section 7
Dissimilatory Sulfate- or
Sulfur-Reducing Bacteria
Genus *Desulfuromonas*
Genus *Desulfovibrio*
Genus *Desulfomonas*
Genus *Desulfococcus*
Genus *Desulfobacter*
Genus *Desulfobulbus*
Genus *Desulfosarcina*

Section 8
Anaerobic Gram-Negative Cocci
Family I. *Veillonellaceae*
  Genus I. *Veillonella*
  Genus II. *Acidaminococcus*
  Genus III. *Megasphaera*

Genus *Desulfotomaculum*
Genus *Sporosarcina*
Genus *Oscillospira*

Section 14
Regular, Nonsporing,
Gram-Positive Rods
Genus *Lactobacillus*
Genus *Listeria*
Genus *Erysipelothrix*
Genus *Brochothrix*
Genus *Renibacterium*
Genus *Kurthia*
Genus *Caryophanon*

Section 15
Irregular, Nonsporing,
Gram-Positive Rods
Animal and saprophytic corynebacteria
(*Corynebacterium*)
Plant corynebacteria
Genus *Gardnerella**
Genus *Arcanobacterium*
Genus *Arthrobacter*
Genus *Brevibacterium*
Genus *Curtobacterium*
Genus *Caseobacter*
Genus *Microbacterium*
Genus *Aureobacterium*
Genus *Cellulomonas*
Genus *Agromyces*
Genus *Arachnia*
Genus *Rothia*
Genus *Propionibacterium*
Genus *Eubacterium*
Genus *Acetobacterium*
Genus *Lachnospira**
Genus *Butyrivibrio**
Genus *Thermoanaerobacter*
Genus *Actinomyces*
Genus *Bifidobacterium*

Section 16
Mycobacteria
Family I. *Mycobacteriaceae*
   Genus I. *Mycobacteria*

Section 17
Nocardioforms
Genus *Nocardia*
Genus *Rhodococcus*
Genus *Nocardioides*
Genus *Pseudonocardia*
Genus *Oerskovia*
Genus *Saccharopolyspora*
Genus *Micropolyspora*
Genus *Promicromonospora*
Genus *Intrasporangium*

Volume 3

Section 18
Gliding, Nonfruiting Bacteria
Order I. *Cytophagales*
   Family I. *Cytophagaceae*
      Genus I. *Cytophaga*
      Genus II. *Sporocytophaga*
      Genus III. *Capnocytophaga*
      Genus IV. *Flexithrix*
      Genus V. *Flexibacter*
      Genus VI. *Microscilla*
      Genus VII. *Saprospira*
      Genus VIII. *Herpetosiphon*
Order II. *Lysobacterales*
   Family I. *Lysobacteraceae*
      Genus *Lysobacter*
Order III. *Beggiatoales*
   Family I. *Beggiatoaceae*
      Genus I. *Beggiatoa*
      Genus II. *Thioploca*
      Genus III. *Thiospirillopsis*
      Genus IV. *Thiothrix*
      Genus V. *Achromatium*
   Family II. *Simonsiellaceae*
      Genus I. *Simonsiella*

Genus II. *Alysiella*
Family III. *Leucotrichaceae*
   Genus *Leucothrix*
Families and genera *incertae sedis* (status of species questionable):
   Genus *Toxothrix*
   Genus *Vitreoscilla*
   Genus *Chitinophagen*
   Genus *Desulfonema*
Family IV. *Pelonemataceae*
   Genus *Pelonema*
   Genus *Achroonema*
   Genus *Peloploca*
   Genus *Desmanthus*

Section 19
Anoxygenic Phototrophic Bacteria
Purple Bacteria

Family I. *Chromatiaceae*
   Genus I. *Chromatium*
   Genus II. *Thiocystis*
   Genus III. *Thiospirillum*
   Genus IV. *Thiocapsa*
   Genus V. *Amoebobacter*
   Genus VI. *Lamprobacter*
   Genus VII. *Lamprocystis*
   Genus VIII. *Thiodictyon*
   Genus IX. *Thiopedia*
Family II. *Ectothiorhodospiraceae*
   Genus *Ectothiorhodospira*
Purple nonsulfur bacteria
   Genus *Rhodospirillum*
   Genus *Rhodopseudomonas*
   Genus *Rhodobacter*
   Genus *Rhodomicrobium*
   Genus *Rhodopila*
   Genus *Rhodocyclus*

Green Bacteria

Green sulfur bacteria
   Genus *Chlorobium*
   Genus *Prosthecochloris*
   Genus *Anacalochloris*

   Genus *Pelodictyon*
   Genus *Chloroherpeton*
Multicellular filamentous green bacteria
   Genus *Chloroflexus*
   Genus *Heliothrix*
   Genus *Oscillochloris*
Genera *incertae sedis*
   Genus *Heliobacterium*
   Genus *Erythrobacter*

Section 20
Budding and/or Appendaged
Bacteria Prosthecate Bacteria

Budding bacteria
   Genus *Hyphomicrobium*
   Genus *Hyphomonas*
   Genus *Pedomicrobium*
   Genus *"Filomicrobium"*
   Genus *"Dicotomicrobium"*
   Genus *"Tetramicrobium"*
   Genus *Stella*
   Genus *Ancalomicrobium*
   Genus *Prosthecomicrobium*
Nonbudding bacteria
   Genus *Caulobacter*
   Genus *Asticcacaulis*
   Genus *Prosthecobacter*
   Genus *Thiodendron*

Nonprosthecate Bacteria

Budding bacteria
   Genus *Planctomyces*
   Genus *Pasteuria*
   Genus *Blastobacter*
   Genus *Angulomicrobium*
   Genus *Gemmiger*
   Genus *Ensifer*
   Genus *Isophaera*
Nonbudding stalked bacteria
   Genus *Gallionella*
   Genus *Nevskia*

Morphologically unusual budding
bacteria involved in iron and manganese
deposition
    Genus *Seliberia*
    Genus *Metallogenium*
    Genus *Caulococcus*
    Genus *Kuznezovia*
Others: Spinate bacteria

Section 21
Archaeobacteria Methanogenic Bacteria
Genus *Methanobacterium*
Genus *Methanobrevibacter*
Genus *Methanococcus*
Genus *Methanomicrobium*
Genus *Methanospirillum*
Genus *Methanosarcina*
Genus *Methanococcoides*
Genus *Methanothermus*
Genus *Methanolobus*
Genus *Methanoplanus*
Genus *Methanogenium*
Genus *Methanothrix*

Extreme Halophilic Bacteria
Genus *Halobacterium**
Genus *Halococcus**

Extreme Thermophilic Bacteria
Genus *Thermoplasma**
Genus *Sulfolobus*
Genus *Thermoproteus*
Genus *Thermofilum*
Genus *Thermococcus*
Genus *Desulfurococcus*
Genus *Thermodiscus*
Genus *Pyrodictium*

Section 22
Sheathed Bacteria
Genus *Sphaerotilus*
Genus *Leptothrix*
Genus *Haliscominobacter*

Genus *Lieskeella*
Genus *Phragmidiothrix*
Genus *Crenothrix*
Genus *Clonothrix*

Section 23
Gliding, Fruiting Bacteria
Order I. *Myxobacterales*
    Family I. *Myxococcaceae*
        Genus *Myxococcus*
    Family II. *Archangiaceae*
        Genus *Archangium*
    Family III. *Cystobacteraceae*
        Genus I. *Cystobacter*
        Genus II. *Melittangium*
        Genus III. *Stigmatella*
    Family IV. *Polyangiaceae*
        Genus I. *Polyangium*
        Genus II. *Nannocystis*
        Genus III. *Chondromyces*
    Genus *incerta sedis*
        Genus *Angiococcus*

Section 24
Chemolithotrophic Bacteria Nitrifiers
Family I. *Nitrobacteraceae*
    Genus I. *Nitrobacter*
    Genus II. *Nitrospina*
    Genus III. *Nitrococcus*
    Genus IV. *Nitrosomonas*
    Genus V. *Nitrospira*
    Genus VI. *Nitrosococcus*
    Genus VII. *Nitrosolobus*

Sulfur Oxidizers
Genus *Thiobacillus*
Genus *Thiomicrospira*
Genus *Thiobacterium*
Genus *Thiospira*
Genus *Macromonas*

Obligate Hydrogen Oxidizers
Genus *Hydrogenbacter*

Metal Oxidizers and Depositors
Family I. *Siderocapsaceae*
  Genus I. *Siderocapsa*
  Genus II. *Naumaniella*
  Genus III. *Ochrobium*
  Genus IV. *Siderococcus*

Other Magnetotactic Bacteria

Section 25
Cyanobacteria
Others
Order I. *Prochlorales*
  Family I. *Prochloraceae*
    Genus *Prochloron*

Volume 4

Section 26
***Actinomycetes* that Divide in
More Than One Plane**
Genus *Geodermatophilus*
Genus *Dermatophilus*
Genus *Frankia*
Genus *Tonsilophilus*

Section 27
Sporangiate *Actinomycetes*
Genus *Actinoplanes* (including
  Amorphosporangium)
Genus *Streptosporangium*
Genus *Ampullariella*
Genus *Spirillospora*
Genus *Pilimelia*

Genus *Dactylosporangium*
Genus *Planomonospora*
Genus *Planobispora*

Section 28
***Streptomycetes* and Their Allies**
Genus *Streptomyces*
Genus *Streptovertillium*
Genus *Actinopycnidium*
Genus *Actinosporangium*
Genus *Chainia*
Genus *Elytrosporangium*
Genus *Microellobosporia*
(The last five genera may be merged
with *Streptomyces*)

Section 29
Other Conidiate Genera
Genus *Actinopolyspora*
Genus *Actinosynnema*
Genus *Kineospora*
Genus *Kitasatosporia*
Genus *Microbispora*
Genus *Micromonospora*
Genus *Microtetrospora*
Genus *Saccharomonospora*
Genus *Sporichthya*
Genus *Streptoalloteichus*
Genus *Thermomonospora*
Genus *Actinomadura*
Genus *Nocardiopsis*
Genus *Excellospora*
Genus *Thermoactinomyces*

Glossary

Adenosine triphosphate (ATP) (add-den'-o-sin tri'-fos-fate). High-energy-rich organic molecule

Agglutination (uh-glue-ten-ay'-shun). The clumping of cells following reaction with antibodies

Algae (al'-gee). Plants with chlorophyll (capable of producing their own food)

Allergen (al'-ur-jen). An antigen that causes an allergic reaction

Allergy (al'-ur-gee). A disease resulting from exposure to an antigen

Amebiasis (a-me-bi'-ah-sis). A disease caused by a protozoan, *Entamoeba histolytica*

Amphitrichous (am-fit'-ri-kus). Bacteria with flagella on both ends

Anabolism (an-ab'-bow-liz-em). Metabolic reactions that result in the biosynthesis of complex cellular materials

Anamnestic (an-am-nest'-tick) **response**. Memory response following antigen exposure in sensitized individuals

Anaphylactic (an-na-fill-lack'-tick) **shock**. A severe allergic reaction that may result in death

Antibiosis (an-tea-buy-oh'-sis). An antagonistic relationship

Antibiotic (an-tea-buy-ot'-tick). Substance produced by microorganisms that inhibit or destroy pathogens during the disease process

Antibody (an'-tea-body). Protein produced by the body in response to foreign antigens

Antigen (an'-ti-gin). A foreign substance that stimulates the production of antibodies

Antiseptic (an-ti-sep'-tick). Chemical disinfectants that are safe to use on living tissues

Antitoxin (an-te-tox'-sin). An antibody that neutralizes a toxin

Arthropod (ar'-throw-pod). A phylum classification of animals including insects, mites, lice, ticks, and fleas

Arthus (ar'-thus) **reaction**. A complex immune skin reaction at the site of repeated injections

Asepsis (a-sep'-sis). Absence of infectious microorganisms on living tissue

Attenuated (uh-ten'-you-ate-ted). A weakened, less pathogenic organism

Autogenous (awe-tah'-gin-us) **vaccine**. A vaccine prepared from a local infection injected back into the same person

Autoimmune (awe-toe-im-mune') **disease**. A disease in which the body produces antibodies to its own tissues

Autotrophs (awe'-toe-trophs). Organisms that obtain carbon from inorganic sources, as from carbon dioxide

Bacillus (buh-sill'-us), *pl* bacilli (buh-sill'-eye). A rod-shaped bacterium; also, *Bacillus* is a genus of aerobic spore-forming rods

Bacteria (back-tier'-ee-uh). Procaryotic, mostly unicellular cells; most primitive organisms

Bactericidal (back-tear-i-side'-all). Bacteria-killing action

Bactericide (back-tear'-i-side). An agent that kills bacteria

Bacteriolytic (back-tear-ee-oh-lit'-tick). A substance that lyses or breaks apart bacteria

Catabolism (ca-tab'-bow-liz-em). Metabolic reactions that break down organic materials into simple molecules

Catalyst (cat'-uh-list). A chemical agents that speeds up a reaction

Catalyze (cat'-uh-lyz). To speed up a reaction

Centrosome (sen'-trow-soam). A eucaryotic cytoplasmic organelle containing two centrioles

Chemolithotrophs (key-moe-lith'-oh-trophs). Organisms that use a chemical source of energy and an inorganic source of nutrients

Chemoorganotrophs (key-moe-or-gan'-oh-trophs). Organisms that use a chemical source of energy and an organic source of nutrients

Chemotaxis (keem-oh-tacks'-sis). Movement of organisms in response to a chemical substance; the attraction of leukocytes to an area of injury is probably due to the release of a chemical substance from the injured tissue

Chemotherapy (key-mow-ther'-uh-pea). The treatment of diseases and infection using chemicals

Chemotrophs (chem'-oh-trophs). Organisms that obtain their energy from chemical sources

Choleragin (kol'-er-ah-gin). The exotoxin produced by *Vibrio cholerae*, which causes cholera

Chromosome (crow'-mow-soam). The genetic material carrying the genes of heredity, containing DNA

Cilia (sill'-ee-uh). Short, hairlike structures that provide for movement; characteristic of Protozoa, class Ciliata

Coagulase (co-ag'-you-laze). An enzyme that clots plasma around the bacteria

Coccus (cock'-cuss), *pl* cocci (cock'-sigh). Spherical or ball-shaped bacterium

Collagenase (co-lodge'-in-aze). An enzyme that breaks down collagen in connective tissue

Commensalism (co-men'-sal-is-um). A relationship in which one member benefits and the other is unaffected in any way

Complement (com'-ple-ment). A blood serum protein group involved in certain antibody-antigen reactions

Cystitis (sis-ti'-tis). An infection of the urinary bladder

Cytology (sigh-tol'-oh-gee). The study of cells

Cytoplasm (sigh'-tow-plaz-um). The protoplasm outside the nucleus of the cell

Cytotoxins (sigh-tow-tok'-sins). Toxic substances that injure certain cells

Dermatophytes (der-mah'-toe-fites). Fungi capable of growing on the skin surface causing ringworm or tinea diseases

Disinfectant (dis-in-feck'-tant). A chemical agent used to destroy pathogens on or within nonliving materials

DNA, deoxyribonucleic (dee-ox'-ee-rye'-bow-nu-clay'-ick) **acid.** The genetic material in the chromosomes

Encapsulate (en-cap'-sue-late). To surround by a capsule

Encephalitis (en-seff-fall-eye'-tis). A disease involving inflammation of the brain

Endemic (en-dem'-ick). A disease present in normal numbers in a community

Endoplasmic reticulum (end-oh-plasz'-mick re-tick'-you-lum). A eucaryotic cell organelle for transport and support

Enterotoxin (en'-ter-oh-tok'-sin). An exotoxin causing damage to intestinal cells producing diarrhea

Enzyme (en'-zym). An organic catalyst

Epidemic (ep-i-dem'-ick). More than the normal number of cases of a disease in a community at a particular time

Epidemiology (ep-i-dem-ee-ol'-oh-gee). The systematic study of epidemics

Eucaryote (you-care'-ree-ot). A cell with a true nucleus

Exotoxin (ek'-so-tock-sin). A toxic substance secreted by a living organism

Exudate (x'-you-date). A viscous secretion containing blood cells and cellular debris from site of inflammation

Facultative anaerobic (fack'-ul-tay-tive an'-air-robe). A microorganism that prefers to live in the absence of free oxygen, but survives in an oxygen environment

Fecal (fee'-cull). Referring to feces or bowel movement

Fibrinolysin (fy-bri-nol'-i-sin). An enzyme that breaks down fibrin clots

Filamentous (fil-uh-men'-tus). Having many threads or filaments

Flagella (fluh-gel'-uh). Protein strands used for movement

Fomes (fo'-meez) or **fomite** (fo'-mite), *pl* fomites (fo'-mi-teez). An object,

such as a book or an item of clothing, that is not in itself harmful but that
is able to harbor pathogenic organisms and thus serve as an agent for
transmission of an infection

Fungi (fun'-ji). Microorganisms that are incapable of producing their own
food and that live on decaying organic material; primitive plants

Fungicide (fun'-juh-side). A substance that kills fungi

Germicide (germ'-uh-side). A substance that kills microorganisms

Gene (jean). The genetic material coding for one polypeptide

Glycolysis (gly-col'-eh-sis). The anaerobic breakdown of glucose to pyruvic
acid or lactic acid with the production of energy

Golgi (goal'-gee). A eucaryotic cell organelle involved in secretion

Haloduric (hey-low-dur'-ick). Surviving in a salty environment

Hapten (hap-ten'). A nonantigenic small molecule that becomes antigenic
when combined with a large molecule

Hemolysin (heem-moll'-uh-sin). An enzyme that breaks down red blood cells

Hepatitis (hep-uh-tight'-us). A disease of the liver, usually caused by a virus

Herpes (her'-peas). A viral disease, causing herpetic lesions in oral or genital
areas.

Heterotrophs (het'-ter-oh-trophs). Organisms that obtain carbon from
organic sources

Histamine (hiss'-tuh-mean). Potent chemical released from cells during some
immune reactions, causing swelling and inflammation

Hyaluronic acid (high-al-your-ahn'-ick). A chemical in connective tissue

Hyaluronidase (high-al-your-ahn'-uh-daze). An enzyme that breaks down
connective tissue

Hypersensitivity (hi-purr'-sense-uh-tive'-it-tea). An antigen-antibody
reaction to foreign proteins in which cell-bound antibodies cause tissue
destruction or inflammation

Hypertonic (hi-per-tahn'-ick). Having a greater osmotic pressure outside the
cell membrane than inside the cell

Hypotonic (hi-po-tahn-'-ick). Having less osmotic pressure outside the cell
membrane than inside the cell.

Immunity (im-mu'-nit-tea). Resistance to disease imparted by the presence
of antibodies

Immunoglobulin (im'-you-no-glob'-you-lyn). The globulin proteins of the
serum and other body secretions, including the humoral antibodies

Immunology (im-mew-noll'-oh-gee). The science that deals with immunity
from disease and the production of immunity

Immunosuppression (im'-you-no-sue-presh'-un). Depression of the immune
response

Infection (in-feck'-shun). The growth of parasitic microorganisms in a host

Innate (in-ate'). Present in an individual at birth

Interferon (in-ter-fear'-ahn). Antiviral, soluble protein substances produced by cells infected with almost any animal virus; interferon is cell-specific and species-specific, but not virus-specific

In vitro (in vee'-trow). In the laboratory, in an artificial environment

In vivo (in vee'-vo). In the living organism

Isotonic (i-so-tahn'-ick). Having the same osmotic pressure inside and outside a cell membrane

Leukocidin (lew-co-side'-in). An enzyme that destroys white blood cells

Lipopolysaccharide (lip'-o-pol-ee-sack'-car-ride). A macromolecule of combined lipid and polysaccharide, often found in gram-negative bacterial cell walls

Logarithm (log'-uh-rhi-thm). Mathematically, the power to which a number must be raised to produce a given number

Lysozyme (lie'-so-zime). The cellular digestive enzyme in lysosomes

Lymphokines (lim'-fo-kines). T-cell secretions after antigenic stimulation

Malaise (mal-az'). A general feeling of illness and discomfort

Mesophilic (mess-so-fill'-ick). Thriving at 30° to 45°C (86° to 113°F)

Mesosome (me'-so-soam). A procaryotic cell organelle involved in cellular respiration

Metabolism (mu-tab'-bow-liz-em). The sum of all the chemical reactions in living cells

Microbial (my-crow'-bee-al). Pertaining to microbes

Microbicide (my-crow'-bi-side). An agent that kills microbes

Microbistasis (my-crow-bi-stay'-sis). The inhibition of growth and reproduction of microorganisms

Microorganism (my-kro-or'-gan-iz-em). Microscopic organisms, usually single cells; sometimes called microbes

Microtubules (my-crow-tube'-yules). Eucaryotic cell organelle involved in support and secretion

Mitochondria (my-tow-con'-dree-uh). Eucaryotic organelles involved in cellular respiration for the production of energy

Monoclonal antibodies (mon-o-clone'-al). Antibodies for a single antigenic determinant produced by hybridoma cells (lymphocytes fused with tumor cells) *in vitro*

Monotrichous (mon-ot'-trick-us). Bacteria with one flagellum

Motile (mow'-till). Having the ability to move

Mutagenic (mu-tuh-jen'-ick). An agent that produces mutations or genetic changes in organisms

Mutant (mu'-tant). An organism that has survived mutation

Mutation (mew-tay'-shun). A change in genetic material and traits that is inherited by offspring.

Mutualism (mew'-chew-al-is-um). A relationship in which both organisms benefit

Necrotoxin (neck'-row-tox'-sin). An exotoxin that destroys certain cells
Neurotoxin (new'-row-tox-sin). An exotoxin that damages nerve tissue
Nosocomial (no-so-com'-ee-ul). An infection acquired during hospitalization
Nucleoid (new'-klee-oid). The nuclear area of procaryotic cells
Nucleolus (new-kle'-oh-lus). The dense portion of the nucleus, containing RNA
Nucleoplasm (new'-klee-oh-plaz-um). The protoplasm inside the nucleus

Oncogenic (on-ko-jen'-ick). Capable of producing tumors
Opportunist (op-poor-tune'-ist). A microbe that causes disease in susceptible individuals
Opsonization (op-son-a-zay'-shun). The engulfment of cells or bacteria by phagocytes, owing to the presence of specific antibodies
Organelles (or-gan-ells'). Discrete structures inside the cell
Osmotic pressure (oz-mah'-tic). The pressure exerted on the cell membrane by the solution inside the cell

Pandemic (pan-dem'-ick). A worldwide epidemic
Parasitism (par'-uh-sit-ism). A relationship in which an organism benefits at the expense of the host organism
Pasteurization (pass-tur-uh-zay'-shun). A process by which heat is used to kill pathogens in foods
Pathogen (path'-o-jen). Disease-causing microorganism
Pathogenicity (path-oh-gin-iss'-city). The ability of an organism to cause disease
Peptidoglycan (pep-tid-o-gly'-can). The rigid component of bacterial cell walls, consisting of polysaccharide chains linked together by peptide chains
Peristalsis (pear-uh-stall'-siss). Waves of contraction passing along tubular organs (particularly the intestine, mixing contents, and moving them along
Peritrichous (pear-ri'-trick-us). Covered by flagella
Phagocyte (faj'-oh-site). White blood cell capable of ingesting foreign particles, including microorganisms
Photolithotrophs (foe-toe-lith'-oh-trophs). Organisms that use light for energy and inorganic chemicals for nutrients
Photoorganotrophs (foe-toe-or-gan'-oh-trophs). Organims that use light for energy and organic chemicals for nutrients
Phototrophs (foe'-toe-trophs). Organisms that use light as their source of energy
Plasmolysis (plaz-moll'-uh-sis). The shrinking of the cell membrane and cytoplasm from the cell wall, causing the cell to shrink
Plasmoptysis (plaz-mop'-ti-sis). A process in which water enters a cell through the cell walls
Poliomyelitis (pole-ee-oh-my-oh-light'-us). A viral disease of nervous system

Polymer (pol'-e-mer). Long-chain molecule consisting of repeated subunits

Precipitin (pre-sip'-it-tin). An antibody to soluble antigen that forms a visible precipitate

Primordial (pry-mor'-dee-al). Early or first in time

Procaryote (pro-kar'-ee-ot). Primitive cells without a true nucleus

Protoplasm (pro'-tow-plaz-um). The semifluid material inside cells

Protoplasts (pro'-toe-plasts). A bacterial cell with no cell wall

Protozoa (pro-toe-zoe'-uh). Single-celled microscopic animals found in water and soil

Psychroduric (sigh-crow-dur'-ick). Having the ability to endure temperatures of $-20°$ to $5°C$ ($-5°$ to $40°F$)

Purine (pure'-reen). A DNA base; adenine or guanine

Pyogenic (pie-oh-jen'-ick). Pus producing

Pyrimidine (perr'-rim-uh-dean). A nucleic acid base; thymine, cytosine, or uracil

Resident flora (flur'-uh). Microorganisms normally found in an area of the human body

Ribosomes (rye'-bow-soams). Organelles necessary for protein synthesis

RNA, ribonucleic acid (rye'-bow-new-clay'-ick). Nucleic acid necessary for protein synthesis

Saprophyte (sap'-row-fight). An organism that obtains its nutrients from dead, decaying organic matter

Sebum (see'-bum). The secretion of the sebaceous (oil) glands of the skin

Serological tests (ser-o-lodge'-eh-cal). Antigen-antibody tests used for diagnostic purposes

Spirochetes (spy'-row-keets). Spiral-shaped bacteria

Sporicidal (spor-uh-sigh'-dull). Having the ability to kill spores

Streptokinase (strep-tow-kine'-ase). An enzyme that helps streptococci to invade the body

Symbionts (sim'-bee-yonts). Organisms living together

Symbiosis (sim'-bee-oh'-sis). A constant relationshp between two or more unlike species of organisms

Synergism (sin'-er-jiz-um). A mutualistic relationship in which organisms accomplish together what neither could do alone

Taxonomy (tax-ah'-no-me). A systematic classification of organisms

Teichoic acid (tie-ko'-ick). A chemical in the cell wall of gram-positive bacteria

Tetanospasmin (tet'-ah-no-spaz'-min). The neurotoxic exotoxin that causes tetanus produced by *Clostridium tetani*

Thermoduric (ther-mow-dur'-ick). Having the ability to survive boiling

Toxigenicity (tox-uh-gen-iss'-city). The ability of a pathogen to produce a toxin, causing damage to the host

Toxin (tok'-sin). A toxic or damaging substance

Toxoid (tok'-soid). An inactivated toxin that can stimulate antitoxin production but not cause disease

Transient flora (flur'-uh). Microorganisms temporarily found in certain area of the body

Tuberculocidal (too-bur-cue-low-sigh'-doll). Killing the bacteria that cause tuberculosis (*Mycobacterium tuberculosis*)

Tyndallization (tin-dull-uh-zay'-shun). A process of boiling and cooling in which spores are allowed to germinate and then are killed

Urethritis (you'-re-thri'-tis). An inflammation of the urethra of the urinary system

Vaccine (vack-scene'). An inactivated agent used to cause the production of antibodies to protect against disease

Vacuoles (vack'-you-oles). Membrane-bound storage spaces in the cell

Vector (veck'-tore). A carrier of pathogenic organisms from one host to another

Virology (vi-rol'-oh-gee). The study of viruses and the diseases they cause

Virucide (vi'-ruh-side). A substance that kills viruses

Virulence (veer'-you-lence). The properties of an organism that make it pathogenic

Virulent (veer'-you-lent). Able to produce disease

Virus (vi'-rus). An infective agent smaller than a bacterium

Selected References for Suggested Reading

Books

Alexander M: Introduction to Soil Microbiology, 3rd ed. New York, John Wiley & Sons, 1982

American Hospital Association: Infection Control in the Hospital, 4th ed. Chicago, American Hospital Association, 1980

Ayliffe GA, Taylor LJ: Hospital-Acquired Infections: Principles and Prevention. Littleton, John Wright-PSG, 1982

Balows A (ed): Manual of Clinical Microbiology, 5th ed. Washington, DC, American Society for Microbiology, 1991

Beaver PC, Jung RC: Animal Agents and Vectors of Human Disease, 5th ed. Philadelphia, Lea & Febiger, 1985

Benenson AS (ed): Control of Communicable Diseases in Man, 15th ed. American Public Health Association, 1990

Block SS (ed.): Disinfection, Sterilization and Preservation, 3rd ed. Philadelphia, Lea & Febiger, 1983

Boyd HC, Payne MJ: Introduction to the Algae, 2nd ed. Englewood Cliffs, NJ, Prentice-Hall, 1985

Boyd RF: General Microbiology, St. Louis, Times-Mirror/Mosby, 1988

Boyd RF, Hoerl BG: Basic Medical Microbiology, 3rd ed. Boston, Little, Brown & Co, 1986

Brock TD (ed.): Milestones in Microbiology. Washington, DC, American Society for Microbiology, 1974

Bryan LE (ed.): Antimicrobial Drug Resistance. New York, Academic Press, 1984

Carr NG, Whitton BA: The Biology of Cyanobacteria. Botanical Monographs, vol. 19. Berkeley, University of California Press, 1982

Castle M: Hospital Infection Control, New York, John Wiley & Sons, 1980

Clayton RK, Sistrom WR (eds.): The Photosynthetic Bacteria. New York, Plenum Press, 1978

Coleman RM, et al.: Fundamental Immunology. Dubuque, IA, Wm. C. Brown, 1989

Creager JG, Black JG, Davison VE: Microbiology: Principles and Applications. Englewood Cliffs, NJ, Prentice-Hall, 1990

Davis BD, et al.: Microbiology, 4th ed. Philadelphia, JB Lippincott, 1990

Difco Manual: Dehydrated Culture Media and Reagents for Microbiology, 10th ed. Detroit, Difco Laboratories, 1984

Evans AS (ed): Viral Infections of Humans: Epidemiology and Control, 3rd ed. New York, Plenum Press, 1989

Faust EC, Beaver PC, Jung RC: Animal Agents and Vectors of Human Diseases, 4th ed. Philadelphia, Lea & Febiger, 1975

Finegold SM, Martin WJ: Diagnostic Microbiology, 7th ed. St. Louis, CV Mosby, 1986

Freeman BA: Burrows' Textbook of Microbiology, 22nd ed. Philadelphia, WB Saunders, 1985

Friedman RM: Interferons: A Primer. New York, Academic Press, 1981

Gerhardt P, et al. (eds.): Manual of Methods for General Bacteriology. Washington, DC, American Society for Microbiology, 1981

Goodfellow M, Mordarski M, Williams S: Biology of the Actinomycetes. New York, Academic Press, 1984

Guari KK: Antiviral Chemotherapy: Design of Inhibitors of Viral Functions. New York, Academic Press, 1981

Holt JG (ed.): Bergey's Manual of Systematic Bacteriology, 1st ed., vol. 1. Baltimore, Williams & Wilkins, 1984; vol. 2 (1985); vol. 3 (1986); vol. 4 (1987)

Hood LE, Weissman IL, Wood WB, Wilson JH: Immunology, 2nd ed. Menlo Park, Benjamin/Cummings, 1984

Hurst A, Gould GW: The Bacterial Spore. New York, Academic Press, 1984

Ingraham JL, Maloe O, Neidhardt FC: Growth of the Bacterial Cell. Sunderland, Sinauer Associates, 1983

Jawetz E, et al.: Review of Medical Microbiology, 17th ed. Los Altos, Appleton and Lange, 1987

Joklik WK, et al: Zinsser's Microbiology, 19th ed. New York, Appleton and Lange, 1988

Lennette EH, et al. (eds.): Manual of Clinical Microbiology, 4th ed. Washington, DC, American Society for Microbiology, 1985

Margulis L: Early Life. Boston, Science Books International, 1982

Mausner JS, Kramer S: Mausner and Bahn Epidemiology. Philadelphia, WB Saunders, 1984

McMurry J: Essentials of General Organic and Biological Chemistry. Englewood Cliffs, NJ, Prentice-Hall, 1989

Mims CA: The Pathogenesis of Infectious Disease, 3rd ed. London, Academic Press, 1987

Myrvik QN, Weiser RS: Fundamentals of Immunology. Philadelphia, Lea & Febiger, 1984

Nester EW, et al.: Microbiology, 3rd ed. New York, Holt, Rinehart & Winston, 1983

Nolte WA (ed.): Oral Microbiology, 4th ed. St. Louis, CV Mosby, 1982

Pelczar MJ, Chan ECS, Krieg NR: Microbiology, 5th ed. New York, McGraw-Hill, 1986

Pratt WB, Fekety R: The Antimicrobial Drugs. New York, Oxford University Press, 1986

Prescott LM, Harley JP, Klein DA: Microbiology. Dubuque, IA, Wm. C. Brown, 1990

Rippon JW: Medical Mycology, 2nd ed. Philadelphia, WB Saunders, 1982

Rose NR, Fahey JL, Friedman H: Manual of Clinical Immunology, 3rd ed. American Society for Microbiology, 1986

Sherris JC (ed): Medical Microbiology, 2nd ed. New York, Elsevier Science, 1990

Smith L deS: The Pathogenic Anaerobic Bacteria, 3rd ed. Springfield, Charles C Thomas, 1984

Standard Methods for the Examination of Water and Wastewater, 15th ed. Washington, DC, American Public Health Association, 1981

Stryer L: Biochemistry, 2nd ed. San Francisco, WH Freeman, 1981

Sutter V, et al.: Wadsworth Anaerobic Bacteriology Manual, 3rd ed. St. Louis, CV Mosby, 1980

Tortora GJ, Funke BR, Case CL: Microbiology, 3rd ed. Menlo Park, Benjamin/Cummings Publishing Co, 1989

Volk WA: Essentials of Medical Microbiology, 4th ed. Philadelphia, JB Lippincott Co, 1991

Watson JD: The Double Helix. Stent GS (ed.). New York, WW Norton, 1980

Watson JD, Tooze J, Kurtz DT: Recombinant DNA: A Short Course. New York, WH Freeman, 1983

Webster J: Introduction to Fungi, 2nd ed. New York, Cambridge University Press, 1980

Wilson ME, Mizer HE, Morello JA: Microbiology in Patient Care, 4th ed. New York, Macmillan, 1984

Wistreich GA, Lechtman MD: Microbiology, 5th ed. New York, Glencoe Press, 1988

Youmans GP, Paterson PY, Sommers HM: The Biologic and Clinical Basis of Infectious Diseases, 3rd ed. Philadelphia, WB Saunders, 1985

Journal Publications

Abraham EP: The beta-lactam antibiotics. Sci Am 244:76–86, June 1981

Ada GL, Nossal G: The clonal-selection theory. Sci Am 257:62–69, 1987

Alt FW, Blackwell TK, Yancopoulos GD: Development of the primary antibody response. Science 238:1079–1088, 1987

Bishop JM: Oncogenes. Sci Am 246:80–92; March 1982

Brill WJ: Biologic nitrogen fixation. Sci Am 236:68–74, 1977

Brunori M, Silvestrini MC, Pocchiari M: The scarpie agent and the prion hypothesis. Trends Biochem Sci 13(8):309–313, 1988

Collier RJ, Kaplan DA: Immunotoxins. Sci Am 251:56–64, July 1984

Cohen SN, Shapiro SA: Transposable genetic elements. Sci Am 242:40, 1980

Dolin R: Antiviral chemotherapy and chemoprophylaxis. Science 227:1296–1303, 1985

Edelson RL, Fink JM: The immunologic function of skin. Sci Am 256:46–53, June 1985

Ferris FG, Beveridge TJ: Functions of bacterial cell surface structures. BioScience 35:172–177, 1985

Fraser DW, McDade JE: Legionellosis. Sci Am 241:82–99, Oct 1979

Godson GN: Molecular approaches to malaria vaccines. Sci Am 252:52–59, May 1985

Haseltine WA, Wong-Staal F: The molecular biology of the AIDS virus. Sci Am 259(4):52–62, 1988

Isenberg HD: Pathogenicity and virulence: Another view. Clin Microbiol Rev 1(1):40–53, 1988

Joiner KA: Complement evasion by baceria and parasites. Ann Rev Microbiol 42:201–230, 1988

Karpas A: Viruses and leukemia. Am Sci 70:277–285, 1982

Kraut J: How do enzymes work? Science 242:533–539, 1988

Leder P: The genetics of antibody diversity. Sci Am 246:102, 1982

Lerner RA: Synthetic vaccines. Sci Am 248:66–74, Feb 1983

Marrack P, Kappler J: The T-cell and its receptor. Sci Am Feb 1986

Marrack P, Kappler J: The T cell receptor. Science 238:1073–1078, 1987

Müller-Eberhard HJ: Molecular organization and function of the complement system. Ann Rev Biochem 57:321–347, 1988

Novick RP: Plasmids. Sci Am 243(6):102, 1980

Parkman PD, Hopps HE: Viral vaccines and antivirals: Current use and future prospects. Ann Rev Public Health 9:203–221, 1988

Payne WJ Jr., Marshall DL, Shockley RK, Martin WJ: Clinical laboratory applications of monoclonal antibodies. Clin Microbiol Rev 1(3):313–329, 1988

Prusiner SB. Prions. Sci Am 251:50–59, Oct 1984

Simons K, Garoff J, Helenius A: How an animal virus gets into and out of its host cell. Sci Am 246:58–66, Feb 1982

Stark A-A: Mutagenicity and carcinogenicity of mycotoxins. Ann Rev Microbiol 34:235, 1980

Steere AC: Lyme disease. N Engl J Med 321:586–596, 1989

Yelton DE, Scharff MD: Monoclonal antibodies. Am Sci 68:510–516, 1980

Answers to Self-test Questions

Chapter 1

Matching Exercises

Historical Milestones of Microbiology
1. Nightingale
2. Koch
3. Pasteur
4. Semmelweis
5. Leeuwenhoek
6. Fracastorius
7. Janssen
8. Tyndall
9. Pasteur
10. Lister
11. Petri
12. Hesse
13. Jenner
14. Koch

Some Types of Microbes
1. indigenous microflora
2. opportunists
3. nitrogen-fixing microbes
4. saprophytes
5. pathogenic
6. iron-utilizing microbes
7. nitrogen-fixing microbes

Theories and Terms
1. sterilization
2. pasteurization
3. sterile technique
4. germ theory of disease
5. biological theory of fermentation
6. biogenesis
7. pure culture
8. spontaneous generation
9. vaccination
10. micrometer (or micron)
11. pathogen
12. fermentation
13. pure culture
14. medium
15. saprophytes
16. contaminant
17. abiogenesis
18. germ theory of disease

True or False (T or F)
1. F
2. F
3. F
4. F
5. F
6. T
7. T
8. F

9. T
10. F

Multiple choice

1. c
2. a
3. b
4. b
5. a
6. b
7. c
8. a

Chapter 2

Matching Exercises

Descriptive terms

1. procaryotes
2. amphitrichous
3. bacilli
4. axial filaments
5. eucaryotes
6. lophotrichous
7. spirilla
8. diplococci
9. procaryotes
10. eucaryotes
11. cocci
12. peritrichous
13. procaryotes
14. staphylococci
15. procaryotes
16. diplobacilli
17. monotrichous
18. streptobacilli
19. procaryotes
20. eucaryotes
21. streptococci

Characteristics of Microorganisms

1. fungi
2. algae
3. protozoa
4. algae
5. chlamydias
6. mycoplasmas
7. *Escherichia coli*
8. rickettsias
9. viruses

Diseases and Microorganisms

1. streptococci
2. rickettsias
3. virus
4. staphylococci
5. mycoplasmas
6. curved rod
7. virus
8. spirochete
9. virus
10. mycobacteria
11. virus
12. chlamydias
13. virus

True or False (T or F)

1. T
2. T
3. F
4. T
5. F
6. F
7. F
8. T
9. T
10. T
11. F
12. T
13. T
14. F

15. T
16. F
17. T

Multiple Choice

1. d
2. d
3. e
4. d
5. c
6. e
7. a
8. b
9. a
10. b

Chapter 3

Matching Exercises

Basic Chemistry

1. atoms
2. ions
3. neutrons
4. ionic
5. covalent
6. metabolism, hydrolysis, dehydration synthesis

Biochemistry

1. glycerol
2. primary
3. DNA, nucleotides
4. polysaccharides
5. enzymes
6. substrate

Match Chemicals

1. a
2. a
3. e
4. b
5. c
6. b
7. a
8. c
9. a
10. b

True or False (T or F)

1. T
2. F
3. T
4. T
5. F
6. T
7. F
8. F
9. F

Multiple Choice

1. c
2. c
3. d
4. d
5. d
6. d
7. b
8. c
9. d
10. a
11. c
12. d
13. b
14. b
15. a
16. d

Chapter 4

Matching Exercises

Nutritional types
1. phototrophs
2. chemotrophs
3. heterotrophs
4. autotrophs
5. chemoorganotrophs
6. chemolithotrophs
7. photoorganotrophs
8. photolithotrophs
9. autotrophs or photolithotrophs
10. autotrophs or photolithotrophs
11. heterotrophs or chemoorganotrophs
12. heterotrophs or chemoorganotrophs

Metabolic Reactions
1. photosynthesis
2. anabolism
3. catabolism
4. aerobic respiration
5. fermentation
6. catabolism
7. anabolism
8. fermentation

Growth Curve
1. lag phase
2. death phase
3. logarithmic growth phase
4. stationary phase
5. logarithmic growth phase
6. logarithmic growth phase
7. logarithmic growth phase
8. death phase

Bacterial Genetics
1. transformation
2. mutation
3. mutation
4. transduction

5. lysogenic conversion
6. conjugation
7. mutagens

True or False (T or F)
1. T
2. T
3. F
4. T
5. F
6. T
7. F
8. T
9. T
10. T
11. T

Multiple Choice
1. b
2. c
3. d
4. d
5. c
6. c
7. d
8. b
9. c
10. c
11. c

Chapter 5

Matching Exercises

Terms
1. fungicidal agent
2. fungistatic agent
3. sepsis
4. antiseptic technique
5. asepsis
6. aseptic technique
7. sterile technique
8. sterilization

9. disinfection
10. pasteurization
11. fungicidal agent
12. antiseptic
13. pasteurization
14. disinfection

Microbial Types

1. barophiles
2. facultative anaerobes
3. obligate anaerobes
4. aerobes
5. halophiles
6. acidophiles
7. alkalophiles
8. psychrophiles
9. thermophiles
10. mesophiles
11. halophiles
12. mesophiles or alkalophiles
13. obligate anaerobes
14. obligate anaerobes

Physical Antimicrobial Methods

1. filtration
2. osmotic pressure
3. sonic waves
4. x-rays
5. ultraviolet rays
6. autoclaving
7. dessication
8. ultraviolet rays

Chemical Antimicrobial Methods

1. isopropyl alcohol
2. ethyl alcohol
3. hydrogen peroxide
4. formalin
5. phenolics
6. mercury salts
7. detergent or soap
8. ethylene oxide

Chemotherapy

1. penicillin
2. broad-spectrum antibiotics
3. Prontosil
4. amphotericin B
5. sulfanilamide
6. antibiotic
7. salvarsan
8. salvarsan
9. penicillin

True or False (T or F)

1. F
2. F
3. T
4. T
5. T
6. T
7. F
8. T
9. F
10. F
11. F
12. F
13. T
14. T
15. T

Multiple Choice

1. c
2. b
3. c
4. d
5. d
6. c
7. c
8. a
9. a
10. c
11. a
12. c
13. e

Chapter 6

Matching Exercises

Symbiotic Relationships
1. pathogen
2. parasite
3. infestation
4. infection
5. symbiotic
6. symbionts
7. mutualism
8. synergism
9. antibiosis
10. antibiosis
11. neutralism
12. commensalism

True or False (T or F)
1. F
2. T.
3. T
4. F
5. T
6. T
7. F
8. T
9. T
10. T
11. T

Multiple Choice
1. d
2. d
3. a
4. d
5. c
6. a
7. b
8. b
9. a
10. e
11. b

Chapter 7

Matching Exercises

Infectious Diseases
1. virulence
2. inflammation
3. infectious
4. infectious
5. contagious
6. communicable
7. inflammation

Types of Disease States
1. local
2. latent
3. asymptomatic
4. acute
5. chronic
6. carrier
7. systemic, generalized
8. primary, secondary

Disease Causation
1. exotoxins
2. capsule
3. hyaluronidase
4. endotoxin
5. coagulase
6. fibrinolysin, streptokinase or staphylokinase
7. hemolysin
8. leukocidin
9. collagenase

Epidemiology
1. pandemic
2. epidemic
3. nonendemic
4. sporadic
5. endemic
6. endemic

7. nonendemic
8. epidemic, pandemic

Reservoirs of Infection

1. arthropods
2. fomites
3. fecal material
4. vectors
5. respiratory pathogens
6. carriers
7. venereal
8. arthropods
9. vectors

True or False (T or F)

1. T
2. T
3. T
4. F
5. T
6. T
7. T
8. F
9. F
10. T
11. T
12. T
13. F
14. T
15. T
16. F
17. F
18. T
19. T
20. F
21. T
22. T
23. F

Multiple Choice

1. c
2. c
3. c
4. a
5. b
6. c
7. b
8. c
9. d
10. c
11. c
12. d
13. c
14. b

Chapter 8

Matching Exercises

Asepsis

1. sterile, sterilization
2. sterile, surgical
3. medical, aseptic
4. sterilization, disinfection, medical
5. sanitation
6. reverse isolation

True or False (T or F)

1. T
2. T
3. F
4. T
5. F
6. F
7. T
8. T
9. T
10. T
11. F
12. T
13. T
14. F
15. T
16. T

17. T
18. F
19. T
20. F
21. F
22. T
23. T
24. T
25. F

Multiple Choice

1. c
2. e
3. d
4. c
5. b
6. d
7. d
8. b
9. d
10. b
11. b
12. b

Chapter 9

Matching Exercises

Resistance Against Pathogens

1. nonspecific
2. bile
3. lysozyme
4. specific
5. indigenous microflora
6. interferon
7. species
8. digestive enzymes
9. innate
10. complement

Immunology

1. serum
2. agammaglobulinemia
3. IgG
4. antigen
5. immunocompetent
6. IgE
7. allergen
8. antitoxins
9. primary response
10. plasma
11. IgM
12. hypogammaglobulinemia
13. complement
14. anamnestic response
15. IgA
16. antibodies
17. anaphylactic response

Immune Response

1. immediate
2. naturally acquired active immunity
3. allergy, immediate
4. artificially acquired active immunity
5. delayed
6. artificially acquired passive immunity
7. autoimmune
8. naturally acquired passive immunity

Antigen-antibody Reactions

1. lysis by complement
2. complement fixation
3. toxin neutralization
4. toxin neutralization
5. agglutination
6. immobilization
7. capsular swelling
8. agglutination
9. precipitation
10. opsonization
11. fluorescent antibody

True or False (T or F)

1. F
2. T
3. F
4. F
5. F
6. T
7. F
8. T
9. T
10. T
11. T
12. F
13. T
14. T
15. T
16. T
17. F
18. T
19. F
20. T
21. F
22. F
23. T
24. F
25. T
26. F
27. F

Multiple Choice

1. a
2. b
3. d
4. a
5. e
6. c
7. d
8. b
9. c
10. b
11. d
12. b
13. d
14. a
15. c
16. b
17. e

Chapter 10

Matching Exercises

Disease and Type of Agent

1. b
2. b
3. b
4. c
5. d
6. c
7. b
8. a
9. a
10. b
11. b
12. b
13. a
14. c
15. b
16. b
17. a
18. a
19. d
20. a

Disease and Synonym

1. b
2. d
3. c

Disease and Etiologic Agent

1. d
2. b
3. e
4. f

5. a
6. k
7. l
8. j
9. m
10. h
11. i
12. j

True or False (T or F)

1. F
2. F
3. T
4. F
5. T
6. T
7. T
8. F
9. T
10. T
11. F
12. F
13. T
14. T
15. F
16. T

17. F
18. T
19. T
20. T
21. F
22. F
23. T
24. T
25. F

Multiple Choice

1. d
2. d
3. d
4. e
5. a
6. d
7. b
8. b
9. c
10. d
11. d
12. c
13. c
14. b
15. a

Index

Page numbers followed by *t* and *f* indicate tables and figures, respectively; those in *italics* refer to major discussions.